ENDODONTICS
KNOW ENDO DO ENDO

Success is Everything
Success Starts with Knowing
Success Comes with Doing
Know Endo Do Endo.

Dr. Pasha

Mentor and Educator

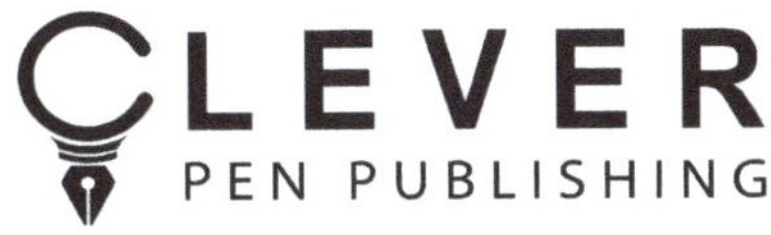

Mumbai

First Edition : 2022

Published by :
CLEVER PEN PUBLISHING
(A joint venture between Bhalani Publishers and National Medical Book House)
D-2 Neelkanth Business Park Co-op. Premises Society Ltd.
Nathani Road, Vidyavihar (West), Mumbai - 400 086.

Mobile : 09867214519

E-mail : cleverpen9@gmail.com

ISBN : 978-93-92215-06-3

Printed & Bound in India.

This Book is Dedicated
to
My Late brother Moula Sabir
Who was rock-bottom to my education
Recently passed away
due to fulminating liver failure.

PREFACE

Being a firm believer in learning by doing, this little volume is the result of 20 years of clinical practice. This book mainly focuses on those who fear, hate and have given up endodontics.

This book enables and guides the readers to Start, Do and Love endodontics by relying more on self potential rather than expensive armamentarium.

Endodontics is competence with oneself rather than a skill, the key is attention.

Do not run behind technology, embrace biology and rely on practice.

ACKNOWLEDGEMENT

Special thanks to -

Dr. Ruchika Oswal for her Support, Help and Encouragement

Dr. Kanksha Bhalani for her Guidance

Thanks to -

1) Dr. Abhilash Dhaytadak

2) Dr. Shantanu Sanjay Sirsath

3) Dr. Shreyash Bagle

4) Dr. Gaurav Sandanshiv

5) Dr. Saurabh Vilas Pakhale

6) Dr. Nitin Waghmare

7) Dr. Kamran Khan

8) Dr. Meghrajhande

9) Dr. Anjum Sharieiff

10) Dr. Mudassir Pasha

11) Dr. Sumit Bhagat

I finally want to thank my lovely wife **Mubarak Jahan** and children **Aasir, Aariz** and **Aarhan** for their continued support and encouragement to follow my dreams.

I would like to take this opportunity to thank **Mr. Rajesh Bhalani, Dr. Kanksha Bhalani, Mrs. Harsha Shah** for his constant support, encouragement and speedily Publication of an excellent quality book.

CONTENTS

1
Investigations

Investigation means collecting data or gathering information by Interrogating, Examining and Testing. Everything starts with proper investigation. Proper investigation guides us to correct diagnosis, correct diagnosis builds confidence and curiosity which are most essential ingredients to perform treatment effectively.

INTERROGATING

It requires patience and interest to uncover patient's true problem. Asking questions, listening and understanding patient's behavior to uncover patient's true problem is the first step to diagnosis.

Medical history

It influences diagnosis, treatment plan and final outcome. It is must to determine the general health of the patient before doing any treatment because it gives lot of information about:

a) Whether the patient is physically and mentally fit for the endodontic treatment.

b) Whether the patient requires antibiotic prophylaxis or any other premedication and special care protocols to follow.

c) Perio-Endo lesions – Endodontic problems of periodontal origin is more common in medically compromised patients

d) Aid in final diagnosis

Some common medical conditions which we encounter in our clinical practice in daily basis include the following:

1) Cardiovascular diseases

Congenital valvular defects, prosthetic valves, patients with recent heart surgery require prophylactic antibiotic therapy to prevent infective endocarditis or sub-acute bacterial endocarditis.

The patients of Ischemic heart disease, patients who have recently undergone angioplasties or coronary artery bypass surgeries are under anticoagulant therapy.

a) Because of additive anticoagulant effect of non-steroidal anti-inflammatory drugs and risk of internal bleeding, opioid analgesics are recommended

b) Because of risk of continuous, bleeding over instrumentation of periodontal regions are avoided

c) Pain of angina pectoris and myocardial infarction radiates to lower jaw

Hypertension - Requires stress reduction protocol. Morning appointments preferred. Make the patient calm, cool and co-operative. Use plain LA (local anesthetic without vasoconstrictor).

2) *Immuno compromised diseases*

Patients suffering from Immuno compromised diseases are more prone to opportunistic infections and require antibiotic prophylaxis to combat delayed wound healing and prevent serious secondary infections.

E.g.:

– Diabetes mellitus
– Patient on prolonged corticosteroid therapy like in certain skin diseases
– Adrenal insufficiency
– Bone marrow suppression
– Leukemia's
– Patient on prolonged immunosuppressant like in organ transplant
– HIV and AIDS
– Radiation therapy

Note: Plain LA is preferred in diabetes mellitus because adrenaline has positive effect on carbohydrate metabolism and increases blood glucose level.

3) *Analgesics medication*

- Patients who are under analgesic therapy to control pain conditions like
- Migraine
- Arthritis
- Chronic pain syndrome. (atypical headache, atypical facial pain)
- Pain killers mask the symptoms of pulpal and periodontal pathology and makes the diagnosis difficult.

4) Pregnancy

Special attention is required especially in first and third trimester with respect to chair position, medication and pain control.

a) Teratogenic drugs like fluoroquinolones, tetracyclines, cephalosporins are contraindicated.

b) NSAIDs like aspirin, ibuprofen, diclofenac, etc. are contraindicated because NSAIDs causes miscarriage, placental tearing and still births.

c) Higher Analgesics like plain paracetamol is preferred.

d) Chair position for the pregnant females should be left lateral decubitus position and semi supine (to avoid pressure on abdomen)

e) High speed films, lead aprons are used to avoid unnecessary radiation exposure to the patient as radiation is hazardous to the developing fetus.

f) Painless RCTs are preferred as compared to extraction of teeth in third trimester of pregnancy.

5) Allergy

History of allergy to any known drug like penicillin, sulpha - containing drugs, NSAIDs, and Chemicals like local anesthetics, eugenol, sodium hypochlorite, latex of gloves, rubber dam should be assessed.

6) Anxiety

History of dental procedure related stress and apprehension is assessed. Stress reduction protocol is followed. If necessary, premedication with anxiolytics and analgesics prescribed.

7) Transmissiable respiratory diseases

TB, common cold, pneumonia, Hepatitis, HIV+ve we have to be careful and cautious, protect from getting infection through saliva, inhalation, blood.

Corona : The emergence of COVID 19 pandemic poses an immense health challenge. As dental care providers we are faced with significant responsibilities both to the dental team and our patient to limit exposure to the virus.

Coronavirus are enveloped single stranded RNA viruses that are zoonotic in nature and cause symptoms ranging from those similar to the normal cold to more severe respiratory, enteric, hepatic, neurological symptoms.

Routes of Transmission:

The 3 most common transmission routes:

1. Direct Transmission (through cough, sneeze or droplet inhalation)

2. Contact Transmission (through oro-nasal-ocular route)

3. Aerosol Transmission

Specific recommendation for dentist to triage patients to decide, what is dental emergency and when and how to schedule such patients.

A) Emergency care: If dental condition leading to impairment of basic functions like breathing and swallowing

Dental Conditions:

- Uncontrolled bleeding
- Diffuse intraoral and extraoral swelling which may obstruct the patient airway or with systemic effects.
- Severe traumatic injury including extraoral tissues which can obstruct airway.
- Level of intervention needed:

  Need immediate care and should be attended immediately

B) Urgent care:

Dental conditions that gravely affect the normal functioning of patient like disabling pain/ infections.

Dental Conditions:

- Irreversible pulpitis
- Primary and secondary symptomatic apical periodontitis
- Acute apical abscess, localized swelling, infections, pericoronitis
- Dental trauma with avulsion
- Level of Intervention:

Pharmacological management and patients to be kept on constant follow up for any worsening of symptoms despite pharmacological management. In case of above, the patient should be scheduled for physical appointment as in emergency care. If symptoms are relieved after pharmacological management; this patient should be scheduled for physical visit.

C) Scheduled care/ Elective care:

Dental Conditions:

- Loss of restoration with no pain
- Dental trauma involving enamel and dentin only
- Replacing temporary filling on endo access opening in patient not experiencing pain.

Level of Intervention Needed:

Such patients should be only tele counselled and may be scheduled as priority when regular dental services are restored.

General Recommendation checklist for dental centers before treating covid19 pandemic:

1. Placed visual alerts for patient's awareness using posters on COVID19 pandemic awareness, cough etiquette and hand hygiene practice.

2. Modify patient exiting patient, waiting area seating arrangement to enforce social distancing of 1-2 meters.

3. Insist on use of alcohol-based hand rub for all upon entry in dental clinic.

4. Provide face mask for all patients prior to consultation.

5. Tissue paper dispenser and foot operated waste bin mandatory in patient waiting room.

6. Mandatory provision hand washing with soap and paper.

7. Avoid usage of commercial split \window air conditioners unless equipped with high efficiency particulate air filters.

8. It is recommended to use natural and mechanical ventilation using fans and exhaust.

Hand hygiene:

Hand washing with soap and water is preferred when hands are visibly dirty or soiled with blood or other body fluids or after using toilet.

Use of alcohol-based hand rubs, when hands are not visibly dirty.

8) Blood disorders like

Iron deficiency anemia, pernicious anemia, sickle cell anemia and leukemia present with paresthesia of oral mucosal tissues which mimics the tenderness or sensitivity of periapical pathology.

Jaw pain of sickle cell anemia mimics the endodontic pain.

9) Bleeding disorders

- Hemophilia
- Thrombocytopenia
- Chronic alcoholism
- Dengue

- Chronic liver diseases
- There is risk of continuous bleeding and hypovolemic shock
- Mild to moderate cases can be managed under anti fibrinolytic agents and using local styptics
- For severe cases co-ordination with hematologist is needed.

10) Hyperthyroidism

- Plain local anesthesia is used
- If needed premedication with sedatives are prescribed

11) Certain systemic conditions like multiple myeloma, sickle cell anemia, hyperparathyroidism present with radiographic changes in jaw bones may be confused with periapical radiolucency.

Past dental history

1) Restorations—large restoration, pulp capping, vital pulp therapy....
2) Root canals
3) History of dental trauma
4) Orthodontic Treatment
5) Dental surgery-extractions, dis-impaction...

Chief complaint

Main reason for patient's visit to the clinic and should be recorded in patient's own words.

History of present illness pain

Extremely unpleasant state of mind and body

Onset (when did the pain start?) and duration of pain (from how long it is there?)

Intensity of pain

Transient, momentary type of pain is due to involvement A-fibers. Continuous, long lasting type of pain is due to involvement of C fibers.

Relieving and aggravating factors of pain

Pain aggravates after taking cold indicates involvement of A delta fibers, pain relieves after taking cold indicates involvement of C fibers.

Nature of pain

Sharp, shooting, pin point, piercing, lancinating-due to involvement of A delta fibers.

Throbbing, Dull aching, stabbing, spontaneous, exacerbating-due to involvement of C fibers.

Location of pain localised or confined to one tooth is due to involvement of A delta fibers.

Diffuse or generalised pain is due to involvement of C fibers.

Nocturnal pain effects of pain on posture bending and lying down, sleep disturbed due to pain indicate involvement of C Fibers.

Referred pain or abandon pain Referred pain is due to the intermingling of 7th,9th and 10th cranial nerves within the nucleus of trigeminal nerve.

Pain of non-odontogenic origin

Non odontogenic pain travel and crosses the midline, most of the time associated with triggering zones and parasthesia.

1) *Maxillary sinusitis* - Heaviness of face, pain aggravates on bending the neck down, history of recurrent rhinitis

2) *Trigeminal neuralgia* - Acute pain associated with trigger zones along course of nerve

3) *TMJ Pain* - Tenderness over the joint, crepitus and altered jaw movements

4) *Migraine* - Watering of eyes, sensitivity to noise and light, nausea

5) *Musculoskeletal pain* - Due to ischemia associated with tenderness of muscles

EXAMINING

Visual inspection

Facial expressions indicate severity of pain and discomfort

Extra oral examination

1. *Swelling:* Indicates infection, is diffused or generalised with systemic manifestations

2. *Facial asymmetry:* Any motor nerve disorders like facial paralysis

3. *Lymph nodes:* Enlarged tender lymph nodes with elevated temperature indicates systemic manifestations of infection like bacteremia, septicemia or toxemia.

4. *TMJ disorders:* Tender muscles of mastication, altered jaw movements, crepitus indicates TMJ pathosis

5. *Neurological disturbances:* Trigger zones and tenderness along the course of nerves indicate trigeminal neuralgia.

TESTING

PULP VITALITY TESTS

> *WHERE THERE IS VITALITY THERE IS SENSITIVITY.*
> *WHERE THERE IS SENSITIVITY THERE IS IMMUNITY.*
> *WHERE THERE IS IMMUNITY THERE IS LIFE.*
> *NO IMMUNITY NO LIFE.*

Sensitivity tests

Vitality of the tooth is determined by its blood supply and sensitivity of tooth is determined by its vital nerve supply, through blood supply tooth retains and maintains its sensitivity. Any tissue said to be vital has to have blood supply, vitality is the life line without which there is no sensitivity (immunity), so sensitivity directly relies on pulp vitality and pulp vitality indirectly depends on sensitivity hence pulp sensitivity tests do not provide us direct evidence, they provide us with indirect evidence. Response to sensitivity tests indicate only the sensory nerve fibers are vital if done attentively and properly they guide us one step closer to diagnosis.

Objective

Assess the health and integrity of sensory neurons of pulp tissue and determine whether the sensory nerve fiber supplying the tooth is vital or nonvital.

To understand pulp sensitivity tests, we need to have essential knowledge about the mechanism of cold and hot conduction through neural pathway.
Pulp has two types of nerve fibres.

1) A-delta fibre   2)   C-fibres

1)   A-delta fibre

Distributed peripherally in the cell rich zone of pulp.

Myelinated and larger in diameter. Conducts impulses very fast.

Mainly responsible for cold sensitivity.

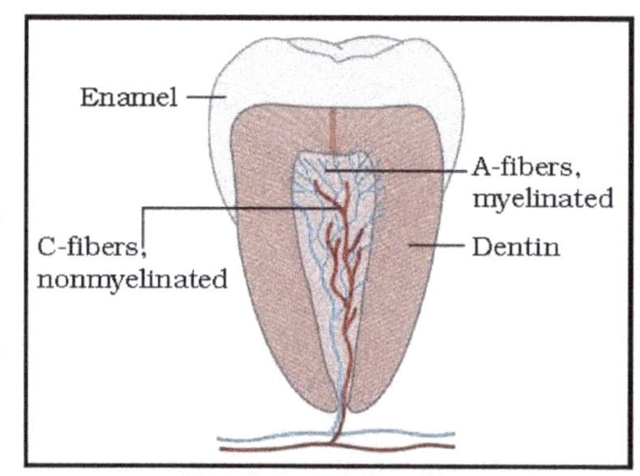

Fig. 1.1 A-delta fibre

Complete loss of cold sensitivity indicates permanent damage of A-Delta fibres and hyper sensitivity to cold is a classic sign of reversible pulp damage.

2. C-Fibres/Core Fibres

Distributed in centre of pulp. Nonmyelinated and smaller in diameter. Conduction of impulses are slow.

Mainly responsible for hot sensitivity.

Hypersensitivity to hot indicates permanent damage to the C-fibres.

Pain aggravates after taking hot and relieves after taking cold is a classic sign of irreversible pulp damage.

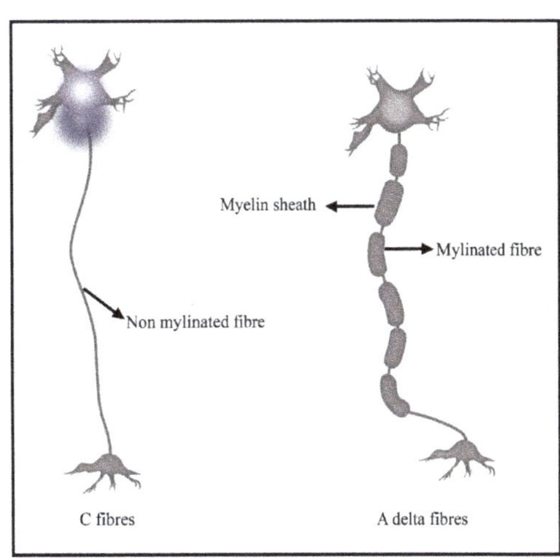

Fig. 1.2 C-Fibres / Core Fibres

Mechanism of cold conduction

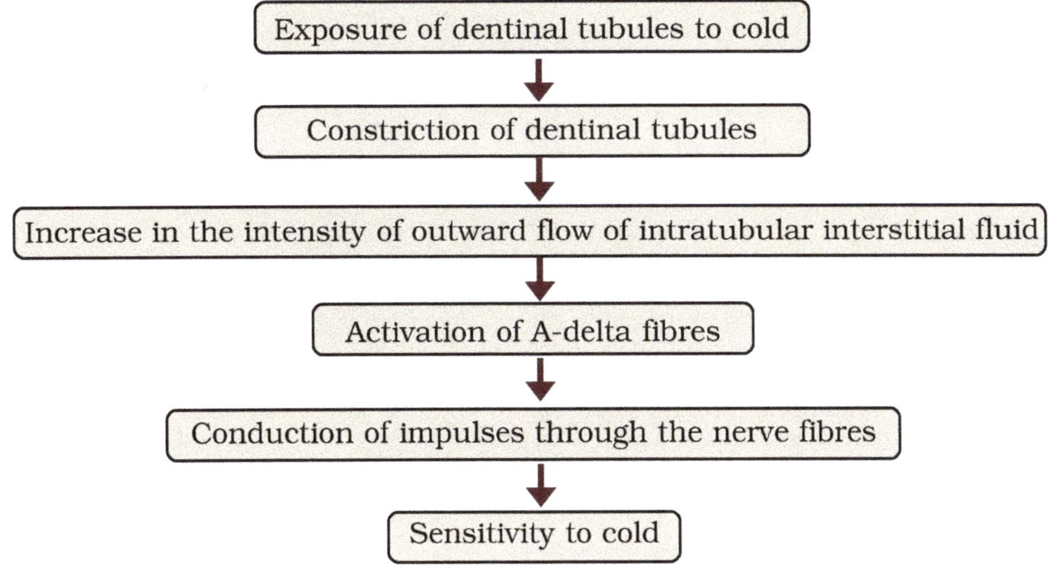

Mechanism of heat conduction

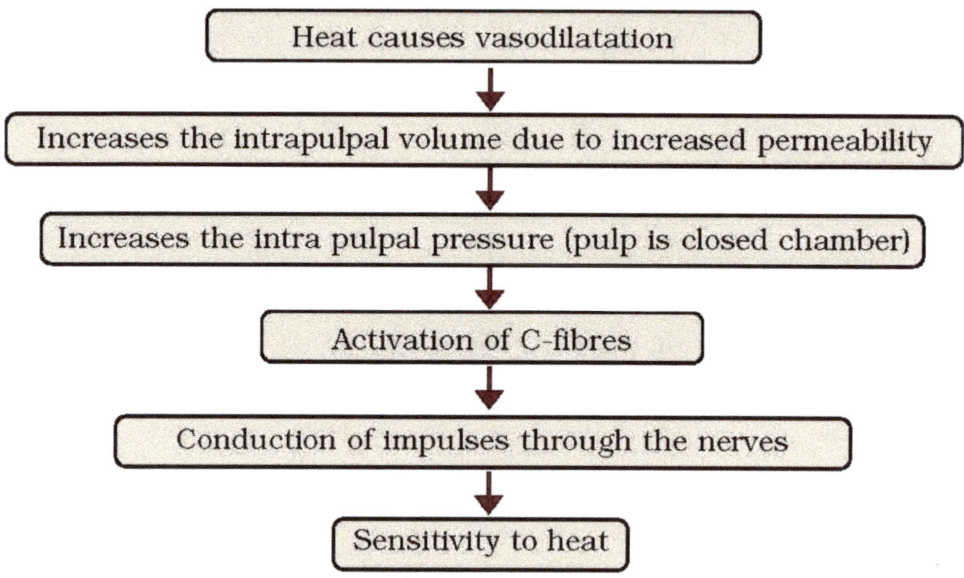

Cold test

Cold test is the primary and basic test. Among sensibility tests it is the only one facet of dental diagnosis which is crucial in monitoring health and integrity of pulp.

It is done by placing cold material on the tooth surface for few seconds, where the enamel is thin. Stimulation of A-delta fibers present in the pulp elicit responses, positive response reflects presence of inflammation and presence of level inflammation superficial or deep. It is initially done on the contralateral and adjacent tooth to gauge the normal response of tooth later on done on the tooth in question. Cold test on tooth with prosthetic crown and restoration is done by placing coldest material on the cervical area of tooth.

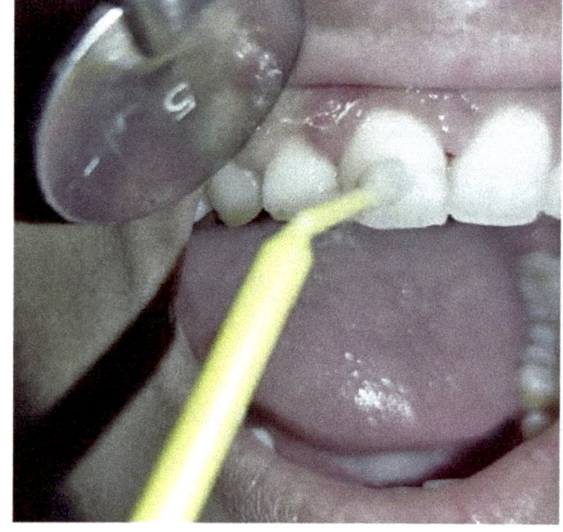

Fig. 1.3: Cold test

Material used

- Cold water
- Ice cube or ice stick
- Refringent spray or dry ice or Carbon dioxide snow
- Ethyl chloride spray

Cold water and ice cube affect the adjacent tooth.

Refringent spray does not affect the adjacent tooth, it is readily available, easy to use and the results are reliable and reproducible

Heat test

It is done only when it's necessary, otherwise patient's history to hyper sensitivity after taking hot coffee or tea suffices the purpose. Heat test does not indicate sensitivity of tooth, it indicates the later stage of inflammation-necrosis of core nerve fibres of pulp. It is done by touching the labial surface of tooth with heated ball burnisher or heated gutta percha. Applying petroleum jelly or vaseline over the tooth surfaces before doing the test prevents the gutta percha or impression compound from sticking to the tooth surface. Care must be taken to prevent permanent damage to the tooth by subjecting the tooth to excessive heat.

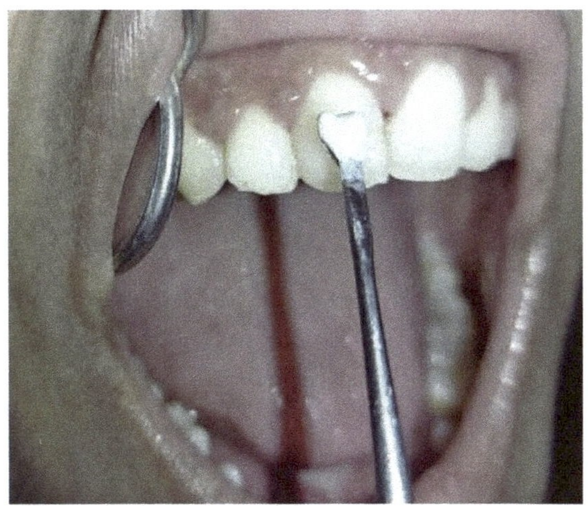

Fig. 1.4: Heat test

Interpretation of cold and heat test

Interpretation in critical patient may respond to cold and heat in the following ways

Response with Mild to moderate sensation 1 to 3 seconds indicates normal healthy pulp.

Response with intense sensation for 4 to 12 seconds which subsides when stimulus is removed indicates reversible pulp damage.

Response with severe sensation for more than 15 seconds to few minutes which lingers even after removal of stimulus indicates irreversible pulp damage.

No response indicates pulp may be non vital or vital.

Electric pulp test

Electric pulp tester is used to conduct this test. The Electric pulp tester designed to stimulate the closest A delta nerve fibers. It does not usually stimulate unmyelinated core fibers because of their threshold the test only indicates the presence of vital nerve. It does not indicate health and integrity of pulp.

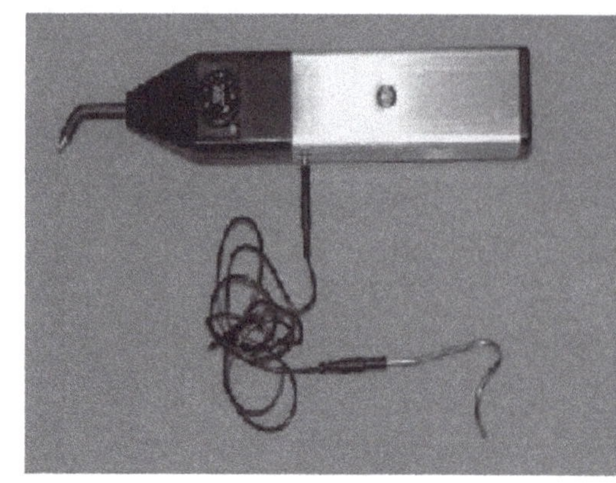

Fig. 1.5: Electric pulp test

Mechanism

Evaluate the blood circulation to the sensory nerves supplying to the pulp and determine whether the sensory nerve fiber supplying to the pulp is vital or non-vital.

Procedure

Explain the nature and diagnostic value of the procedure in detail to the patient. The test initially performed on the adjacent and contralateral tooth to gauge normal response of tooth. Isolate and dry the control tooth and tooth to be tested, test area must be kept dry to avoid false positive results. Check for the electric pulp tester function and coat tip of electric probe with conducting medium usually tooth paste which acts as electrolyte helps in conduction of electric current. Patient be informed about the sensations of warm and tingling felt during testing. Selection of site and proper placement of probe is critical to ensure accurate response from the tooth. An area of high neural density is chosen like buccal cusp tips of posterior teeth, incisal edges of anterior teeth where enamel is thin or absent, for anterior teeth incisal third of labial surface and for posterior teeth middle third of facial surface is chosen. Place the coated tip in close contact with tooth surface care should be taken so that the electrode (probe tip) or electrolyte (tooth paste) not in contact with adjacent gingival tissue or any restoration in the tooth. Once the probe is in contact with tooth the lip clip is directly placed inside the oral cavity. The lip clip clamp is attached to the cheek or buccal mucosal if lip clip is not used direct the patient to hold the end of probe to complete the circuit. Once the circuit is completed turning the rheostat slowly at first very low intensity current is introduced in to the tooth. This avoids excessive stimulation and discomfort. Later intensity of stimulus increased steadily at preselected rate. The patient is instructed to remove his or her hand from the end of probe when warm sensation or tingling is felt the readings from probe are recorded. Each tooth should be tested two or more times and an average result is noted.

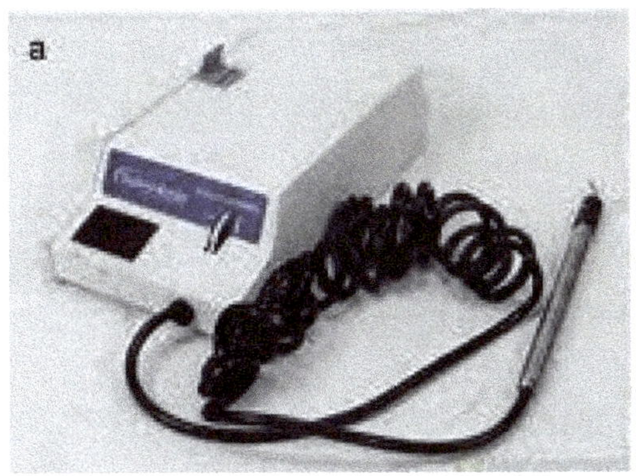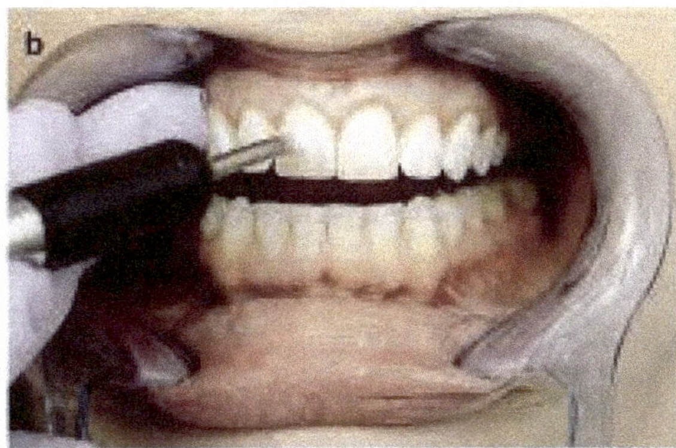

Fig. 1.6:

Interpretation

No response indicates = Pulp necrosis.
Responding low currents indicate = Reversible pulpitis.
Responding high currents indicate = Irreversible pulpitis.

Drawbacks of electric pulp test

The following conditions cause incorrect results.

False positive results

- Although sensory nerve fibers are non-vital, sensory sensations are felt by the patients.

- The following conditions may give rise to false positive results.

- Contact of electrolyte or electrode with adjacent gingival tissue or any metal restoration in tooth can conduct electric current and give rise to false positive results.

- Contamination of testing area with saliva and tissue fluids due to poor isolation and inadequate drying can conduct electric current and results false positive outcome.

- In patients with high anxiety

- In teeth with moist gangrenous necrosis

- Gases or liquefied products within the pulp can conduct electric current and give rise to false positive result.

- In multirooted teeth

- The sensory nerve fibers may be viable in one or more root canals and necrosed in other canals. The vital nerve fiber transmits electric impulses and give rise to false positive result.

False negative results

- Although sensory nerve fibers are vital no sensory sensations are felt by the patients.
- In teeth with extensive restorations and pulp protecting bases there is hindrance to transmission of electric current leading to false negative results.
- In teeth with calcific or fibrotic obliteration of pulp there is obstruction to passage of electric current.
- Patients on premedication with drugs like NSAIDs, tranquilizers, sedatives
- Patients with high pain threshold.

Trauma

In traumatic injuries of tooth like luxation sensory innervations are damaged, vascular supply remain intact. Within two weeks of injury due to functioning of true vitality pulp, the pulp is in physiologic state of shock, behave differently and give false negative result, the phenomena is called stunting of pulp. Hence pulp sensitivity and pulp vascularity tests are contraindicated within 2 weeks of teeth injuries.

Recently erupted immature tooth wide open apex

Poor passage of electric current due to incomplete development of nerve supply to tooth give rise to false negative results.

Pulp vascularity tests

True blood supply to the tooth depends upon health and integrity of microvasculature of pulp tissue rather than its sensory nerve supply. Pulp vascularity tests assess the health and integrity of microvasculature within pulp tissue and provide direct evidence of actual blood flow to the pulp tissue therefore pulp vascularity tests are considered to be more accurate in determining the vitality of tooth.

Objective

Determines the blood circulation of the tooth by finding the presence of moving red blood cells within the microvasculature of pulp tissue.

Doppler principle

Shift in the frequency of light occur that is encountered by dynamic object.

Laser doppler flowmeter

A beam containing infra-red light wave lengths 633nm and 780nm made to incident on to the tooth by securing fiber optic probe against tooth buccal surface.

The light beam from fiber optic probe transmits through the hard tissues of tooth as the beam encounters a circulating red blood cells within the microvasculature of pulp tissue, the incident beam scatters /absorbs and undergoes shift in its frequency.

Note: according to doppler principle when light encounters a stationary object it does not get scattered/absorbs and undergoes shift in its frequency.

The shift in the frequency of incident beam results in reflection of incident beam which is recorded by the microprocessor of sensor the output of which corresponds to the number and velocity of red blood cells.

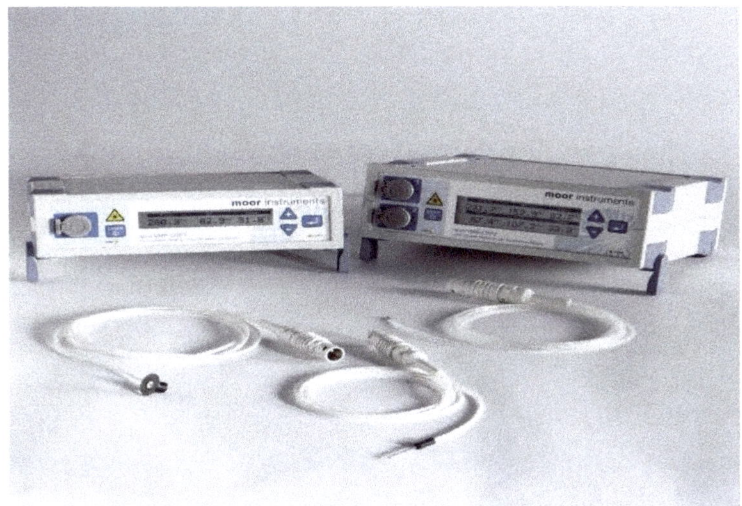

Fig. 1.7:

Indications

In children

Laser doppler flowmetry is a suitable method to test pulp vitality because sensibility tests are not reliable in children because they are subjectively rely upon patient's response.

In teeth with moist gangrenous necrosis particularly when referred is present

Laser doppler flowmetry is a suitable method to test pulp vitality because gases or liquefied products within the pulp can conduct thermal stimulus and give rise to false to positive result.

In traumatic injuries of teeth

Laser doppler flowmetry is a suitable method to test pulp vitality in traumatic teeth because sensitivity tests are contraindicated due to stunting phenomena of pulp. Laser doppler flowmetry performed at 4 weeks following trauma give accurate results.

In recently erupted immature tooth with wide open apex

- Laser doppler flowmetry is a suitable method to test pulp vitality in recently erupted immature tooth with wide open apex, sensitivity tests are inaccurate due to incomplete development of nerve supply to tooth.
- In teeth with extensive restorations and pulp protecting bases
- Patients on premedication with drugs like NSAIDs, tranquilizers, sedatives
- In teeth with calcific or fibrotic obliteration of pulp
- In patients with high anxiety
- Patients with high pain threshold

Advantages

Patient satisfaction is great

Eliminate the need for application of an unpleasant stimulus like cold , heat, electric current allows the painless diagnosis of pulp vitality of tooth.

Objective test

Need not rely upon patient responses particularly very useful in children whose responses are unreliable.

Non- invasive test

- Its non -invasive nature promote patient co -operation and acceptance.
- Reliable and Reproducible.
- Accurate test to check vitality.

Limitations

- Technique sensitive subtle moments of tooth or sensor results in artifacts and inaccurate readings cannot be used in patients who cannot refrain from moving or tooth be tested cannot be stabilized.
- Medications used in cardiovascular diseases can affect the blood flow pulp and can give rise to wrong results.
- In traumatic injuries of teeth laser doppler meter tests should be performed at 4 weeks following trauma.
- Costly device for use in a dental clinic.

Pulse oximetry

Pulse oximetry is a noninvasive method for monitoring a person's oxygen saturation. Though its reading of peripheral oxygen saturation is not always identical to the more desirable reading of arterial oxygen saturation (Sao) from arterial blood gas analysis, the two are correlated well enough that the safe, convenient, noninvasive, inexpensive pulse oximetry method is valuable for measuring oxygen saturation in clinical use In its most common (transmissive) application mode, a sensor device is placed on a thin part of the patient's body. Usually a fingertip or earlobe, or in the case of an infant, across a foot. The device passes two wavelengths of light through the body part to a photodetector. It measures the changing absorbance at each of the wavelengths, allowing it to determine the absorbances due to the pulsing arterial blood alone, excluding venous blood, skin, bone, muscle, fat, and (in most cases) nail polish. Reflectance pulse oximetry is a less common alternative to transmissive pulse oximetry. This method does not require a thin section of the person's body and is therefore well suited to a universal application such as the feet, forehead, and chest, but it also has some limitations.

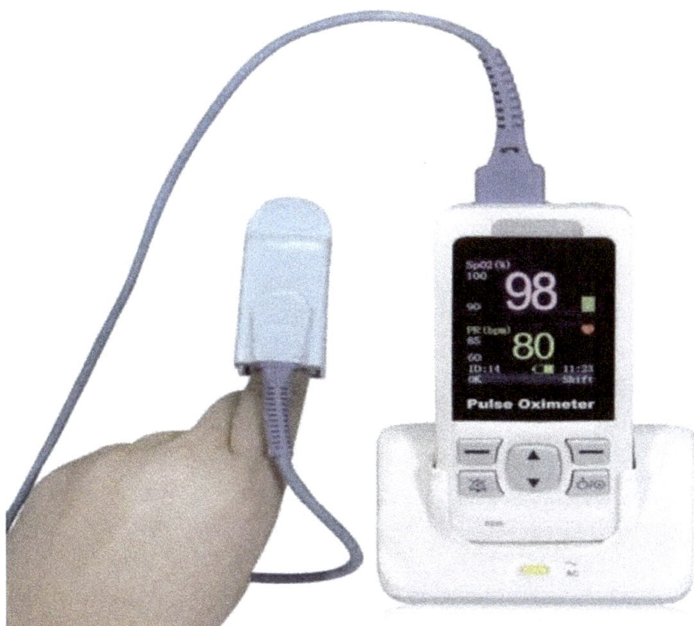

Fig. 1.8: Pulse oximeter

Function:

A blood-oxygen monitor displays the percentage of blood that is loaded with oxygen. More specifically, it measures what percentage of hemoglobin, the protein in blood that carries oxygen, is loaded. Acceptable normal ranges for patients without pulmonary pathology are from 95 to 99 percent. For a patient breathing room air at or near sea level, an estimate of arterial po, can be made from the blood-oxygen monitor "saturation of peripheral oxygen (Spo) reading.

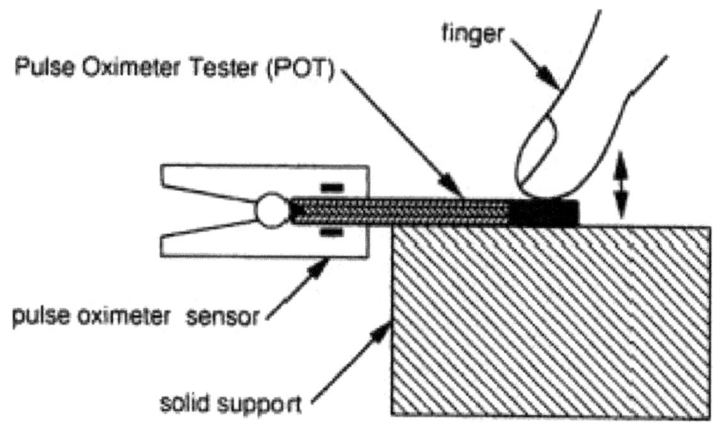

Fig. 1.9: Parts of Pulse oximeter

Indication:

A pulse oximeter is a medical device that indirectly monitors the oxygen saturation of a patient's blood (as opposed to measuring oxygen saturation directly through a blood sample) and changes in blood volume in producing a photoplethysmogram that may be further processed into other measurements.

Advantages:

Pulse oximetry is particularly convenient for noninvasive continuous measurement of blood oxygen saturation. Pulse oximetry is useful in any setting where a patient's oxygenation is unstable, including intensive care, operating, recovery, emergency and hospital ward settings, pilots in unpressurized aircraft, for assessment of any patient's oxygenation, and determining the effectiveness of or need for oxygen, or the amount of oxygen being used by a patient. Although a pulse oximeter is used to monitor oxygenation, it cannot determine the metabolism of A pulse oximeter probe applied to a person's finger in room air, since it can result in hypoventilation going undetected . Because of their simplicity of use and the ability to provide continuous and immediate oxygen saturation values, pulse oximeters are at critical importance in emergency medicine and are also very useful for patients with respiratory or cardiac problems. Portable battery-operated pulse oximeters are useful for pilots operating in non-pressurized aircraft above 10,000 feet (3,000 m) or 12,500 feet (3,800 m) . Portable pulse oximeters are also useful for mountain climbers and athletes whose oxygen levels may decrease at high altitudes or with exercise. Some portable pulse oximeters employ software that charts a patient's blood oxygen and pulse serving as a reminder to check blood oxygen levels.

Limitations:

Pulse oximetry solely measures hemoglobin saturation, not ventilation and is not a complete measure of respiratory sufficiency. It is not a substitute for blood gases checked in a laboratory, because it gives no indication of base deficit, carbon dioxide levels, blood pH, or bicarbonate. Most of the oxygen in the blood is carried by hemoglobin; in severe anemia, the blood contains less hemoglobin, which despite being saturated cannot carry as much oxygen. Erroneously low readings may be caused by hypoperfusion of the extremity being used for monitoring (often due to a limb being cold, or from vasoconstriction secondary to the use of vasopressor agents), incorrect sensor application highly calloused skin, or movement (such as shivering), especially during hypoperfusion. If there is insufficient blood flow or insufficient hemoglobin in the blood (anemia). tissues can suffer hypoxia despite high arterial oxygen saturation. Since pulse oximetry measures only the percentage of bound hemoglobin, a falsely high or falsely low reading will occur when hemoglobin binds to something other than oxygen.

Periodontal status tests: Periodontal status tests are performed when pulpal infection is not confined to the root and has reached the periodontal area.

Palpation test

It is done by applying gentle pressure at the apices of teeth with the index finger on the facial and lingual surfaces of upper teeth and only facial surfaces of lower teeth. Presence of tori and exostosis on the lingual surfaces of lower molars may give false positive result.

It is done to detect

a)   Tenderness

b)   Sensitivity

c)   Draining sinuses

d)   Crepitus

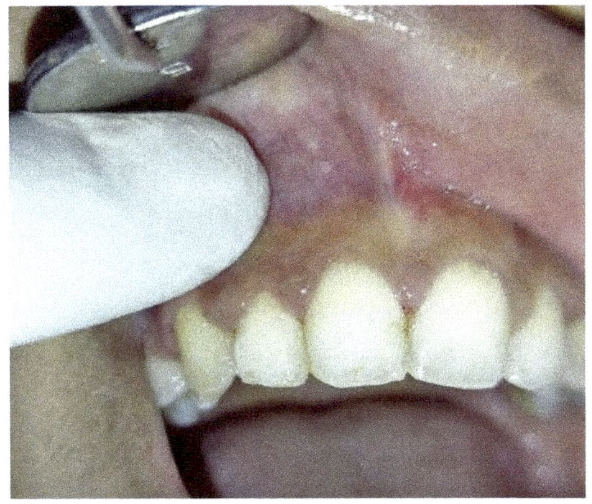

Fig. 1.10: Palpation test

Palpation test routinely done before incision and drainage of abscess to assess the consistency and dimensions of abscess.

Percussion test

The basis of this test is activation of proprioceptors present in periodontium by pressure. Normal tooth requires more percussion pressure to elicit pain while abnormal tooth requires gentle pressure to elicit pain. It is most commonly done, simple and most reliable method to assess the periodontal status of tooth.

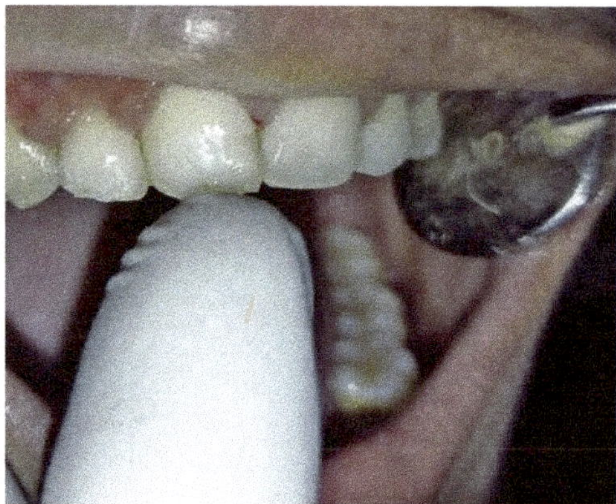 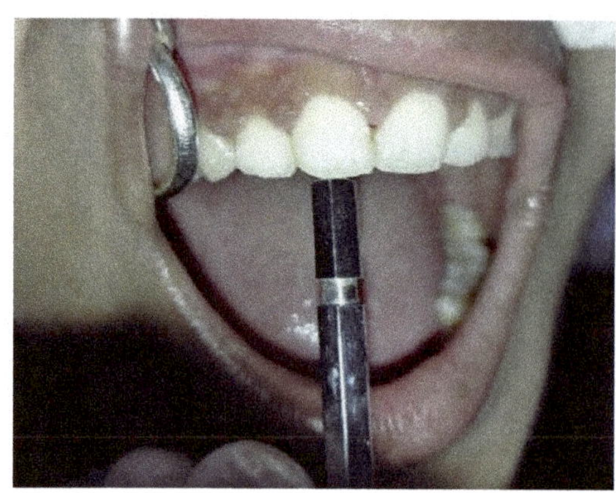

Fig. 1.11: Percussion test

It is done randomly by applying gentle pressure on the occlusal or incisal surfaces of teeth initially with index finger and later on with back of the instruments. Pain on vertical percussion indicates periapical pathology. Pain on lateral percussion indicates para radicular pathology. Multi rooted tooth should be percussed over each cusp. Positive response on mild digital percussion indicates acute inflammatory conditions.

Note: Care must be taken while performing percussion test in pain sensitive patient or while percussing sensitive tender tooth, percussion pressure must not exceed beyond the patient tolerance.

Biting test

It is done if patient complains of pain on mastication to detect cracks or leaky restorations. Instruct the patient to bite down on cotton swab or handle of the instrument and release. If patient complains of pain on releasing indicates crack or leaky restoration. Pain is due to deflection of cusps and increase in the outward flow of intratubular interstitial fluid and activation of pain pathway through the stimulation of A Delta nerve fibers. Pain on biting indicates periodontal pathology.

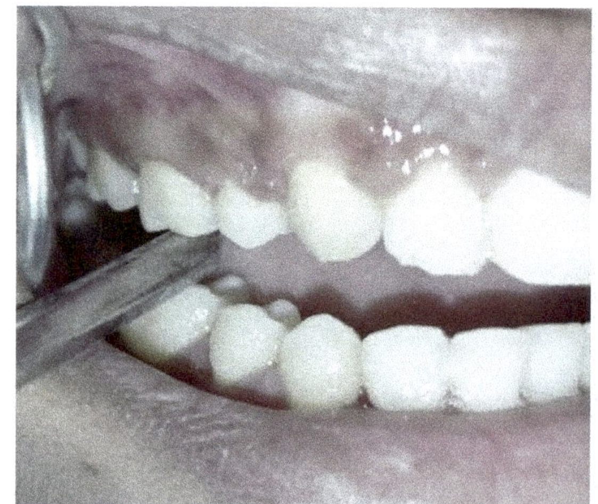

Fig. 1.12: Biting test

Transillumination test

This test helps to identify longitudinal crown fractures because a fracture will not transmit light. Transillumination produces contrasting dark and light areas at the fracture site.

A Fiber optic wand may be positioned directly on the exterior surface of the tooth so that a high intensity light passes through the crown perpendicular to the long axis of tooth detecting decay, cracks and fractures.

Fractures and cracks appear as thin hair like translucent lines passing through the tooth in longitudinal direction.

This test is helpful in identifying

I.   Interproximal decay

II.   Decay under old restoration

III. Helpful in assessing the pathologic calcifications.

IV.   Helpful to detect orifices.

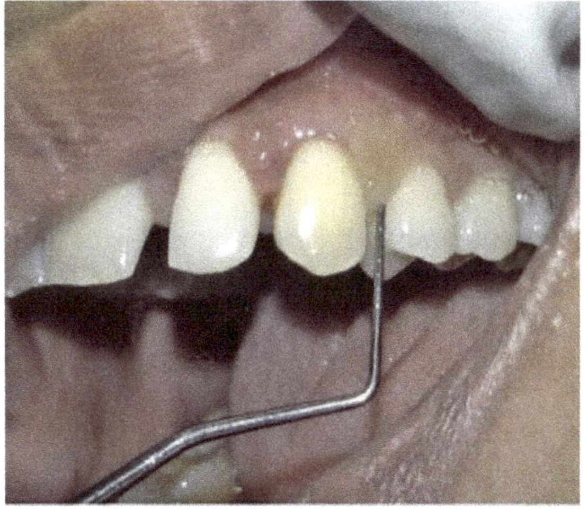

Fig. 1.13: Transillumination test

Periodontal probing

This test gives lot of information about the health of the periodontium. It is done by walking the probe around the gingival sulcus of tooth to detect periodontal pockets and quality of interproximal restorations. The presence of narrow pockets indicates periodontal pathology of pulpal origin. (endo perio lesions). Presence of wide pockets indicate pulpal pathology of periodontal origin. (perio endo lesion). Narrow pockets are wider apically and narrow cervically, wide pockets are narrow apically and wider cervically. Age of the patient is very important while assessing the pocket because 4 to 5 mm of pocket in older

Fig. 1.14: Periodontal probing

patient is normal. Periodontal probing test is very useful in detecting vertical fracture, sinus tracts and rarely even large lateral canals that are open into periodontal ligament space. It is also helpful to assess the presence of developmental grooves. Example palato- gingival groove in upper incisors. Multirooted teeth should be carefully probed to determine furcation involvement.

Mobility test

It is done to assess the stability of tooth within the bone. It gives the evidence of loss of periodontal support due to trauma or infection. The degree of periodontal break down depends upon the severity of infection or intensity of trauma. This test gives significant information in cases of acute alveolar abscess, infected radicular cyst, periapical granuloma and phoenix abscess. It is done by moving the involved tooth Bucco-lingually in the socket gently with help of handle of two instrument or two index fingers.

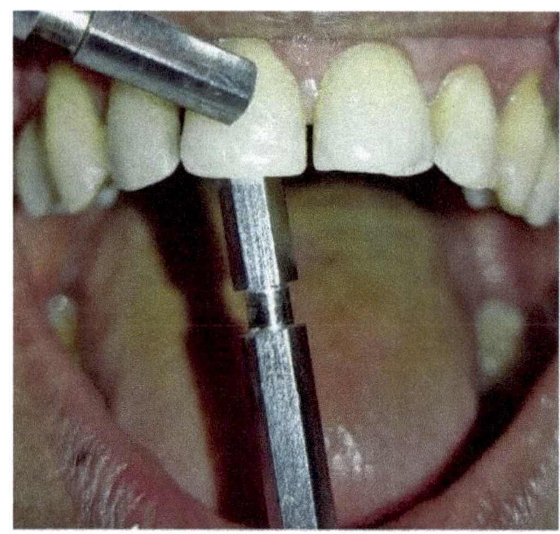

Fig. 1.15: Mobility test

Bucco lingual movement of tooth within 0.1 to 0.3 mm is considered to be normal, more than 0.3 mm is considered to be abnormal.

Vertical depressibility indicates acute Alveolar abscess. or accumulation of more pus in the periapical area. It is done by applying vertical pressure on the occlusal or incisal surface of tooth in apical direction and noticing vertical movement if any.

Selective anesthesia test

Due to absence of adequate proprioceptors in the pulp, the nature of pain of pulpal origin is generalized and referring whereas due to the presence of adequate proprioceptors in the periodontal ligament the pain of periodontal ligament origin is localized and specific.

Though achieving single tooth anesthesia without anesthetizing the adjacent tooth has been questioned. The selective anesthetic test is a remarkable tool in identifying the source of infection in the following situations:

- When patient has difficulty in identifying the offending tooth.
- When routine tests have failed to identify the source of pain.

Pre-requisite

Patient must have pain at the time of test.

Selective tooth anesthesia test

Based on other test results and clinician judgement most posterior (distal) tooth is anesthetized by precisely giving intraligamentary injections (course of nerve supply is from distal to mesial)

If pain subsides - The correct tooth has been diagnosed

If pain persist - The tooth mesial to it is anesthetized and continue to do so until the correct tooth is diagnosed.

Selective arch anesthesia test

It is carried out by giving nerve blocks. Superior posterior alveolar nerve block and infra orbital nerve block in maxilla and inferior alveolar nerve block in mandible.

After giving inferior alveolar nerve block if pain subsides - the source of pain is in the mandible. If pain persists the source of pain may be in maxilla.

If pain persists after anesthetizing both upper and lower arches the pain is of non-odontogenic origin.

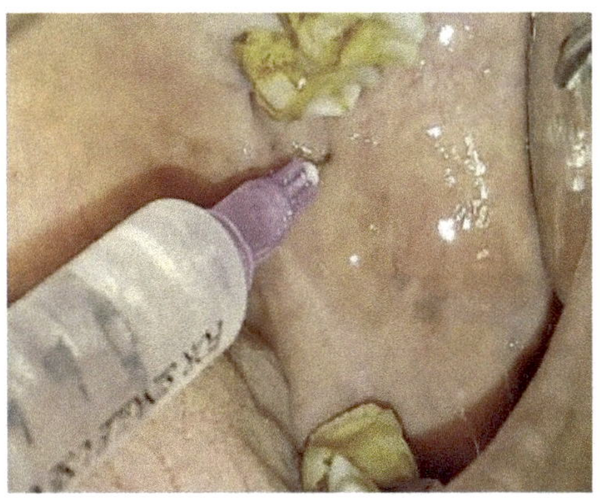

Fig. 1.16: Selective tooth anesthesia test

Fig. 1.17 : Selective arch anesthesia test

Test cavity

It is the final test to diagnose the vitality of a tooth when all other tests have failed to identify the offending tooth.

Sites

Lingual surfaces of anterior.

Occlusal surfaces of posteriors

After explaining the nature of test to the patient in detail drill through the enamel to the dentino enamel junction of an unanesthetized tooth in question at high speed with adequate water coolant, if patient complains of sensitivity or pain immediately stop drilling; the tooth has been diagnosed as vital, end the procedure by filling the tooth with appropriate filling material. On conversely, if patient does not complain of pain, the drilling is continued to the pulp chamber and routine root canal treatment is done.

Note: Test cavity test does great iatrogenic damage to the tooth.

Radiography

The discovery of X-rays in 1895 by Sir Wilhelm Conrad Roentgen was an incredible era in the history of medicine. The first intraoral radiograph was taken by Edmond kells in 1896 since then radiographic imaging technique has been the most important and crucial for the diagnosis, treatment plan and management of wide variety of dental procedures.

Introduction

One cannot imagine doing root canal treatment without using intra oral periapical radiographs. Though IOPAs shadow two-dimensional image (apico-coronal and mesio-distal) of three-dimensional dental anatomy (apico-coronal, mesio-distal and Bucco-lingual) they play core role in determining the diagnosis, treatment plan and evaluation of prognosis. Radiographs are the axial around which all the procedural steps revolve. Minimum 3 good quality IOPAs are required throughout the treatment procedure. IOPAs should be of full length and cover at least 4 mm of periapex area. For upper and lower posterior teeth, the X-ray cone should be directed from distal to mesial direction to move mesial roots of lower and mesio buccal roots upper away from furcation and prevent overlapping of buccolingual roots or buccolingual canals. For anterior teeth, the X-ray cone should be directed from mesial to distal direction to rule out presence of any extra canal or abnormalities in a buccolingual plane.

Main advantage of IOPAs are simple to use and less expensive. If done with attention there is less chances of distortion. Care must be taken to control dose dependent over exposure to prevent health hazards.

Pre-operative radiographs

Taken prior to treatment to identify and detect

1) Caries lesions close to pulp or involving pulp.
2) Large caries lesion involving furcation area.
3) Proximal caries and root caries.
4) Pulp calcification.
5) Pulp stones.
6) Pulp fibrosis.
7) Crown to root angulations.
8) Fractures.
9) Number of roots, number of canals, size and shape of canals.
10) Complex anatomy of tooth.
11) Congenital anomalies of tooth   .
12) Double curvatures and dentinal wedges.

13) Periapical status in periapical diseases of tooth.
14) Position of apical foramina.
15) Curvature and branching of root canals.
16) Size and shape of pulp chamber.

Operative radiographs

Taken during the treatment to assess, evaluate and determine:

1) Working length.
2) Perforations.
3) Blockages.
4) Instrument separation.
5) Apical seal of master gutta percha cone to avoid under obturation and over obturation.

Post-operative

Taken after the treatment to assess and evaluate the prognosis:

1) To detect voids and improperly condensed canals.
2) To detect under and over obturations.
3) To detect extrusion of sealers in periodontal area.
4) To detect missed complex root anatomy.
5) To assess resolving periapical radiolucency in periapical pathologies like acute and chronic periapical abscess, Pyogenic granuloma, Infected periapical cyst.

Methods

Film based imaging

X-ray film has an emulsion made of silver halide crystals and Sulphur compounds and a base made of polyester polyethylene terephthalate which is protected by an overcoat.

Film based imaging consists of X-ray interaction with electrons in the film emulsion that is film must be exposed to an x/ray radiation source then we through chemical processing transfer latent image in to visible one. Film based imaging requires fairly narrow exposure factors to produce a diagnostic quality radiograph. Film is a relatively inefficient radiation detector and thus requires relatively high radiation exposure and also image resolution is not adequate so specifying exact nature of tissues in field of interest is difficult.

X-ray films are available in various sizes for use in different areas. Films used for periapical view come in three sizes which can be chosen according to area of usage. The other films available are for occlusal view, panoramic view and cephalometric view in order of increasing size.

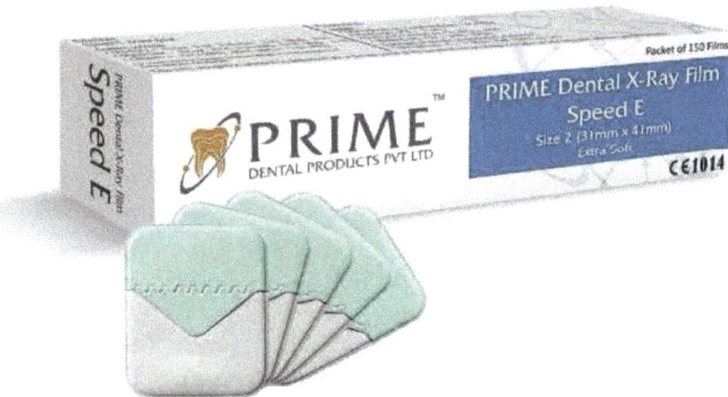

Fig. 1.18:

Advantages

- Film size is similar to beam size
- Films cover larger area
- High speed or faster films are used to reduce the radiation exposure
- Initially inexpensive
- Portable
- Can be viewed by all

Disadvantages

- Films are relatively insufficient radiation detectors and thus require relatively high radiation exposure
- Film has limited exposure latitude less detailed contrast
- Time consuming processing requires developing fixing and drying
- Requires dark room
- Loss of quality due to errors in processing
- Requires physical handling and storage
- Radiographic image cannot be adjusted once it is made

Digital radiography

Digital imaging is the result of X-ray interaction with electrons in the electronic sensor it incorporates computer technology in the capture, display, enhancement and storage of direct radiographic images. uses digital X-ray sensors to replace X-ray film.

Enhancement and modification of various properties of radiograph like brightness, contrast, density, magnification (zoom) linear mesurements, pseudocolouring, rotion helps in better diagnosis.

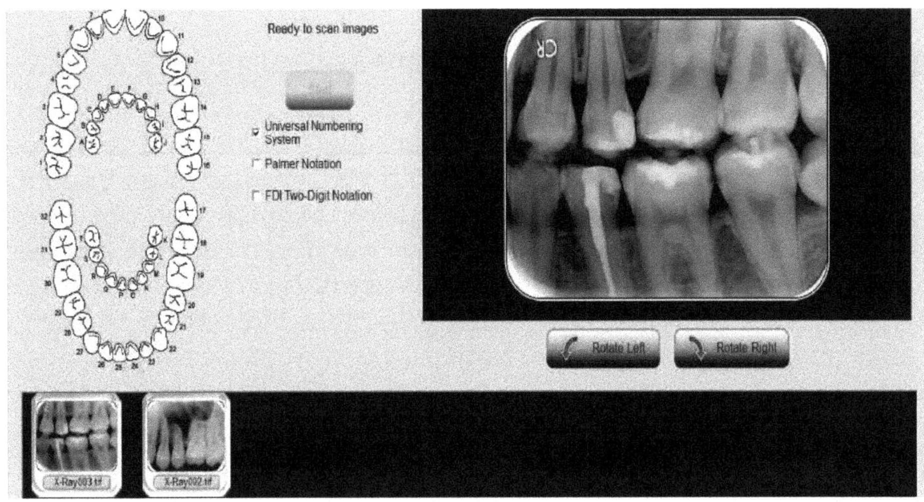

Fig. 1.19:

Advantages

- Superior gray scale image
- Less radiation exposure as frequency of exposing is less
- Instant exposure and viewing of image
- More information on image
- Easy documentation
- Enhancement of image
- Eliminates dark room
- Films and chemical processing no longer needed
- Aid in patient education
- Images can be transferred electronically
- Lower per image cost

Disadvantages

- Initially expensive
- Sensor is bulky in size
- Sensor size is smaller than beam size
- Sensor covers smaller area compare to film
- Non portable
- Difficulty in tender mobile tooth

Imaging techniques

Paralleling technique or long cone technique

It is the method of choice for intraoral radiography. It is the most intraoral radiographic technique can be achieved effectively by using digital sensor. In order to achieve parallelism, it is necessary to place receptor more lingual to the structures where there is adequate depth to place receptor. The use of receptor holding devices help us to standardize and execute this technique but attention to the relationship of the receptor to the objects of interest of critical to successful outcomes. Rigid sensor initially more difficult to place may result in more errors and can cause more discomfort for the patient. To overcome these problems rigid receptor should be placed closer to the mid line to aid proper placement and to reduce discomfort.

Principle

X-ray receptor is supported parallel to the long axis of the tooth and the central X-ray of the X-ray beam is directed at right angles to the teeth and receptor.

The film or sensor must be placed parallel with the being radiographs, the X-ray beam must be directed at right angles to the tooth and receptor.

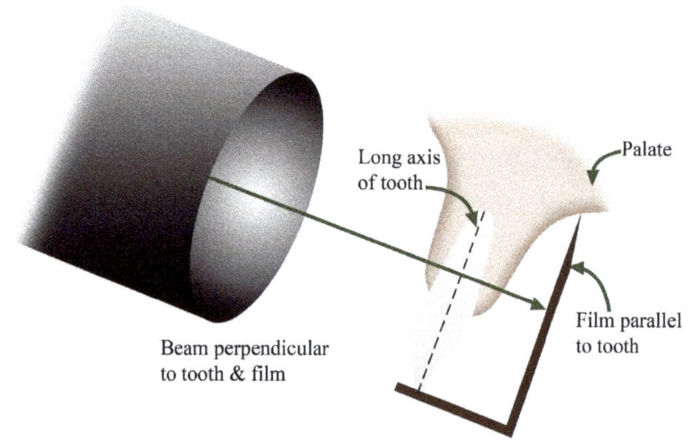

Fig. 1.20:

Advantages

Parallel technique should be always attempted before other techniques because parallel technique is superior to bisecting angle technique in producing more optimal images and in reproducing apical anatomy of the tooth.

Better dimensional accuracy – the paralleling technique results in less distortion of the image of the teeth. (The shape of the teeth and the relationship of the teeth to surrounding structures is more accurate).

Least distortion and less superimposition of apices of maxillary molars with zygomatic process.

Reproducibility: ability to take two or more radiographs of a given tooth at different time intervals and producing an image of same/near to same characteristics, especially useful in evaluating the healing of large lesions.

Procedural steps

- Proper infection control of intraoral sensor
- Placement of sensor in the patient mouth on a conventional film holder
- Paralleling technique is preferred as exposure technique
- Radiation exposure of sensor with conventional radiographic unit
- Digitalized conversation of analog image into computer
- Display of digital image in to computer monitor for diagnostic purpose of current procedures

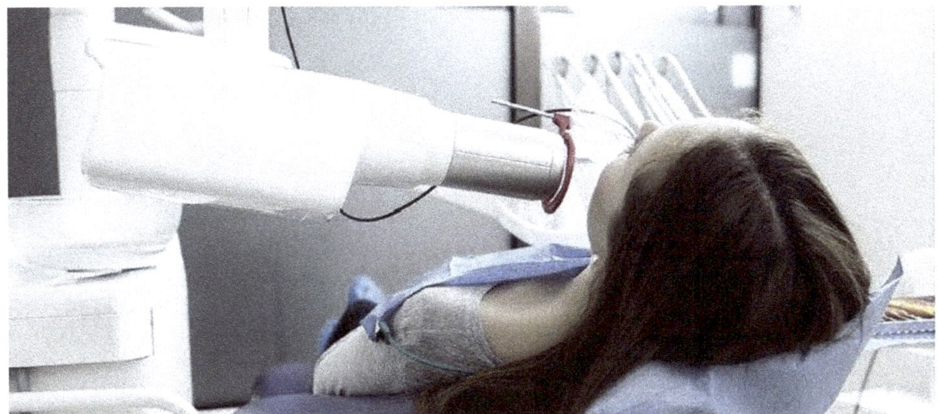
Fig. 1.21:

Bisecting angle technique or short cone technique

This technique is not routinely used in endodontics; It is useful alternative technique when receptor placement cannot be achieved due to patient trauma or anatomical abstractions .

Principle

Bisecting angle technique is accomplished by placing the receptor as close to the tooth as possible the central ray of X-ray beam should be directed perpendicular to an imaginary line that bisects the angle formed by the long axis of the tooth and plane of the receptor.

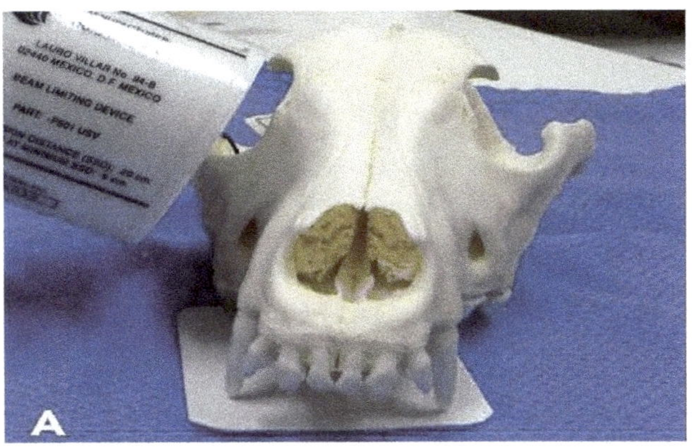

Fig. 1.22:

Indications

1) Anatomical abstraction like
   - Presence of tori or exostosis
   - Presence of shallow palate or low palatal vault
   - Presence of shallow floor of mouth
   - Presence of short frenum
   - Edentulous and /or narrow arches

2) Patient Trauma
   - Tender mobile teeth
   - Painful mobile teeth

Advantages

- Quick and More comfortable because receptor is placed against the tooth as close as possible the receptor does not impinges on the tissues
- Film holder is not mandatory
- No anatomical restrictions

Disadvantages

- Too flat angulation produces elongations and too acute angulations produces shortening.
- Deformation of the film results in distortion of the images

Limitation

Produces less optimal images because the receptor and teeth are not in same vertical plane

Indications

1) Anatomical abstraction like
   - Presence of tori or exostosis
   - Presence of shallow palate or low palatal vault
   - Presence of shallow floor of mouth
   - Presence of short frenum
   - Edentulous and /or narrow arches

2) Patient Trauma
   - Tender mobile teeth
   - painful mobile teeth

SLOB rule

Major drawback of conventional radiography is two-dimensional reproduction of three-dimensional entity radiograph provides visualization of anatomy under examination in the mesiodistal and apicocoronal plane while affording very little appreciation in the third (buccolingual) dimension.

A technique used to determine the buccal or lingual location of object and to determine the spatial relation of the object by shifting X-ray tube head mesially or distally, (the direction of the beam must be opposite to the way tube head is moved), is called tube shift technique also known as

- Cone shift technique
- Clarks technique
- Buccal object rule

Principle

The image of any buccally oriented object appears to move in the opposite direction from a moving X-ray source. contrarily the image of any lingually oriented object appears to move in the same direction as a moving X-ray source. Same lingual and opposite buccal"

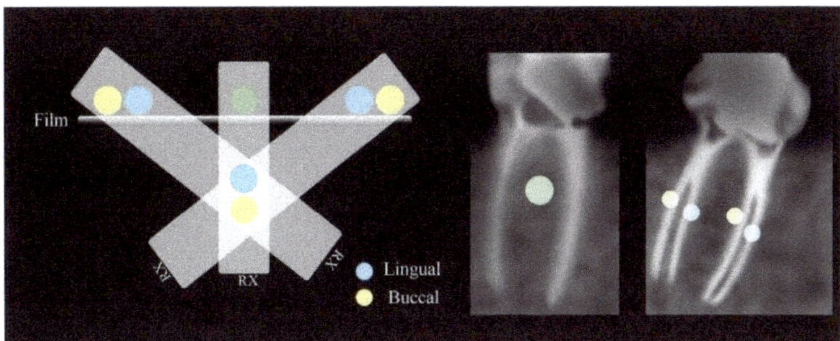

Fig. 1.23: The buccal object rule

Indication / Application

1) Separation and identification of superimposed canals.

Usually when we are doing root canal treatment of lower molars or maxillary first premolars, we have two canals that are superimposed to each other and we don't know which canal is buccal and which canal is lingual because we are viewing at two-dimensional image of three-dimensional object. When we have two canals on top of each other inside one root we split, separate and identify which canal is which by applying <u>Slob</u> rule.

When tube head is shifted mesially the mesio lingual canal (lower molars) palatal canal (upper first premolar) will also be shifted mesially (in same direction as the shifted tube head).

Mesio buccal canal (lower molar) buccal canal (upper first premolar) shifted distally (in the opposite direction as the shifted tube head).

2) Movement and identification of superimposed structures

Example: Zygomatic process which often obscures apices of maxillary molars

3) Determination of working length

Helpful to determine the full working length especially in single rooted teeth with two canal example mesial roots of lower molars and lower lateral incisors.

4) Determination of curvatures

Helpful to determine the acute curvature of the roots multirooted teeth especially buccal roots of upper molar.

5) Determination of faciolingual location separated instruments, impacted tooth, pathosis and foreign bodies

Example : Impacted canine.

6) Identification of undiscovered canals examples mb2 canal in maxillary molars, disto-buccal canal in lower canals

7) Location of calcified canals

8) Application of technique allows to distinguish between various types of resorptions

Example: Internal resorption or extrarenal resorption

9) Helps to determine buccolingual portion of fractures and perforative defects

10) To locate foreign bodies and to locate anatomical land marks in relation to root apex such as mandibular canal

Disadvantages

Decreased clarity

Changing the horizontal or vertical angulations of tube head lead to change in the direction of central beam relative to object and film that results in blurring of images. The more the change in angles less will be the clarity of images.

Superimposition of structures.

Objects that ordinarily have a separation on parallel radiographs may be with cone shift move relative to each other and become super imposed.

Example: Roots of maxillary molars.

Mesial and distal angled radiographs move the palatal root over the distobuccal or mesio-buccal reducing ability to distinguish apices clearly.

Limitations of conventional radiography

Compression of three- dimensional structures

Conventional radiography provides no depth information because conventional radiographs compress three dimensional structures on two-dimensional image. The radiograph provides a visualization of the anatomy under examination in the mesiodistal and apical coronal plane whilst affording very little appreciation of structures in the buccolingual dimension.

The compression of third dimensional anatomy associated with conventional radiographs often hinders an accurate appreciation of the spatial relationship of a tooth's roots to anatomy and any associated periapical lesions.

Example: True assessment of the spatial relationship of the roots of the teeth to their surrounding anatomical structures in three dimensions such as inferior alveolar canal, mental foramen and maxillary sinus cannot be achieved.

Even multiple radiographs with different horizontal or vertical angulations do not always guarantee complete detection of all the relevant structures or the pathos'.

Anatomical complexities the extent of resorptive lesions as well as iatrogenic procedural errors may not be truly appreciated.

Evaluation of the root to theoretical plate and thickness of cortical plate for presurgical evaluation is extremely difficult as the diagnostic information is missing in the third dimension.

Geometric distortion

The geometry of area being assessed is rarely reproduced with complete accuracy using conventional intraoral radiograph.

Due to the divergent nature of the X-ray beam during imaging and the unavoidable separation between the image receptor and the object a minimum 6% magnification of the object being radiographed can be expected in the final image even when the paralleling procedure is executed perfectly. Geometric distortion of image may also occur due to lack of proper orientation of the film/sensor to the long axis of tooth.

Anatomical superimposition

Reduced clarity and loss of details due to superimposition of underlying anatomical structures like zygomatic process, maxillary sinus, mandibular canal etc.

Anatomical noise

Anatomy in the area of interest during conventional radiographic may impair visualization of the object under investigation and complicate interpretation of the radiograph, these anatomical interferences can vary in radiodensity and are referred to as anatomical noise.

Anatomical noise caused by feature of overlying alveolar bone such as the cortical plate trabeculae and marrow spaces.

Temporal perspectives

The cases in which a particular area or tooth need to be compared over times assess the development or progression of a disease. The radiographs should be standardized with respect to the X-ray beam angle the distance between the object and the image receptor (film)and all of the radiation exposure parameters.

Poorly standardized radiographs may result in a misinterpretation of disease onset or progression. Chronic inflammatory tissues cannot be differentiated from healed fibrous tissues.

Considerable amount of bone loss should occur for being visible on the radiograph.

Plain radiographs have false positive rate of 4%.

Plain radiographs have false negative rate of more than 30%.

CBCT

Also known as

- Dental volumetric tomography.
- Cone beam volumetric tomography
- Dental computed tomography
- Cone beam imaging

Abstract

Since the discovery of X-ray in 1895 by Sir Wilhelm Conard Roentgen, Germany. Diagnostic imaging turned out to be more refined owing to addition of various imaging techniques with complex physical principles. In 1967 the limitations of classic conventional radiography overcome by introduction of computerized axial scanning by Godfrey house field which later on developed into CT scanning in 1972.

In 1990 Tachibana Matsumoto first reported use of CT in endodontics however owing to its high radiation exposure, high cost and limited availability the use in endodontic limited and also could not be justified. In 1997 with the independent works of Arai in japan Mosso in Italy, quantitative radiology produces first CBCT in 2001 FDA licensed first CBCT for use in USA.

Introduction

CB - A beam of divergent X-rays forming cone

CT – A technique involves in imaging of layers or slices

Slice is the cross section of the body which is scanned for the production of three-dimensional CT or CBCT images.

BCT is modification of traditional CT scanning

In CT slices are acquired first then reconstructed to create volume whereas in CBCT the volume is acquired first then slices are reconstructed from the volume.

Definition

Cone beam computed tomography is an extra oral modern digital imaging technique specifically designed for the use on the maxillofacial skeleton to provide accurate high quality undistorted three -dimensional image of an area under examination.

Principle

An x-ray beam in cone or pyramidal shape collimated through an area of interest on to the detector. The X-ray source and sensor of CBCT system rotates around the patient head between 180-360° for a few seconds. This single rotation captures multiple sequential projections of images around the area of interest. This results in a cylindrical or spherical volume of data described as the field of view (FOV).

In routine clinical practice an experienced clinician working with microscope would be expected identify the canals in majority of cases therefore routine use of CBCT for every case is not justified.

CBCT in endodontics require high detail and resolution to appreciate the intricacies of root canal system and periodontium. High image resolution comes at the cost of higher patient radiation exposure, potential benefits of CBCT must be balanced with comparatively higher levels of risk from radiation exposure cases must therefore be assessed on an individual basis to determine whether the addition information from scan will be beneficial in influencing the management of case.

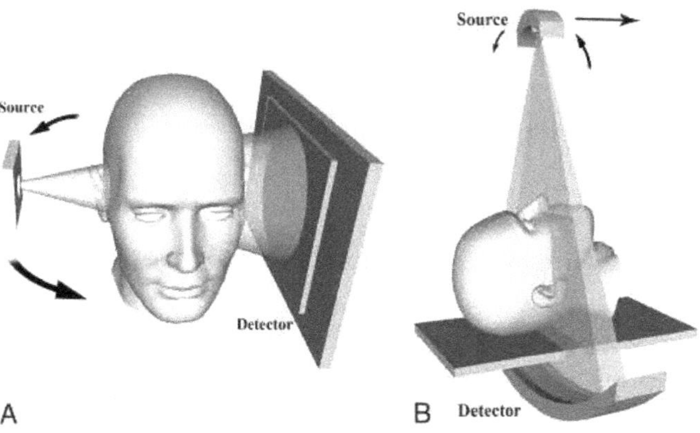

Fig. 1.24:

How CBCT works

The single rotation captures the planned data (180 -1024 2D images) this raw data is collected and analyzed by the sophisticated software of scanner, with the help of digital imaging the analyzed and processed data converted into two - dimensional picture elements called pixels. The spatial resolution of 2D image is determined by the individual picture elements (pixels)

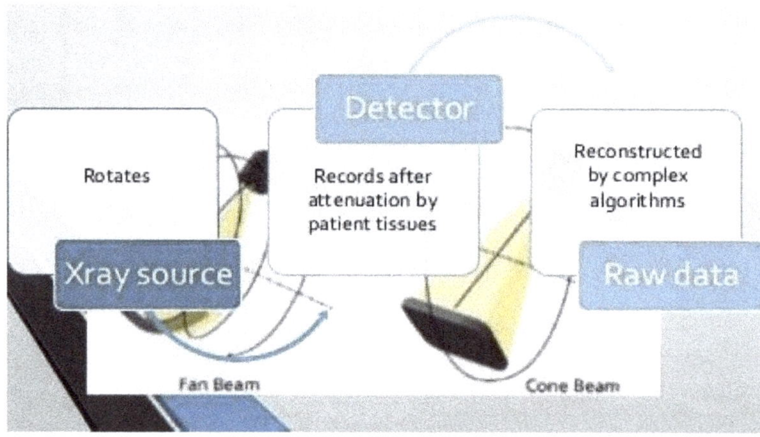

Fig. 1.25:

Pixel

Pixel are minute areas composed of picture elements. These picture elements are united and formatted with the help of digital software to form two-dimensional radiographic image with the help of CBCT based algorithms. The pixels are converted into voxels just as a digital radiograph subdivided into pixel, the CBCT images are composed of voxels.

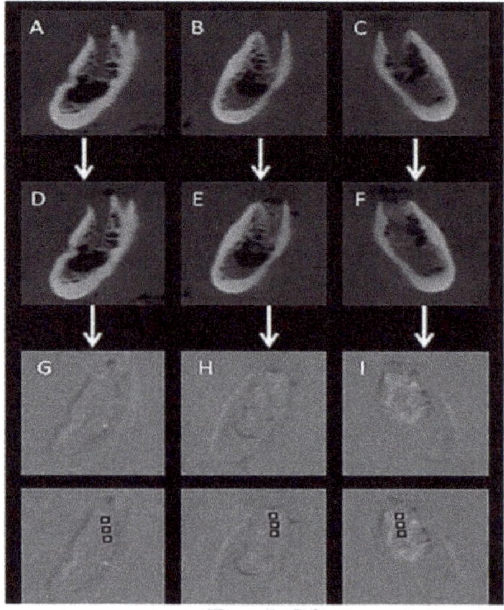

Fig. 1.26:

Voxel

A voxel is a three-dimensional pixels. CBCT images are composed of voxels just as a digital radiograph composed of pixels. Voxels are isotropic (cubic in nature similar in all Dimensions) the spatial resolution of the CBCT images determined by individual volume elements (voxels) the principal determinant of voxel size is pixel size of the detector hence the size of the voxel corresponds to the size of the pixel detector. Smaller the field of view smaller will be the pixel and voxel size better will be the spatial resolution.

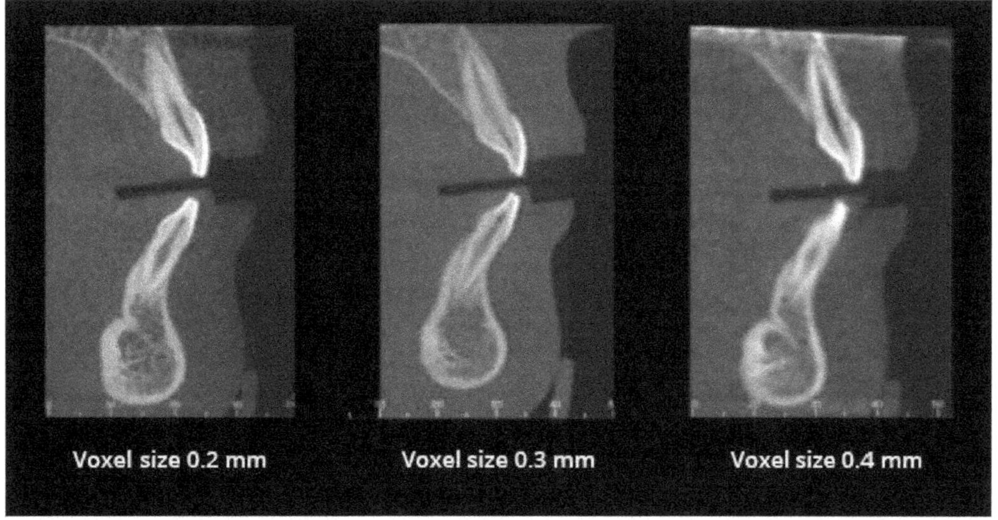

Fig. 1.27:

Field of view or scan volume

- It is the amount of anatomical area that will be irradiated in a single scan to obtain spherical or cylindrical data volume.

Size of the FOV field of view depends upon the following

- Detector shape and size

- Collimation ability of primary beam

- Beam projection geometry

- Scan time and exposure time

- CBCT beam can be pulsatile the patient is often exposed

- To radiation for only small portion of overall scan time that is actual exposure time markedly less than the scanning time. The average scan time may vary from 7 to 30 seconds. It also varies if half rotation or full circle rotation is used lesser the scan time lesser will be the motion artifacts

- Standard exposure time is 3-4 seconds
- Patient exposure time depends upon the following
- Presence of pulsatile X-ray beam
- Size of the image field
- Patient position

Imaging may be performed with patient seated, supine, or standing the patient head is positioned and stabilized between the X-ray generator and detector by a head holding apparatus.

Seated units are most comfortable artifacts due to substile movement of head less compared to standing units requires small surface area /physical footprint. Supine unit equipment require larger surface area/physical footprint. The artifacts due to substile movement are more in standing units.

Procedure

Patient selection

CBCT utilizes ionizing radiation, patient exposure to radiation is higher compared to other types of radiological imaging techniques so CBCT must not be used routinely for endodontic diagnosis or screening or for screening in the obscene of clinical signs and symptoms. Each CBCT examination should be tailored to the individual patient and their diagnostic needs. There must be justification of exposure to the patient so that total potential diagnostic benefits are greater than individual determined radiation exposure.

Selection FOVs

Every effort should be made to reduce the effects of radiation doses for endodontic specific tasks using smallest possible FOVs and voxel size recommended. Restricted or small FOVs provides high detail and resolution of limited region which is required to appreciate the intricacies of root canal system and periodontium hence best suited for endodontic use.

Only small FOV CBCT are recommended for the diagnosis and management of endodontic problems for the following reasons.

increased spatial resolution to improve the accuracy of endodontic specific tasks such as visualization fine details or small tasks reduces the exposure to the patient.

1) Reduce the volume of exposed tissues
2) Effective radiation dose is reduced
3) Reduces the scatter and improves the image quality.
4) Smaller volume to be interpreted saves time

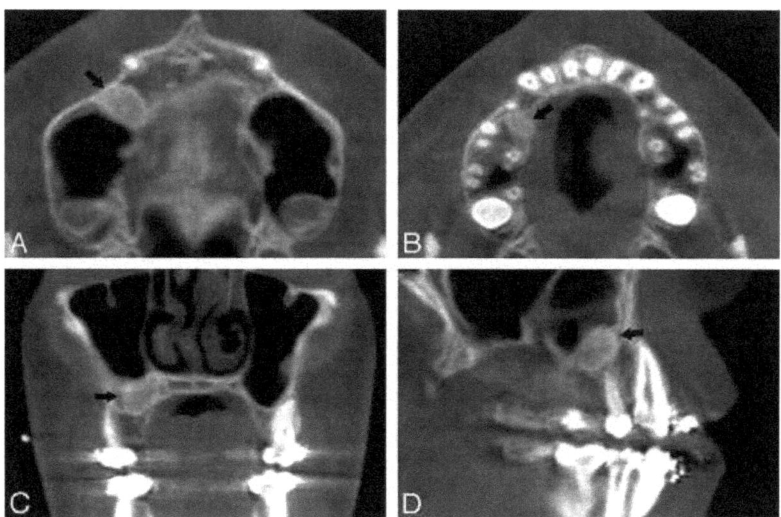

Fig. 1.28:

Patient preparation

personal protection barrier like lead aprons and thyroid collars must be provide to the patients to protect from unnecessary radiation exposure and its hazardous effects.

Special protection protocols must be followed to prevent hazardous effects of high radiation in children, pregnant women, patient with thyroid disorders.

Head stabilization

Head is positioned and stabilized between the X-ray generator and detector by a head holding apparatus made of chin cups and lateral head support to prevent subtle head movements. Subtle head movements degrade image quality, head holding apparatus is made of chin.

Alignment

Alignment of an area of interest with X-ray is critical in imaging.

The X-ray beam is aligned and collimated such that only the area of interest irradiated producing specific volume of data appropriate and relevant to the patient needs.

Facial topographic reference planes plane Frankfort horizontal or intra oral reference occlusal plane aligned with external laser light position.

Imaging protocols

A set of technical exposure parameters is developed to produce images of optimal quality with least amount of radiation exposure to the patient; these include Resolution, Kvp, ma, Acquisition time in seconds and Radiation dose.

Imaging

During imaging the C arm or gantry rotate around a patient head to acquire multiple sequential projection images in one complex scan around area of interest. The data are analyzed and reconstructed using CT based algorithm to create a volume of data which can be viewed in three planes.

Advantages of using CBCT

3D reconstruction: -Three-dimensional visualization of the region of interest is obtained in sufficient to localize teeth and adjacent anatomy in a manner which is simply not achievable with conventional intraoral, panoramic and cephalometric images. This application can be theoretically used to reconstruct intra and extra oral images, the uses range from profiling root canals to visualizing facial fractures in all 3-dimensions buccolingual, mesiodistal and apical coronal thus this three-dimensional volume rendering technology allow the clinicians to come up with faster more accurate and diagnosis, treatment plans and evaluations.

Enhancement of images

Enhancement of images include zoom, magnification, window /level adjustments and text or arrow annotations can be applied, curser-driven measurement algorithms provide the clinician with an interactive capability for real-time dimensional assessment. On screen measurements are free from distortion and magnification.

Image accuracy

Provides images of highly contrasting structures, superior gray scale resolution of 256 colors of gray in comparison with 16 – 25 shades of gray on conventional film and is therefore particularly well suited for the imaging of osseous structures of the craniofacial area.

Multiplanar reformation. Interactive display modes applicable to maxillofacial imaging.Custom image reformatting to provide optimal visualization from different angles and perspectives

Rapid scan time. Produces a complete volume of image in a single scan rotation compare to fan beam CT only produces a single slice image per scan. Rapid scan time reduces motion artifacts, reduces radiation exposure.

Comfortable and improves patient satisfaction

Dose-reduction: - Based on the type of radiograph being taken radiation can be reduced by as much as 3-4 or more time as conventional CBCT offers distinct FOV sizes variation imaging mode and the possibility to select the volume size. According to the diagnosis allow dental professionals to obtain excellent image resolution and minimize the risk of radiation for patients..

Beam limitation: - Through collimation reduces and limit the radiation to the area of interest.

Filtration: - Addition of filters to the airspace around face can clarify the soft tissue profile if original image was poor.

Patient- education: - patients will have a much better experience when coming to your office usually dentists use 2D images to visualize 3D pictures patients cannot read 2D scans, taking a CBCT image and immediately explaining finding as the patients view condition on an operatory monitor, patients can clearly see and understand the issues they are having and it improves acceptances of treatment options and plans.

Teleradiology: -The digital image file can further send colleagues for review

Example via email

Easy to use

Taking a cone beam scan is almost the same as taking a panoramic X-ray. The image is displaced at the chair-side immediately post exposer CBCT system allow the dentists to convert CBCT images in to other formats such as panoramic or cephalometric images.

Environmentally friendly: - No processing chemicals are used or disposed.

High patient satisfaction: - convenient painless and more time saving.

Darkroom is no longer needed: -So it is economically convenient; now this space can be used for other more useful purpose in dental office.

Cheaper

Cheaper compare to CT scanner, A brand new CT scanner cost 5 times more than a brand-new cone-beam CT. Latest smaller size CBCT systems reduces footprint.

Disadvantages

1) Artifacts - motion artifacts are distortions in the image caused due to subtle patient movements during scanning present as double contours.Streaking artifacts caused due to scatter and beam hardening appear as streaks and dark bands between two dense structures.

2) Cost –It is expensive

3) Medicolegal-Ability to manipulate the images for fraudulent purposes.

4) High Dose (more radiation exposer to patient)-more radiation exposure compared to conventional radiographic techniques and less radiation exposure to CT scanning.

5) Availability limited to hospitals and medical radiology practices, medico-legal considerations exist with this modality.

6) Inability to accurately represent the internal structure of soft tissues and soft tissue lesions.

When to consider a CBCT scan-General guidelines

CBCT is considered when regular conventional radiography is not sufficient. though CBCT is an invaluable tool in detection and diagnosis in endodontic conditions there are substantial missing links regarding its efficiency and benefits to the endo problems. Appropriate utilization of this technology result in more efficient patient management. In routine clinical practice an experienced clinician working with microscope would be expected to identify the canals in majority of cases therefore routine use of CBCT for every case is not justified.

CBCT in endodontics require high detail and resolution to appreciate the intricacies of root canal system and periodontium. High image resolution comes at the cost of higher patient radiation exposure, potential benefits of CBCT must be balanced with comparatively higher levels of risk from radiation exposure cases must therefore be assessed on an individual basis to determine whether the additional information from scan will be beneficial in influencing the management of case.

A CBCT scan may only be considerd after the following

1) Comprehensive clinical examination and history.

2) Appropriate conventional radiograph taken and assessed.

3) The benefits of the CBCT scan must outweigh the risks

4) The ALARA principle "As low As Reasonably Achievable".

5] New information to aid the patient

6] Not be repeatedly routinely

7] Diagnosis with lower radiation imaging is questionable

8] Through clinical evaluation report should be made

9] Should not be done for soft tissue assessment

10] Use small doses where you can

11] Resolution compatible with adequate diagnosis yet low radiation

12] Small FOV for Denton alveolar regions and teeth

Indications /application of CBCT in endodontics

Cone beam computed tomography overcomes the limitation of conventional radiography. Therefore, the potential benefits of this imaging system in endodontics, where the anatomy being assess is complex, are vast.

Diagnostic and detection of periapical pathology

Cone beam computed tomography is significantly more specific and sensitive in the diagnosis of Periapical pathology in presence of contradictory (nonspecific) signs and / or symptoms than conventional radiography. CBCT has the ability to detect small areas of periapical pathos's, can reveal bone defects of cancellous bone and cortical bone separately.

Periapical bone destruction of apical periodontitis associated with endodontic infection can be identified using CBCT. Prior to being appear on two dimensional radiographs, the prevalence of apical periodontitis was found to be significantly higher when using CBCT in comparison with conventional radiographs. CBCT may also be used to confirm the absence of odontogenic etiology therefore assist in the diagnosis of non-odontogenic causes of pain.

Assessment of potential surgical sites

CBCT technique is enhancing endodontic surgical case management and preventing the potential for iatrogenic damage, Preoperatively better analyze and relate the position and orientation of the specific roots undergoing the surgical procedure to surrounding vital anatomical structures like maxillary sinus, the inferior dental nerve canal and the mental foramen.

Assessment and management of dental trauma

The exact nature and extent of the injuries to the teeth and the alveolar bone can be assessed accurately by eliminating anatomical noise and image compression. Horizontal root fractures, resorptive defects such as internal or external resorption and alveolar fractures are readily observed and differentiated. Current evidence indicates CBCT scans cannot reliably detect small cracks or incomplete vertical root fracture; only give information about lateral bone resorption associated with vertical root fractures, a CBCT would therefore not be indicated.

The degree and direction of displacement associated with luxuriation injuries can be evaluated using CBCT. Finally, patients are likely to find extraoral CBCT imaging technique far more comfortable than tolerating intraoral sensor holders especially when teeth are mobile or fractured or there are soft tissue injuries.

Diagnosis, assessment and management of root resorption

Teeth affected by a root resorption have a poor prognosis if the causative lesions are not treated.

Although intraoral imaging techniques can be helpful in localizing root resorption. CBCT has been shown to be significantly more sensitive in detecting resorptive lesions the buccolingual extent of the resorptive lesion into canal or periodontal ligament can more easily assessed. CBCT assessments can provide the true size and position of all resorptive defects and distinguishes different types of resorptions in the region of interest therefore preoperative CBCT scans should be performed on all teeth with resorptive lesions that are potentially treatable.

Calcified canals

Canal sclerosis or calcification is a common challenge in adequately disinfecting the canals. Magnification and illumination are essential tools for the identification and treatment of calcified canals or sclerosed canals. CBCT be of minimal benefit in assisting with location of these canals as the resolution is significantly less than periapical radiographs.

Assessment of treatment complications

Useful to assess complications such as separated files and perforations, CBCT will provide information about root canal morphology to determine if the separated fragment can be retrieved or bypassed, perforation on a buccal or lingual aspect may also be more clearly assessed with CBCT to determine most appropriate management technique. Valuable tool when additional information is needed in postoperative assessment of extrusion of sealers, over obturations.

Assessment of root canal anatomy and morphology

Each tooth demonstrates variety of canal configurations, the internal and external morphological features are variable and complex, several classification have been proposed to define the various types of canal configurations that occur commonly, the lack of knowledge regarding this can result in inadequate instrumentation and consequent failure of root canal treatment. An experienced clinician working with microscope would be expected to identify canals, root curvatures, anomalies within the canals examples obstructions, narrowing , bifurcation and pulp stones in majority of cases therefore routine use of CBCT is not justified.

Cone beam computed tomography has been shown to be reliable tool to accurately assess root canal anatomy and morphology cases with unusual root formations such as dense in dente, dense-evaginates, C-shaped molars, multirooted premolars may benefit from CBCT scan.

Presence of additional roots or canal "distolingual roots in mandibular molars, second mesiobuccally(mb2) canal maxillary molars", Root curvature and anomalies within the canals themselves examples obstructions, narrowing, bifurcation and pulp stones).

The availability of this information preoperatively reduces the chances of the aberrations or mishaps during root canal treatment.

To confirm the causes of nonodontogenic pathology and to determine the extent of the lesion and its effects on surrounding anatomical structures.

Provide information exact location of apical foramina especially when root apices are resorbed.

A case where the root canal treatment was performed to a good standard and has still failed may require CBCT imaging before endodontic orthograde retreatment to assess and determine missed extremely complex anatomy which went unidentified and untreated during conventional treatment.

Limitations

The spatial resolution is lower than that of conventional radiograph, spatial resolution of film is 15-20-line pairs /mm where as CBCT images have 2 -line pairs /mm however CBCT technology is improving and resolution is improving.

Contrast resolution of CBCT limited by high scatter radiation during image acquisition, divergence of X-ray beam and in-built flat panel detector related artifacts. If the objective of examination soft tissue only, using CBCT would not serve the purpose.

Scatter and beam hardening

When the CBCT X-ray beam encounters a very high density object, such as enamel or metallic restorations such as sliver amalgams, metal posts, metal crowns or even gutta percha the beam scatter and the low energy photons in the beam are absorbed by structure, as result the mean energy of the beam increases which is referred to beam hardening, scatter and beam hardening can cause significant radiographic artifact sufficient to compromise details of root canal anatomy and relevant pathos's such as root resorption and root fractures. If this scatter and beam hardening is within or close to the tooth being assessed the resultant image will be of minimal diagnostic use.

Higher radiation dose of CBCT as compare to conventional radiographic techniques limits its usage to very specific situations.

Cannot diagnose caries adjacent to metal restoration as far as proximal and pit and fissure caries is concerned the research is limited.

Current evidence indicates CBCT scans cannot reliably detect small cracks or incomplete vertical root fracture.

Patient related factors

- Age young growing children

- Radio sensitivity

- Pregnancy

- History of heavy radiation exposure

- Research on the treatment out comes related to CBCT application in endodontic practice is needed for full-fledged support regarding its uses.

2
Diagnosis

> KNOWLEDGE ILLUMINES THE MIND
> THE MORE WE KNOW, THE MORE LIGHT THERE IS.
> WHEN IT COMES TO EFFECTIVE ENDODONTIC DIAGNOSIS,
> PERCEPTIONS ARE PRAYERS AND CLARITY IS WORSHIP.

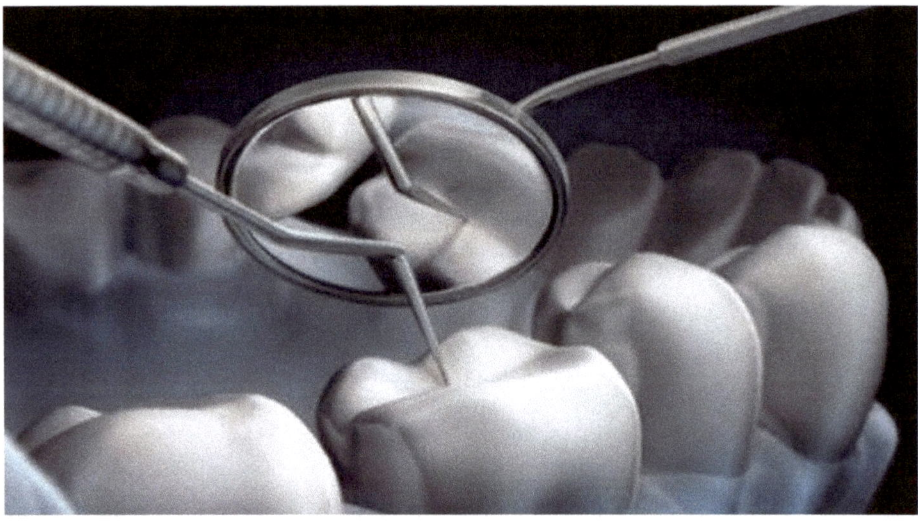

Fig. 2.1:

INTRODUCTION

- Effective and quality endodontics starts with correct diagnosis. The correct diagnosis is made by analyzing and interpreting data gathered from investigations with clear perceptions and right knowledge.

- Clear perceptions are developed over time only with knowing, the more we know the more light there is.

- Knowing is developed over time with accumulating essential knowledge by doing. So, we humans learn by Doing. The only things which make our endodontic diagnosis perfect is practicing more and learning by mistakes.

PULPAL PATHOLOGY

Reversible pulpitis

Mild to moderate inflammation of pulp due to exposure of dentin. May also be due to abnormal occlusal contacts.

- Also known as dentinal pain.
  Pain is due to involvement of A-delta fibers
  On inspection involved teeth may have caries, large restorations, improper, occlusal contacts, cracks or fracture of crowns.

- The pain is sharp, localized, short and momentary.

- Pain aggravates after taking cold and disappears immediately after the removal of stimuli.

- Response to low current electric pulp test.

- Tender on percussion is negative.

  Radiographs revels depth and extension of caries or restorations.

Management

Insulation or covering of exposed dentin with restorative material such as glass ionomer cements, composites, bio dentin and bio ceramic materials.

Correction of abnormal occlusal contacts if due to improper occlusal contacts.

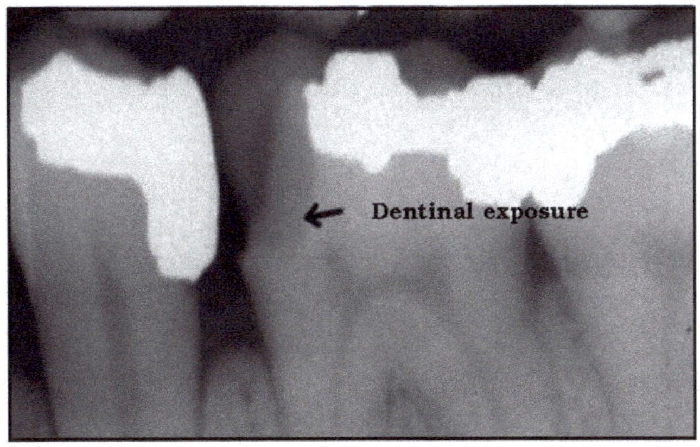

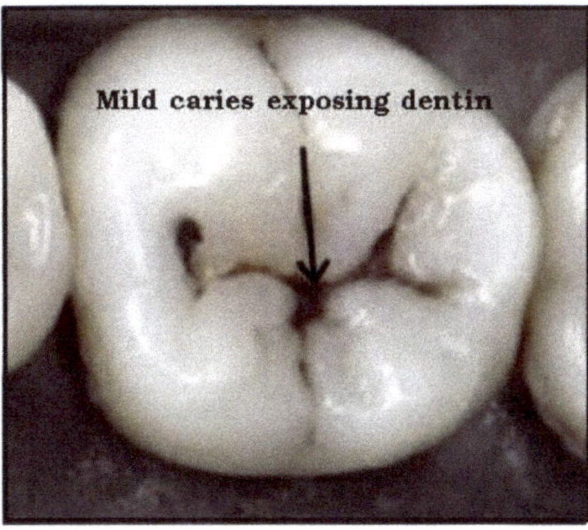

Fig. 2.2: Reversible pulpitis

Irreversible pulpitis

Partial or Total permanent damage of pulp tissue due to caries, trauma or reversible pulpitis. On examination involved teeth may have deep caries or large restorations.

Tender on percussion is positive.

- Response to high current electric pulp test.
- Pain is due to involvement of C-fibers.
- Nature of pain is spontaneous, continuous, referring, long duration, severe as if tooth is under constant pressure.
- Pain aggravates after taking hot and persist even after removal of stimuli may be for minutes.
- Pain relieves after taking cold and is the classical sign of irreversible pulpitis.
- Pain exacerbates on changes in posture, *e.g.*, bending or lying down.

Radiographs revels radiolucency (caries) involving pulp or secondary Caries beneath restorations.

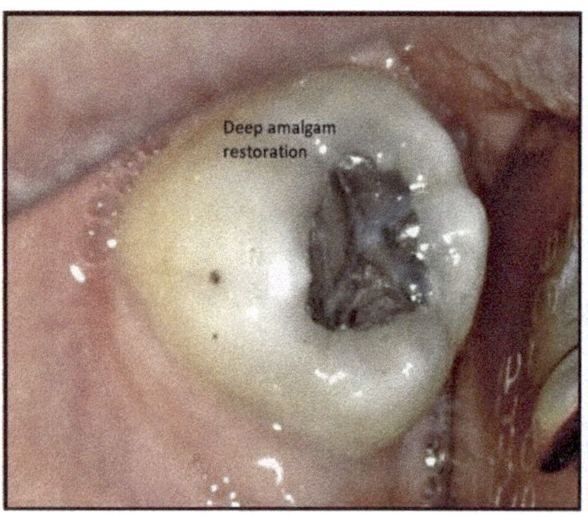

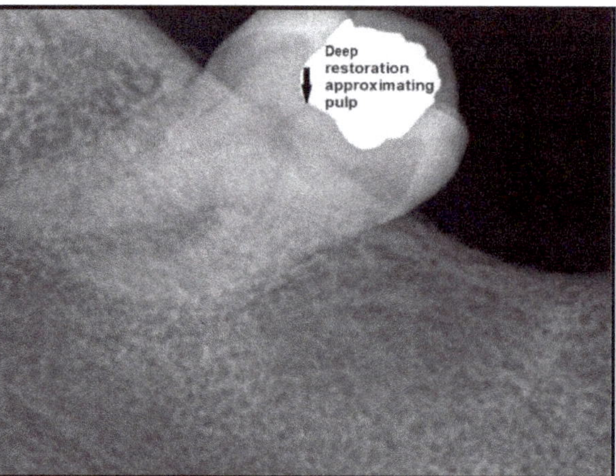

Fig 2.3: Irreversible pulpitis

Management

Root canal treatment

Asymptomatic irreversible pulpitis

History of recent trauma.

Asymptomatic.

Slight discoloration of tooth or dull appearance of crown

Response to high current electric pulp test.

Most of the time discovered through full mouth radiographs by chance.

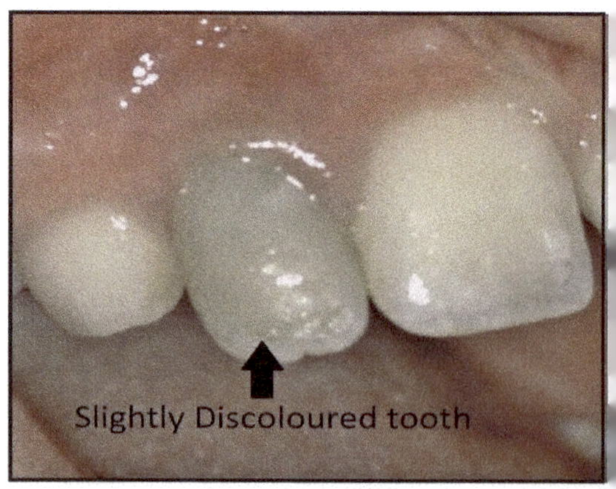

Fig. 2.4: Pulp necrosis

Management

It is incapable of healing unless irreversibly damaged pulp tissue is removed

Pulp necrosis

- May be symptomatic or asymptomatic.
- Non responding to electric pulp test.
- Teeth with multiple canals may show mixed response due to only one canal have necrotic pulp
- History of trauma

Clinical feature

Discoloration or opaque appearance of tooth.

Radiograph

Shows normal appearance or slight widening of periodontal ligament space

Management

Root canal treatment.

Chronic hyperplastic pulpitis

Commonly associated with lower molars.

Seen in children and young adults.

Due to long standing, low grade

Infection (irritation) of young pulp.

Discomfort during chewing

Pulp polyp (granulation tissue seen in crown portion of tooth).

Tissue may bleed easily due presence rich vascular supply.

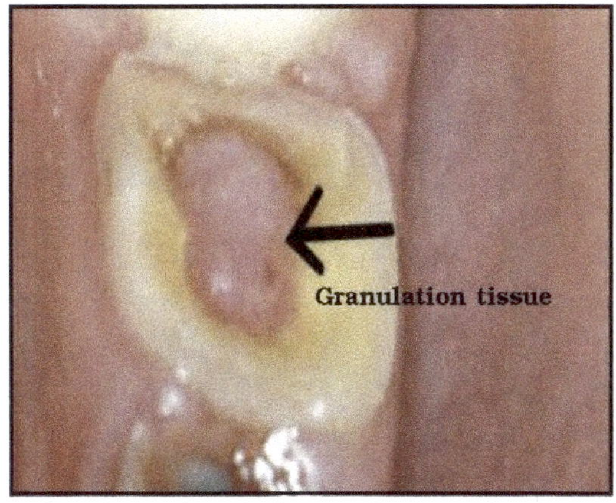

Fig. 2.5: Chronic hyperplastic pulpitis

Radiographically

Open cavity with direct access to pulp chamber

Management

Root canal treatment.

Reinforcing and strengthening of tooth with fiber post and flowable composite restorations.

If needed crown lengthening

Finally cover the restored tooth with prosthetic crown

Note

When very minimum amount of tooth structure is left which is unfavorable for restoration as seen in late stages of chronic hyperplastic pulpitis extraction is considered.

Internal resorption

Resorption of pulp chamber and root canals.

It initiates in the pulp and initially affects the internal or pulpal surface of dentin hence it is called internal resorption.

It is less common compared to external resorption, sometimes it may get confused with external cervical resorption.

Commonly seen in maxillary and mandibular central incisors.

Etiology

Auto immune in origin

Etiopathogenesis

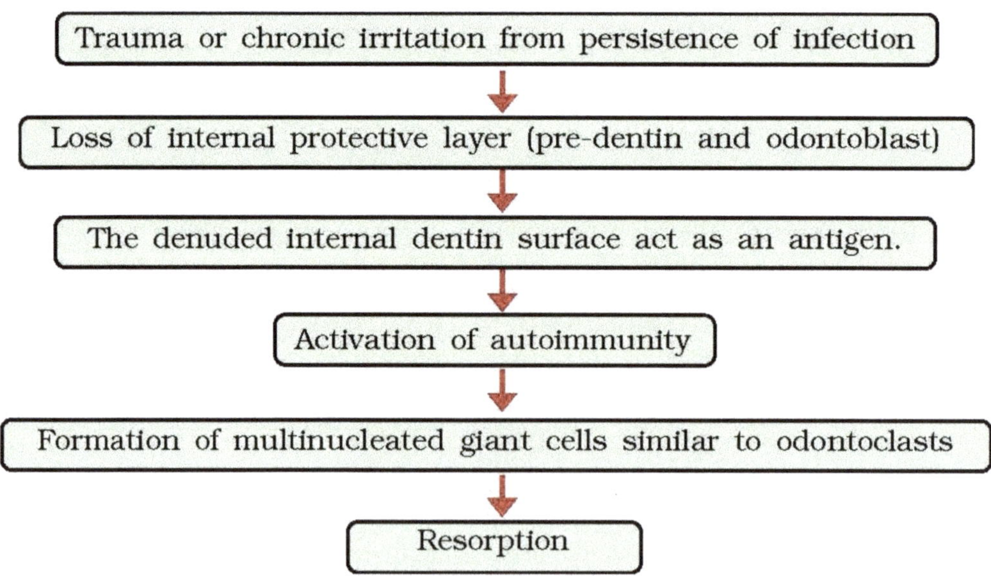

Clinical features

Initially pink spot appears in the cervical portion of labial surface of crown later the pink spot gradually increases in size to involve the whole labial surface of the crown.

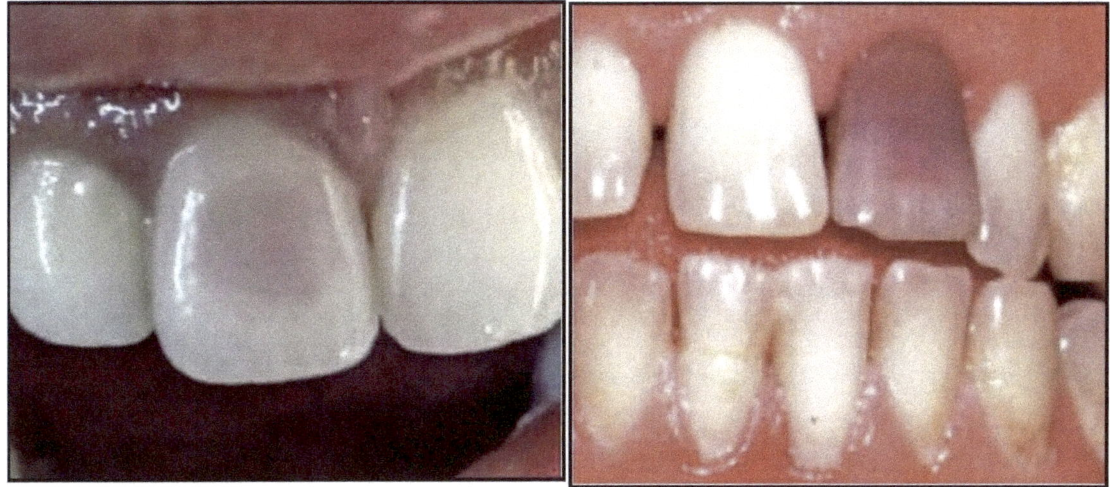

Fig. 2.6: Internal resorption

Radiographically

Ovoid to round shape radiolucency in crown and root portion of tooth. The margins are smooth clearly defined. The walls of the root canal may appear to balloon out, radiolucency confined to root and crown.

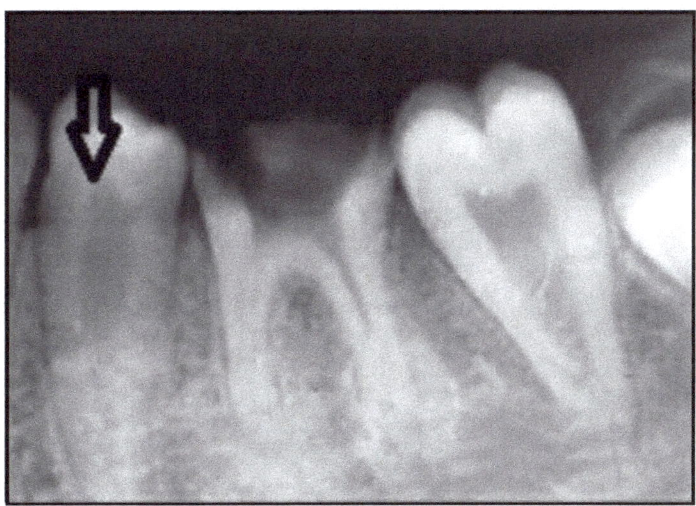

Fig. 2.7: Ovoid shaped radiolucency in crown and root portion

Management

- Removal of pulp stops the internal resorption process/Root canal treatment.

- Obturation with warm gutta percha fills the resorptive lacunae completely.

- In tooth with open apex and large resorptive lacunae obturation with MTA is recommended to seal open apex and resorptive defect effectively.

- If resorptive defects are perforated MTA recommended to repair and seal the perforations.

Definition

CRACKED TOOTH SYNDROME

The term used to describe the minute unapparent cracks running through the tooth which leads to recurrent discomfort, sensitivity and pain on relieving biting pressure is called cracked tooth syndrome.

It is one of the most common misdiagnosed conditions in dental practice.

Incidence

This condition is commonly seen in mandibular first molars between the age group 35 and 50 years.

Mandibular First molars are the first teeth to erupt in the oral cavity hence more prone to decay and extensive restoration.

Wedging of mesio palatal cusp of upper molars upon lower molars may lead to uneven stress distribution and causes cracks.

Predisposing factors

Existing restoration in the teeth.

Ageing (The elasticity of dentin decreases with age).

Maturation defects of tooth (formation of microcracks during defective mineralization and calcification) or due to incompletion of fusion.

Parafunctional habits (bruxism, nail biting).

Causes

1. Trauma from occlusion
   Eccentric contacts.
   Deep bite.
   Increased vertical dimension of occlusion Cusp to cusp contact.
   Over bite and decreased over jet.
2. Defective and highly placed restorations.
3. Large extensive restorations.
4. Cyclic forces due to occlusal disharmony.

Aetiopathogenesis

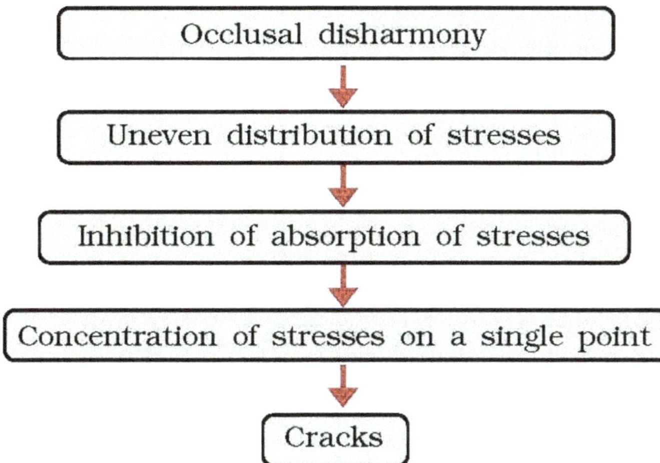

Pathophysiology of pain

On biting

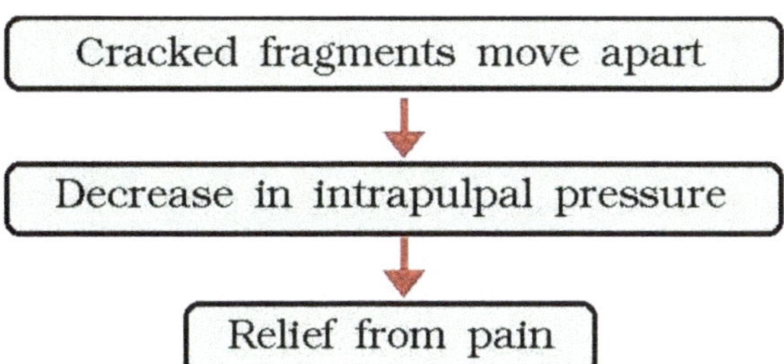

On relieving biting pressure

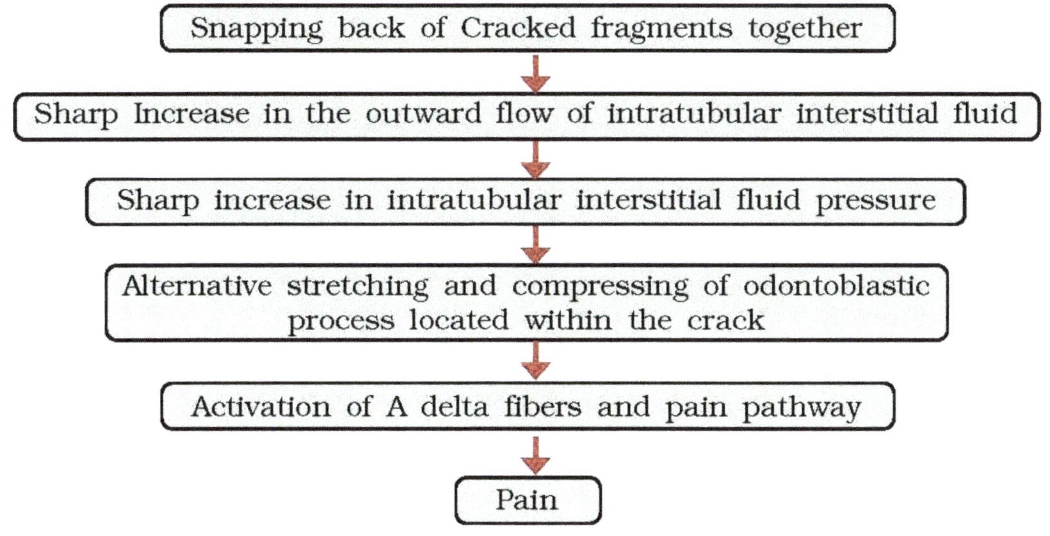

Symptoms

- Discomfort
- Sensitivity to cold and sweet
- Pain on relieving biting pressure
- May be absence of sensitivity to hot

TYPES

Type 1: Cracked crown syndrome

Incomplete, multiple, micro cracks confined to enamel and dentin without involving pulp. The quantity, dimension and direction of the crack are unknown and the cracks are scattered, judged to be look like spider web.

The signs and symptoms are very vague and complex and may be confused with pain of sinusitis, atypical facial pain, neurologic pain.

Diagnosis is extremely difficult.

Treatment: Prosthetic crowns

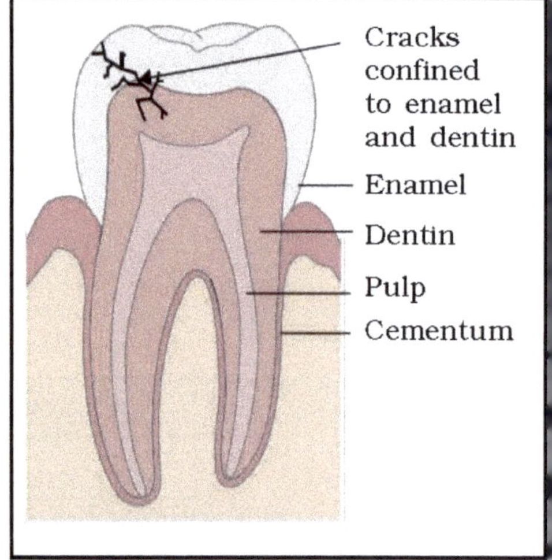

Fig. 2.8: Type 1-Cracked crown syndrome

Type 2

Complete, minute cracks propagating deep through the dentin to involve pulp.

The signs and symptoms are severe compared to type 1.

Diagnosis is relatively easy compared to type 1 because the cracks appear as translucent line on transillumination test.

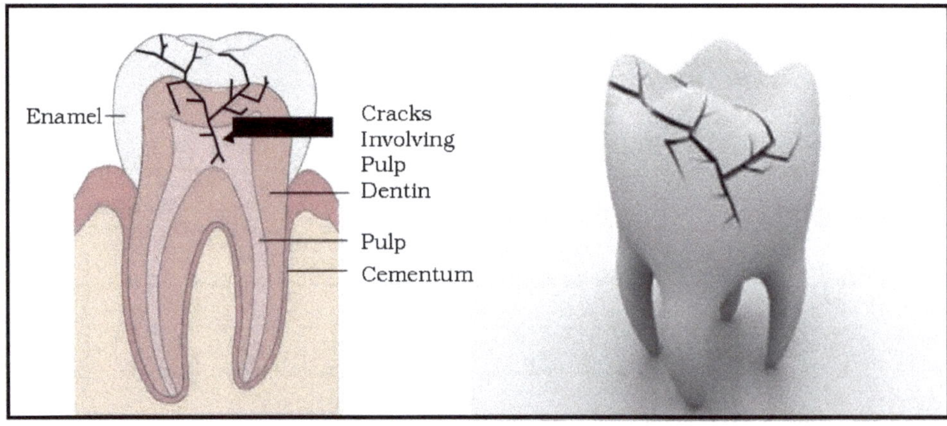

Fig. 2.9: Type 2 - Cracks involving pulp

Treatment

Root canal treatment followed by prosthetic crown.

Type 3

Sometimes complete cracks may propagate further deep into the root through cementum and dentin towards periodontium.

May be associated with periodontal defects. Diagnosis relatively easy compared to type 1 and type 2, cracks appear as hair like translucency on radiographs.

Treatment

Periodontal therapy to correct periodontal defects.

Root canal treatment followed by prosthetic crown.

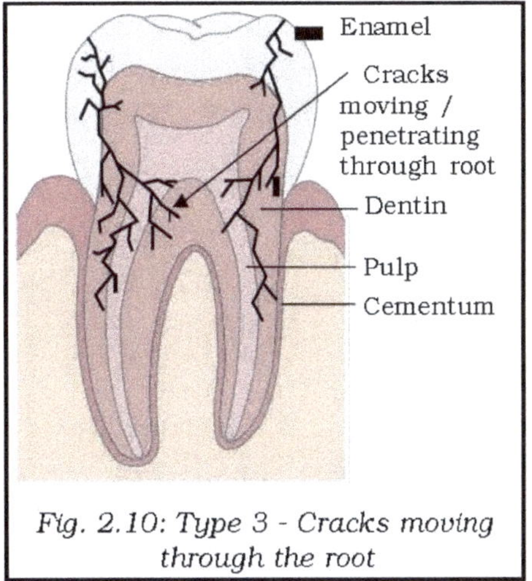

Fig. 2.10: Type 3 - Cracks moving through the root

Diagnosis

Bite test - Positive
Pain on relieving biting pressure

Transillumination test – Positive
Translucent line running through the tooth

Pulp vitality tests – Positive
Sensitivity to cold
Presence of vital nerve

Microscopic detection

Radiographic examination.
Hair like translucency running through the tooth

Management

Treatment of underlying cause –
- Orthodontic correction of malocclusion.
- Correction of highly placed defective restorations.

- Covering the large extensive restoration with prosthetic crowns.
- If pulp is involved root canal treatment followed by covering the tooth with Prosthetic crown.

Diagnosis

Bite test - Positive

Pain on relieving biting pressure

Transillumination test – Positive

Translucent line running through the tooth

Pulp vitality tests – Positive

Sensitivity to cold

Presence of vital nerve

Microscopic detection

Radiographic examination.

Hair like translucency running through the tooth

Management

- Treatment of underlying cause –
- Orthodontic correction of malocclusion.
- Correction of highly placed defective restorations.
- Covering the large extensive restoration with prosthetic crowns.
- If pulp is involved root canal treatment followed by covering the tooth with Prosthetic crown.

RETROGRADE PULPITIS

Backward spread of infection from periodontium to pulp leading to inflammation of pulp is called retrograde pulpitis. It may be reversible or irreversible.

Types

Reversible retrograde pulpitis

Irreversible retrograde pulpitis

Reversible retrograde pulpitis

It occurs after periodontal therapy (sub gingival scaling, root planning and curettage) due to cut off of blood supply to the pulp through accessory canals and influx of microorganisms in to the pulp. It is self-limiting does not require treatment.

Irreversible retrograde pulpitis

This condition is commonly seen in immune compromised patients with acute aggressive periodontitis where vascular supply to the pulp through apical foramina is compromised.

Etiopathogenesis

Potential route of reverse spread of infection is may be through apical foramina which is principal and most direct route of communication between pulp and periodontium. May also spread through open dentinal tubules, lateral canals, furcal canals and resorption lacunae.

Ingress of Micro-organisms and their by-products from the periodontal infection

↓

Through or via open dentinal tubules, lateral canals, apical foramen, accessory canals, resorption canals

↓

Into the immune compromised or vascular compromised pulp

↓

Retrograde pulpitis

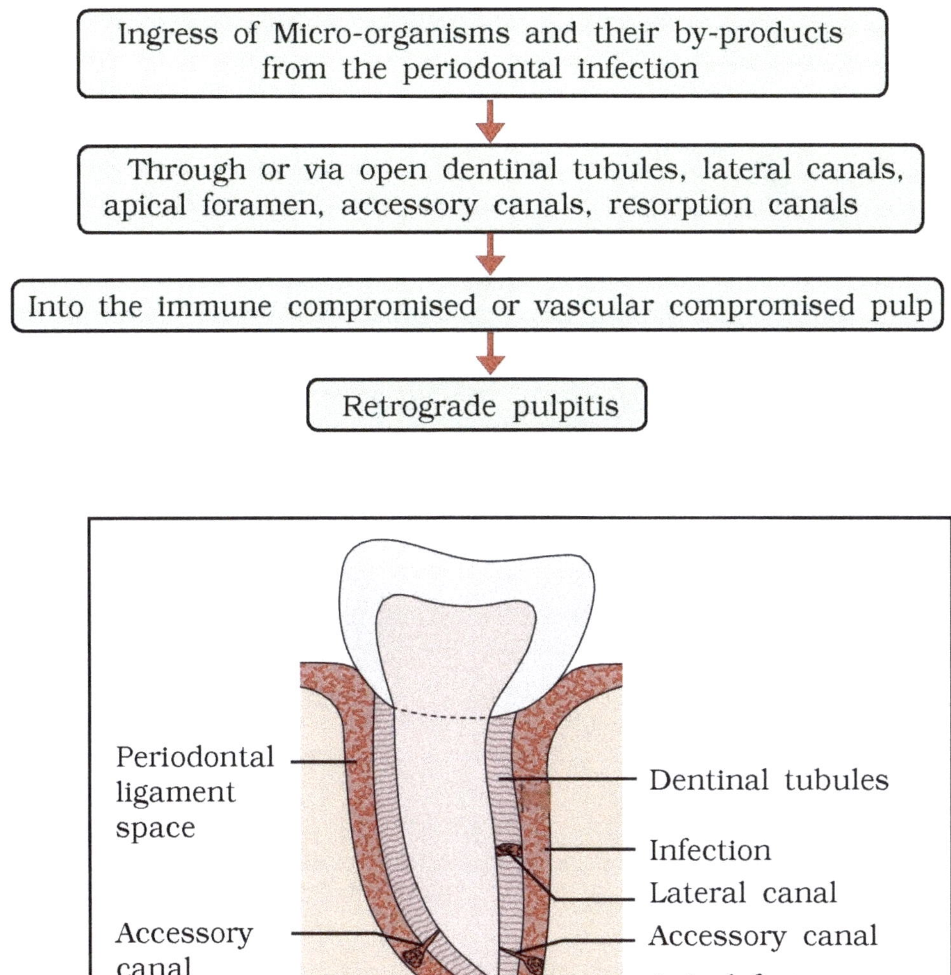

Fig. 2.11: Retrograde pulpitis

Predisposing factors

- Presence of open dentinal tubules.
- Developmental anomalies like palato-gingival groove and microcracks.
- Perforations.
- Vertical root fractures.
- Internal resorption.
- External resorption.
- Aggressive periodontal therapy where cementum is absent or thin.

Clinical features

- Intact crowns without decay or extensive restorations.
- Signs and symptoms of both periodontitis and pulp necrosis.
- Swollen gum.
- Extensive loss of epithelial attachment.
- Mobility of tooth.
- Deep Pocket formation Pus discharge.
- Fistulous tract
- Mild to moderate pain and tenderness

Palpation test -positive

Presence of peri-radicular abnormality

Vitality test

Thermal sensitivity tests are positive.

Percussion test- positive

Presence of peri-radicular inflammation
Percussion on lateral pressure is positive

Periodontal probing test

Wide pockets which are broader cervically and narrow apically. Fistulous tract may be present.

X-ray

Vertical bone loss

Periapical radiolucency

Systemic disease

Blood investigation for immune compromised diseases like uncontrolled diabetes mellitus, adrenal insufficiency, bone marrow suppression may be present

Management

Treatment of immune compromised disease

Periodontal therapy

Root canal treatment

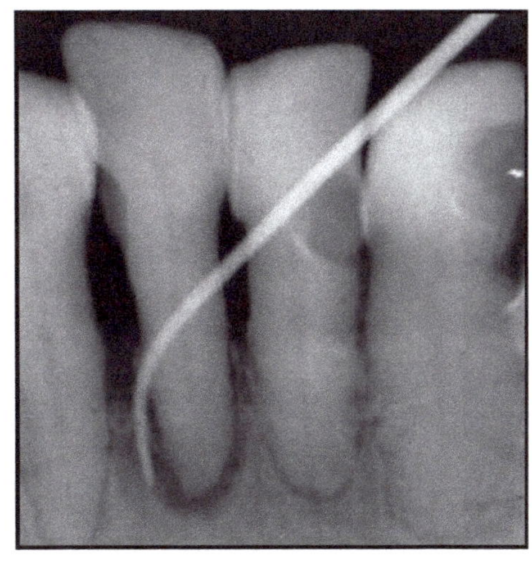

Fig. 2.12. Retrograde pulpitis

PERIODONTAL PATHOLOGY

Acute apical periodontitis

Acute apical periodontitis associated with vital tooth

Inflammation of the apical periodontal ligament is mainly due to abnormal occlusal contacts.

Etiopathogenesis

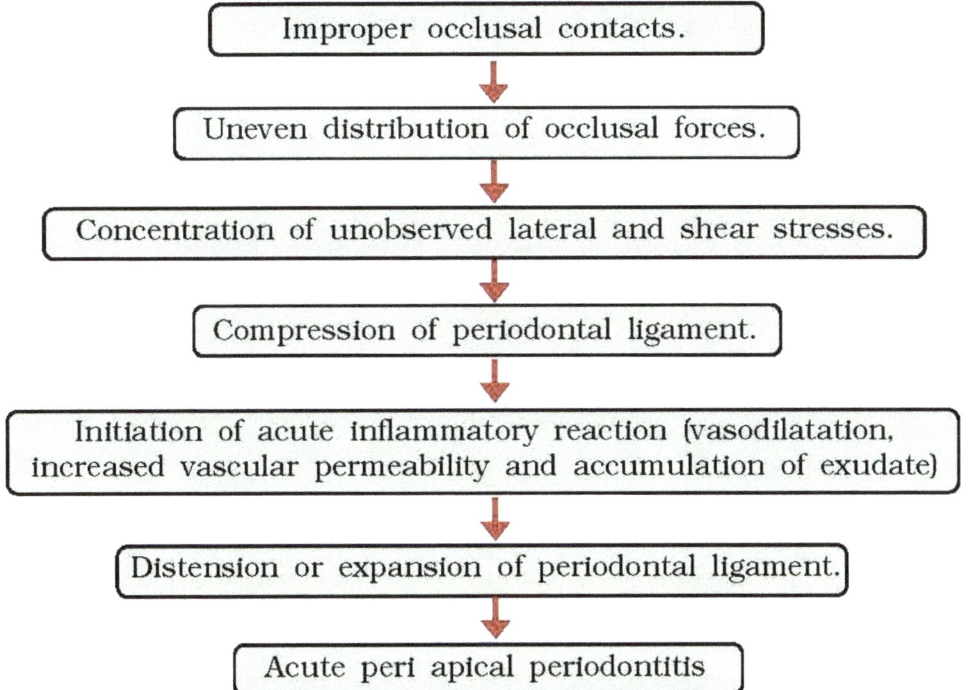

Clinical features

- Patient complains of severe sharp Pain.
- Pain on mild percussion is positive.
- Pain on chewing.
- Tooth may feel extruded.

Radiographically

Normal anatomic structures or Widening of periodontal ligament space.

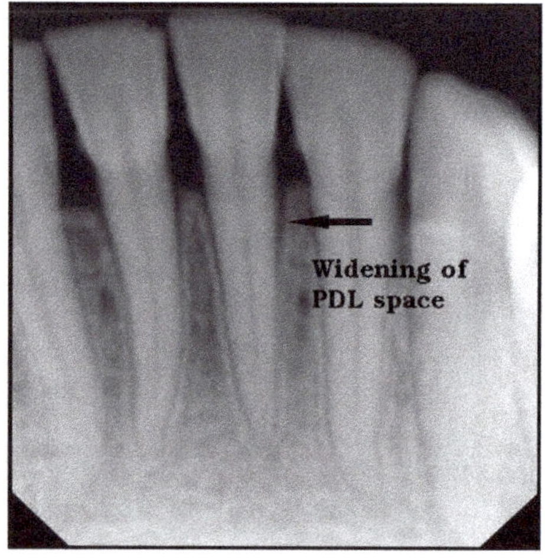

Fig. 2.13 : Apical periodontitis associated with antheviar vital tooth

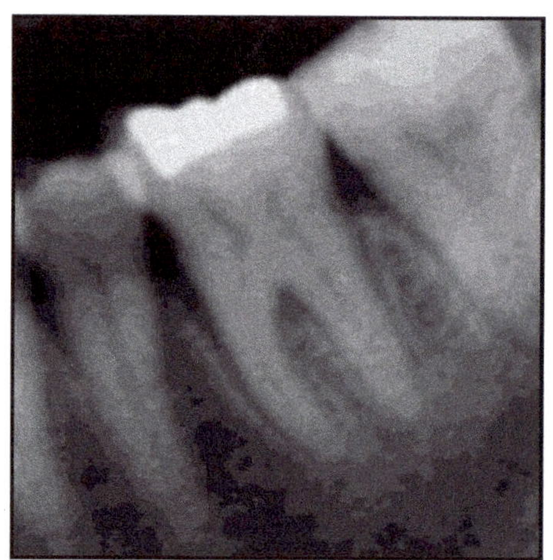

Fig. 2.14: Apical periodontitis associated with vital tooth

Treatment

- Removal of offending agent.
- Apical periodontitis associated with pulpal pathology (non vital tooth)
- It is sequel to pulpal diseases
- Infiltration of bacteria from pulp to the periapical area.
- Diffusion of bacterial toxins and byproducts from pulp to the periapical area.

Etiopathogenesis

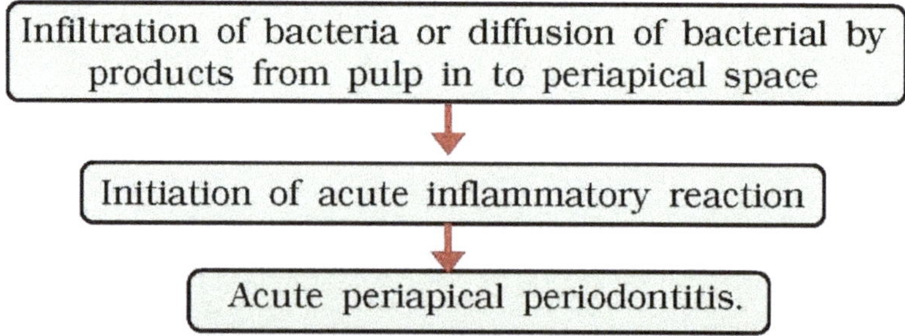

Clinical features

- Singns and symptoms are similar to irreversible pulpitis
- Pain on percussion is positive
- No swelling.
- Pain on biting
- Cold may relieve the pain
- Heat may exacerbate the pain.

Radiographs

- Caries involving the pulp or secondary caries beneath the restorations.
- Widening of periodontal ligament space.
- Break in the continuity of lamina dura.

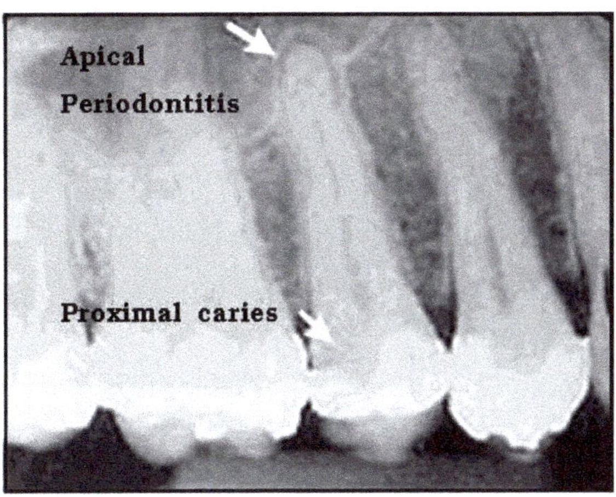

Fig. 2.15: Apical periodontisis associated with non vital tooth

Management
Root canal treatment

Acute periapical abscess

- It is a progressive sequelae of periapical periodontitis
- Pain is severe throbbing in nature due to localized collection pus.
- Initially swelling is small as infection progresses swelling becomes more pronounced.
- Overlying mucosa is tender and sensitive.
- Pain on percussion is positive.
- Tooth feel elongated or extruded and exhibits mobility.

Radiographically

Break in continuity of lamina dura and slight widening of periodontal ligament space.

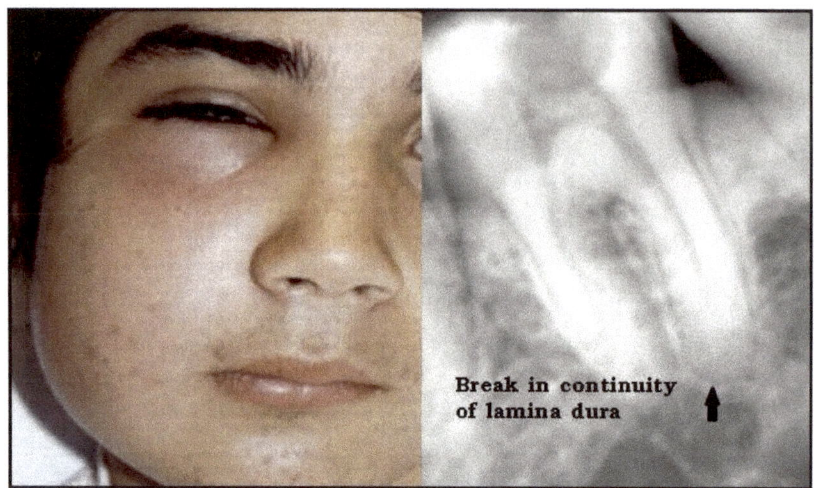

Fig. 2.16: Acute periapical absecess

Complications

If left untreated   may lead to the following

a)   Chronic alveolar abscess

b)   Cellulitis (canine space infection, buccal space infection)

Management

Root canal treatment

Chronic periapical abscess

It is a natural sequelae to untreated acute periapical abscess.

The involved teeth have large caries lesions, extensive restorations, discolored or fractured crowns.

Causes

Due to long-standing low-grade irritation of periapical tissues from extended infection of pulpal diseases.

Clinical features

● Mild or no pain, Asymptomatic chronic periapical abscess detected only during routine radiographs.

- Pain on percussion is positive.
- May have bony swelling.
- Draining sinus track may be present, it is due to burrowing of abscess through bone and soft tissues.
- Shows no response to thermal sensitivity tests and electric pulp vitality test.

Radiographically

Break in continuity of lamina dura and widening of periodontal space Ill-defined radiolucency.

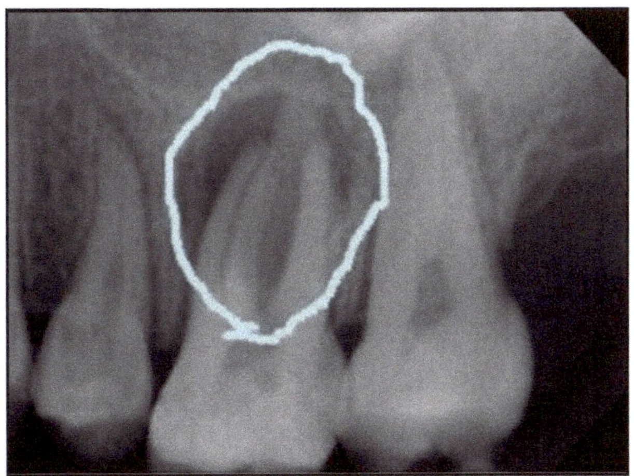

Fig. 2.17: Ill defined radiolucency

Management

Root canal treatment

Periapical granuloma

- Localized mass of granulation tissue around the root apex of non-vital tooth.
- Mostly asymptomatic detected during routine radiographs.
- Soft tissue overlying the mucosa may be tender.
- On radiograph well defined or poorly defined radiolucency and widening of periodontal ligament space.
- Resorption at the tip of root apiece may be seen.

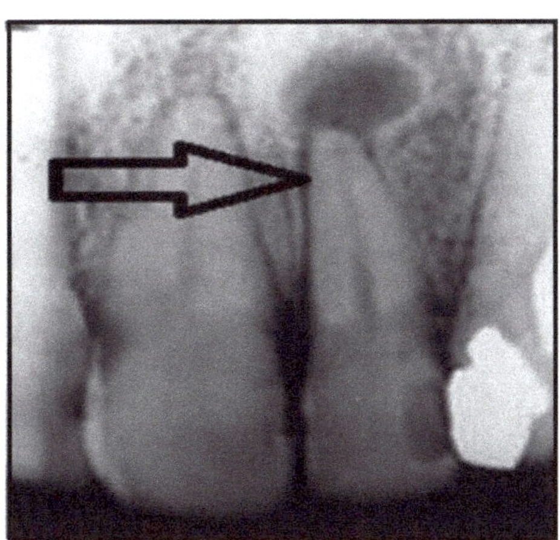

Fig. 2.18: Widening of periodontal ligament

Periapical cyst

- Always associated with non-vital tooth, the crown of involved tooth is deeply discolored or fractured.
- Males are commonly affected.
- More commonly seen in maxillary anterior region.
- If cyst is large malalignment, spacing and mobility of teeth may be present.
- On palpation cracking sound may be present.
- The involved tooth is asymptomatic usually discovered on routine radiographs.
- Bony swelling may be present.

Clinical feature

Discoloration of crown is seen

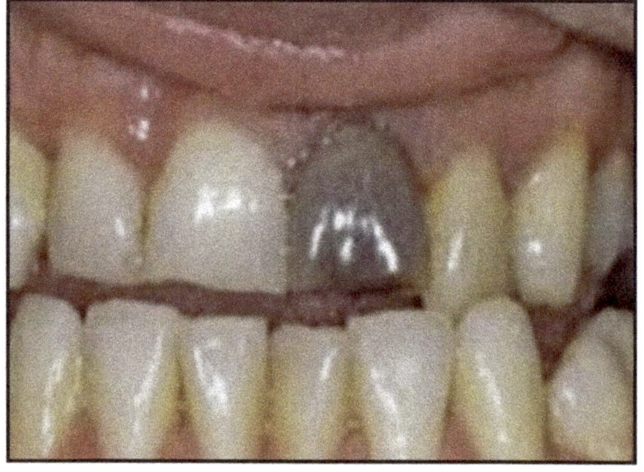

Fig. 2.19: Discoloration of crown

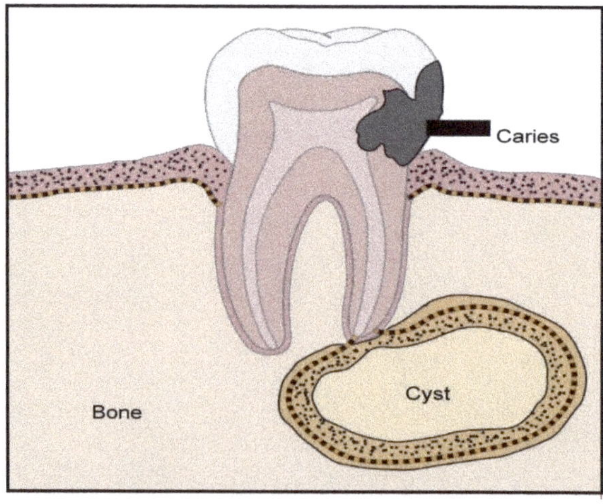

Fig. 2.20: Periapical cyst

Radiographically

Well defined radiolucency surrounded by radioopaque border, radiolucency is larger than periapical granuloma or chronic periapical abscess. Divergent roots are seen if cyst is large.

Loss of lamina dura.

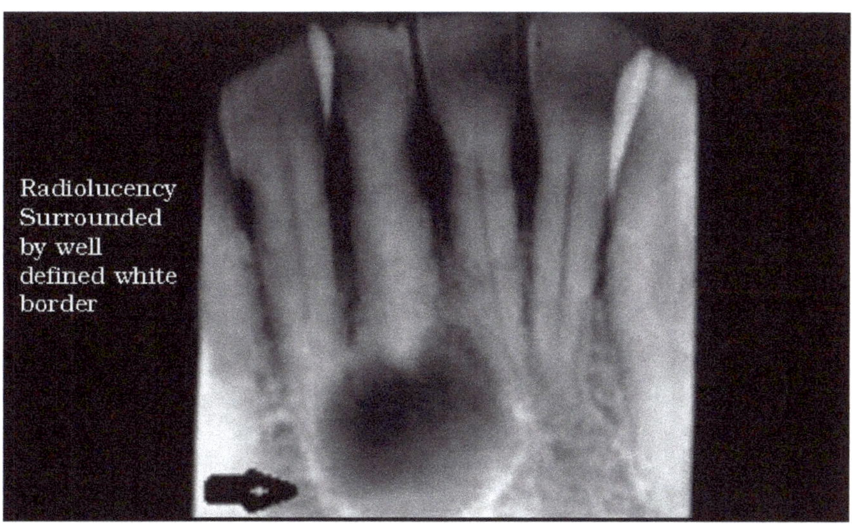

Fig. 2.21: Periapical cyst

Management

- Root canal treatment
- Apicoectomy

PHOENIX ABSCESS

Most of the time associated with non-vital tooth

Definition

An acute exacerbation of long standing asymptomatic chronic lesion of tooth.

or

Sudden eruption of acute inflammatory reaction in chronic asymptomatic lesion of tooth.

Pathogenesis:

Mechanism 1

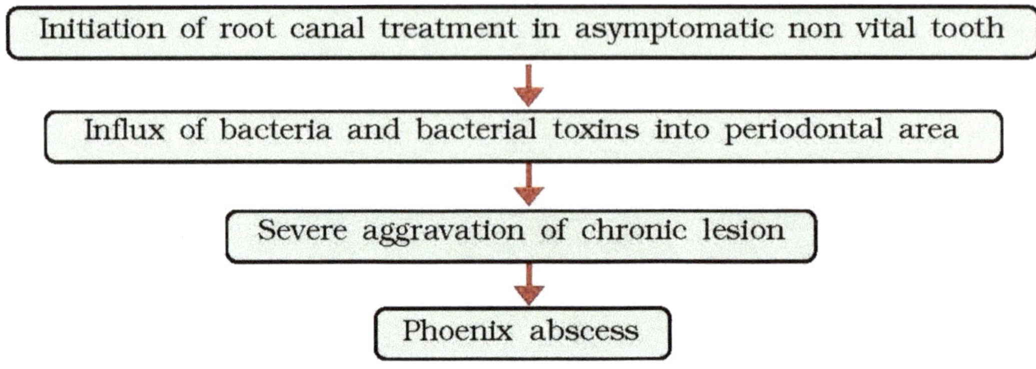

Mechanism 2

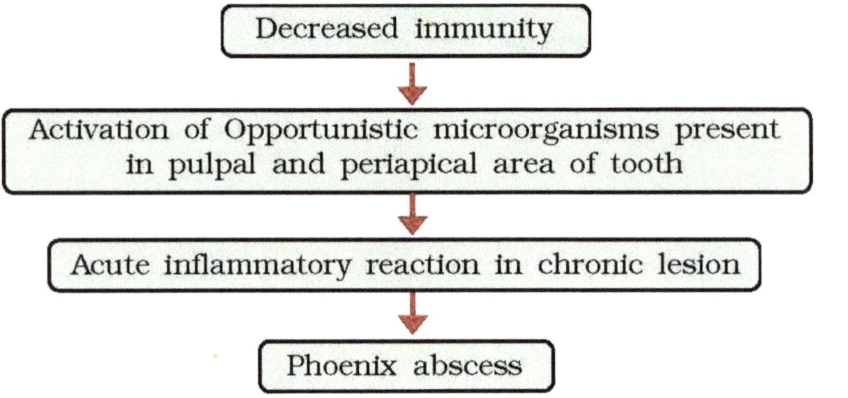

Clinical features

General symptoms fever, weakness, malaise, lymphadenopathy.

- Pain is severe
- Swelling.
- Pain on percussion is positive
- Extruded tooth and mobile tooth.

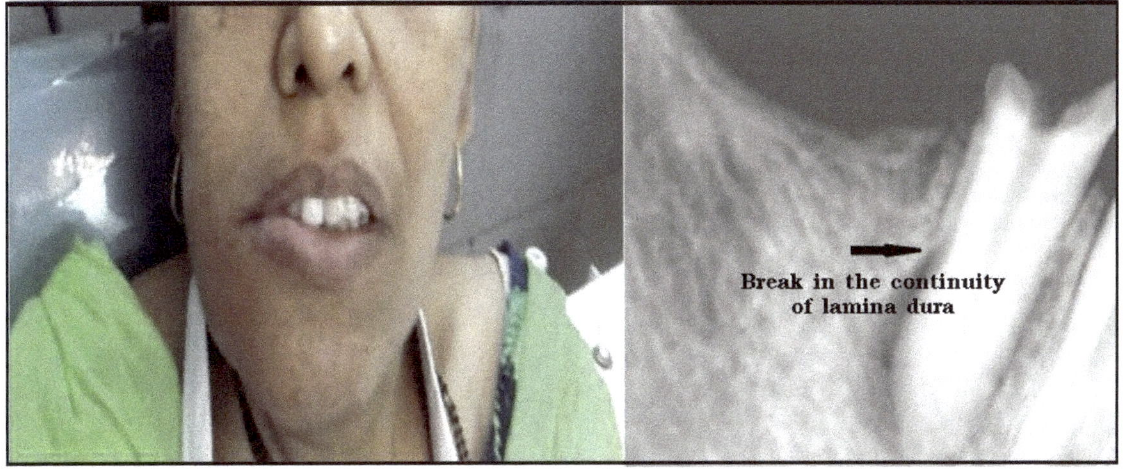

Fig. 2.22: Phoenia Abscess

Radiographically:

Well defined radiolucent area

Break in the continuity of lamina dura

Treatment

Root canal treatment.

TOOTH RESORPTION

Gradual dissolution of hard tissues of tooth is called tooth resorption

It may be physiologic as seen in natural shedding of deciduous teeth or may be pathologic as seen in tooth due to trauma or continuous irritation.

The outer surfaces of roots of the teeth are protected by pre-cementum and cemento-blasts and the inner surface of pulp cavity is protected by pre-dentin and odontoblasts. If these protective layers get denuded, the stripped tooth surface behaves as antigen or foreign body and body's immune system start producing antibodies against it, and this leads to the formation of multinucleated giant cells against body's own cells (autoimmune response.).

Classification

Depending upon nature

Physical

Pathologic

Depending upon anatomy or site of initiation

Internal (initiates in pulp)

External (initiates in periodontium)

Depending upon location, external resorption further classified into –

1) Cervical
2) Lateral
3) Apical

Depending upon aetiology

1) Transient
2) Infective
3) Replacement
4) Coerce

Aetiology

Local causes

Trauma

Chemicals

Example:

- Bleaching agents
- Persistent pulpal and periapical infections.
- Continuous pressure from impacted tooth, excessive orthodontic forces, odontogenic cysts and tumors

Systemic causes

- Paget's disease
- Hyperparathyroidism
- Hypo-phosphatemia
- Hypothyroidism Acromegaly
- Dwarfism

Etiopathogenesis of resorption

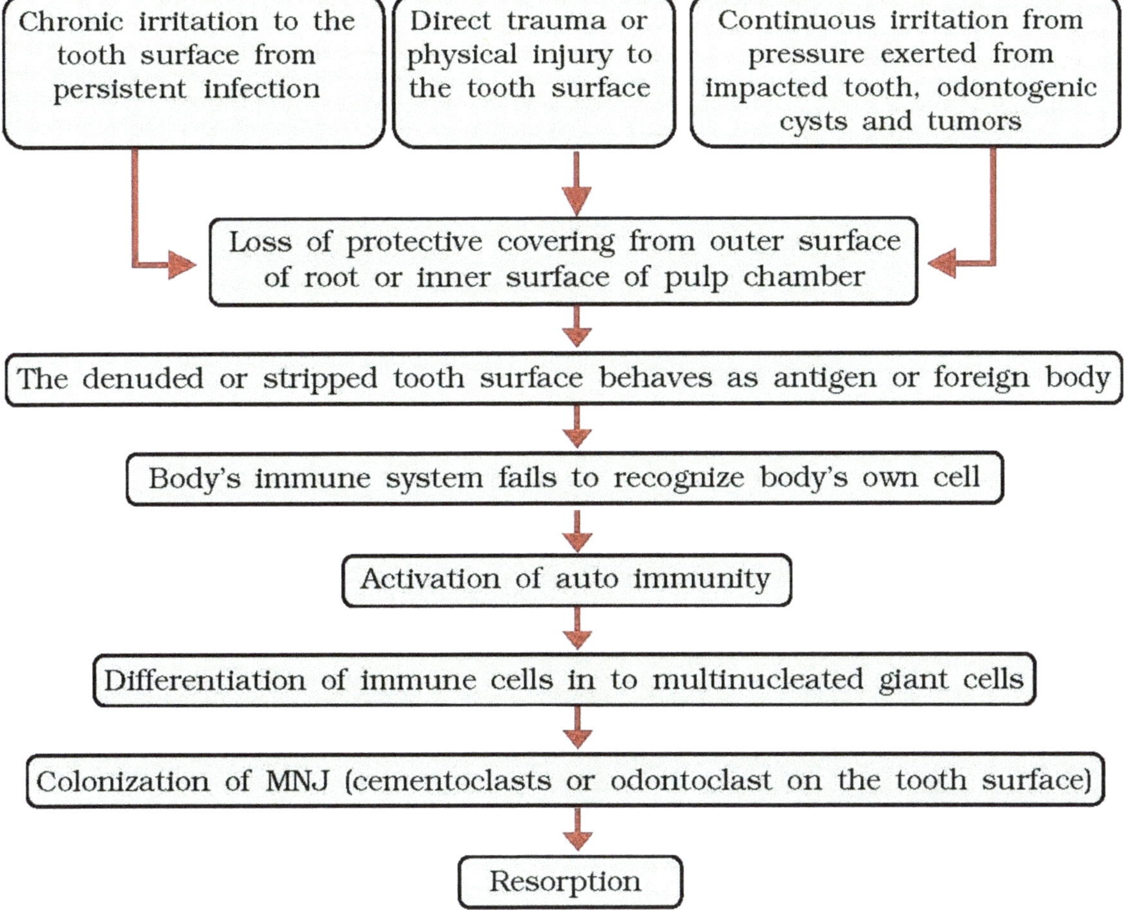

Complications of resorption

Undetected and untreated cases of resorption lead to the following:

- Weakening of tooth.
- Discoloration of tooth.
- Retrograde pulpitis.
- Loss of tooth
- Crooked teeth

Management

Since the exact etiology is unknown early detection and prevention is the best treatment for resorption.

EXTERNAL RESORPTION

The resorption which starts in the periodontium and initially affects the external root surface of tooth is called external resorption.

Types of external resorption

Transient resorption

Mild surface resorption which heals spontaneously. It often occurs after periodontal therapy (sub gingival scaling, root planning and curettage) and orthodontic treatment

Treatment

It is self-limiting, requires no treatment.

Cervical resorption

Occurs due to injury to the periodontium below the attachment epithelium at the cervical 1/3 of root. It is invasive in nature relatively uncommon.

Also occurs following the orthodontic treatment, orthognathic surgery.

Causes

Trauma
Internal bleaching

Radiographic feature

Irregular and tunnel shaped radiolucency around the root canals at cervical 1/3.

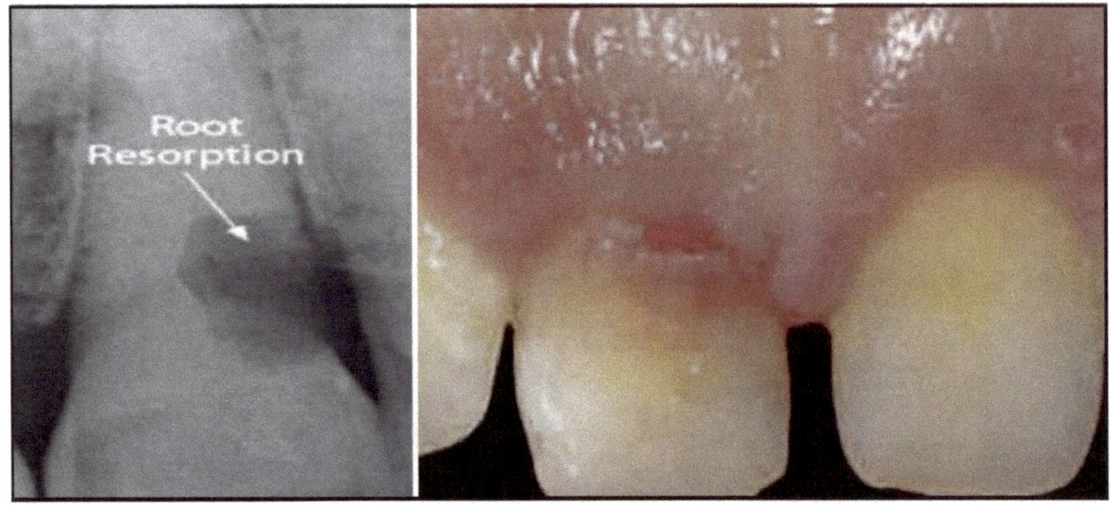

Fig. 2.23: Cervical resorption

Treatment

Surgical exposure of the defect by raising the flap and thorough curettage of granulation tissue and restore the defect with adhesive cements.

Root canal treatment.

Infective resorption

Due to pulp necrosis, there is seepage of microorganisms and their by-products into the periodontium through apical foramina, accessory canals, lateral canals and furcal canals leads to persistence of infection in periodontium. This persistence of infection especially in periapical area causes resorption of root tip; this is called as infective resorption.

Example:

Resorption of root tips in chronic alveolar abscess and infected periapical granuloma.

Replacement resorption or ankylotic bone resorption

Occurs in two conditions

1) Occurs in the intruded tooth following severe trauma, vertical force causes the crushing of apical periodontium and death of periodontal ligament cells. Due to this root surface comes in direct contact with bone. This results in gradual replacement of dead periodontal cells and space by bone leading to dentoalveolar ankylosis. With time the whole root gets gradually resorbed and gets replaced by the bone and hence the term "replacement resorption". Ankylosis follows resorption hence ankylotic resorption.

Replacement resorption or ankylotic bone resorption

Occurs in two conditions

1) Occurs in the intruded tooth following severe trauma, vertical force causes the crushing of apical periodontium and death of periodontal ligament cells. Due to this root surface comes in direct contact with bone. This results in gradual replacement of dead periodontal cells and space by bone leading to dentoalveolar ankylosis. With time the whole root gets gradually resorbed and gets replaced by the bone and hence the term "replacement resorption". Ankylosis follows resorption hence ankylotic resorption.

2) In avulsed tooth if the reimplantation is delayed for more than 3 hours, the cells of the periodontal ligament die; due to this root surface comes in direct contact with bone and this results in slow replacement of root by surrounding bone. This is known as dentoalveolar ankylosis. With time the whole root gets gradually resorbed and gets replaced by the bone and hence the term "replacement resorption".

Ankylosis follows resorption hence ankylotic resorption.

Clinical features

- Tooth appear firm in the socket
- Tooth may be in infra occlusion
- Metallic sound is heard on percussing the ankylosed tooth.

Radiographic features

- Periodontal ligament space is absent
- Roots appear short

Coerce resorption

- It is external tooth resorption, occurs due to continuous pressure.
- Can also be observed during eruption of permanent dentition
- Example upper and lower canines and lateral incisors

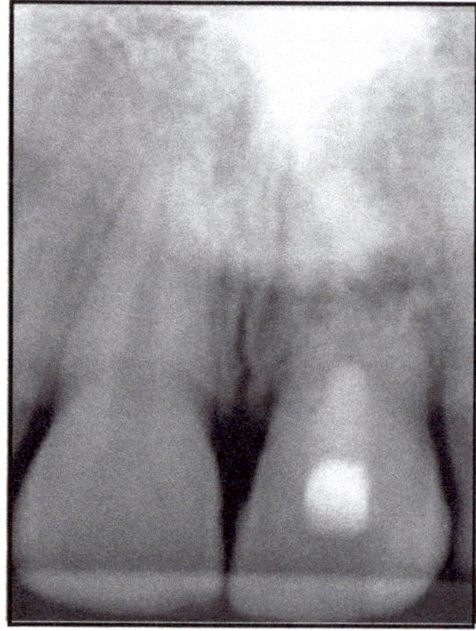

Fig. 2.24: Replacement resorption

Causes

- Pressure from impacted tooth.
- Expansion pressure from cysts.
- Impingement from odontogenic tumors.

X-ray

Moth eaten appearance

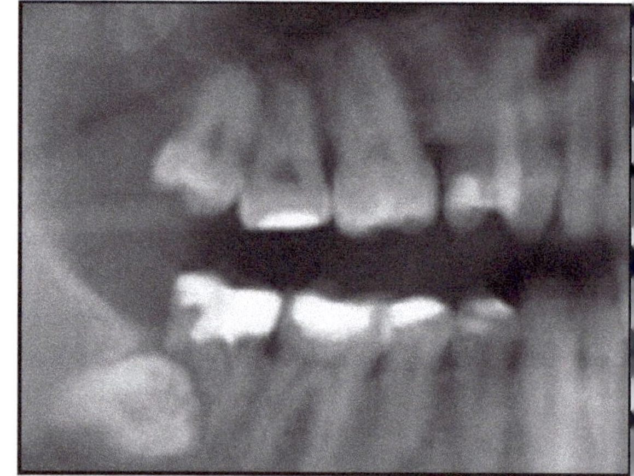

Fig. 2.25: Coerce resorption

Treatment

Resorption tends to be arrested when the underlying cause is removed.

Internal resorption

(for detailed description refer the chapter pulpal pathology)

HOT TOOTH

The tooth in which anesthesia is difficult to achieve is called hot tooth. It may be due to local causes or general causes.

Local causes

1)   Acute alveolar abscess.
2)   Acute irreversible pulpitis.
3)   Phoenix abscess.
4)   Cellulitis (chronic abscess with swelling)
5)   Space infection

Etiopathogenesis

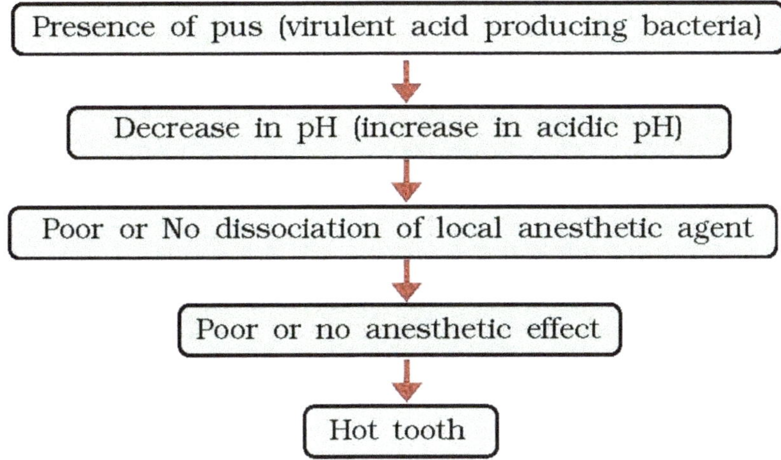

Management

Pain control

a)   Pre medication with sedatives or tranquillizers
b)   Intramuscular injection Dynapar-AQ 75 mg/ml
c)   Intramuscular injection Gentamicin 40 mg/ml

Anesthesia

4% Articaine is more potent than 2% lidocaine. Surface anesthesia with lidocaine spray or ointment Local anesthesia by nerve block.

Infiltration anesthesia.

The mucosa covering the abscess is infiltrated, the needle should be tangential to the mucosa so that the needle should not penetrate through the abscess and visible through the transparency of tissues.

Incision and drainage

- (where there is pus let it out)

- Prepare the surface of abscess with betadine solution.

- Make incision on the most dependent surface of the abscess to encourage drainage with the help of no. 11 blade.

- Apply gentle pressure to allow the purulent material to drain-out and finally gently insert a small curved artery forceps to break up loculations.

General causes

Mechanism 1

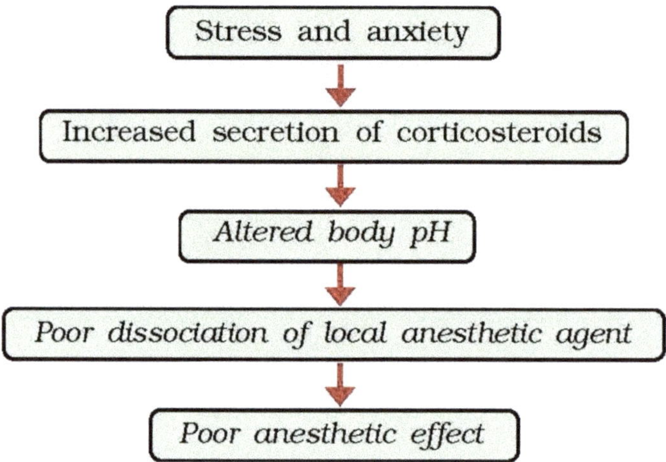

Mechanism 2

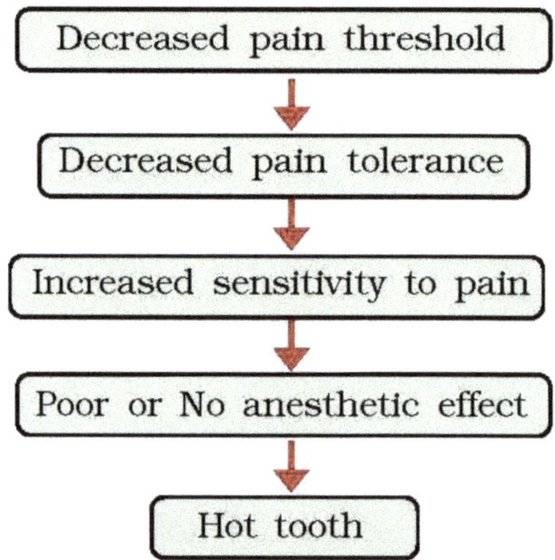

Management

1) Our approach should be kind, calm, tranquil and confident.

2) Positive professionalism: make the patient aware that pain free effective treatment will be done.

3) Premedication with analgesics, anxiolytics and sedatives.

4) Antibiotic prophylaxis to control infection.

5) To achieve effective anesthesia intra pulpal, Intra-ligamentary, intraosseous injections are used.

3
Treatment Planning

PLANNING IS THE FOUNDATION TO EVERYTHING.

PLANNING PROMOTES DECISIONS. DECISION FACILITATES ACTIONS.

THERE IS NO SUBSTITUTE TO ACTIONS.

ACTION LEADS TO OUTCOMES

Treatment planning starts with correct diagnosis. Every patient is different, every case is different. Some are simple, some are complex and few are complicated so we have to stream line our efforts and actions accordingly.

Planning means organizing the course of action. It saves lot of time and energy as it guides us one step closer to success.

Indirect pulp capping

1) Tooth with hard, non-progressive sterile caries close to the pulp.

2) Deep dentinal caries close to the pulp without involving pulp.

3) Gross caries lesion may or may not be associated with sensitivity.

4) Traumatic fracture involving enamel and dentin nearing pulp exposure but not exposing the pulp.

5) Deep dentinal exposure close to the pulp but not exposing the pulp.

Direct pulp capping

Pin point accidental or mechanical exposure during crown cutting or restorative procedures:

1) Pin point Caries exposure of pulp less than 0.5 mm in immature young permanent tooth when there is high chance for favorable response.

2) Pin point caries exposure of pulp less than 0.1 mm in young permanent tooth when there is high chance for favorable response.

Note: Caries exposure through affected dentin not infected dentin. If caries exposure occurs through infected dentin pulpotomy or root canal treatment should be considered :

3) Pin point traumatic pulp exposure due to deep dentinal fractures reported within 12 hours in asepsis state that is in dry condition without contamination.

4) Pin point traumatic pulp exposure in immature young permanent tooth due to deep dentinal fractures reported within 48 hours in asepsis state that is in dry condition without contamination.

5) Few chosen cases of deciduous teeth nearing their exfoliation.

Exfoliation period is within 6 months.

PULPOTOMY

Superficial pulpotomy

- Part of the infected/affected pulp is removed.
- Mechanical exposure less than 1 mm.
- Traumatic exposure less than 1 mm if reported immediately in dry condition.
- Caries exposure lees than 1mm in immature permanent tooth.

Total or coronal pulpotomy

- Total coronal pulp is removed.
- Reversible pulpitis and a very few selected cases of early irreversible pulpitis in immature young permanent tooth.
- Carious exposure of pulp less than 2 mm in primary tooth.
- Carious exposure of pulp less than 2 mm in immature young permanent tooth.
- Mechanical exposure of pulp greater than 1 mm in young permanent tooth.
- Traumatic exposure of pulp less than 2 mm in young permanent tooth due to enamel dentin fractures reported within 24 hours of injury.
- Tooth with soft non arrested, aggressive carries close to the pulp.

Pulpotomy and apexogenesis

- Traumatically exposed immature young permanent vital tooth.
- Caries exposure of immature young permanent vital tooth.
- Luxation of immature young permanent vital tooth.
- Iatrogenic injuries of immature young permanent vital tooth.
- In young permanent vital tooth with wide open apex.

Pulpectomy and apexification.

In young permanent non vital tooth with wide open apex

1) Calcium hydroxide apexification
2) MTA apexification

Pulpectomy and Revitalizations via blood clot (natural obturation via blood clot)

1) Non vital incompletely formed immature permanent tooth with following features:

- Short roots

- Wide open apex

- Thin fragile root walls

- Blunder buss canals

2) Non vital immature tooth with congenital anomaly where conventional root canal treatment is not possible *e.g.*, dense invaginatus or dense in dente.

3) Immature avulsed tooth.

ROOT CANAL TREATMENT

Single visit RCT

Diseases of the pulp without periapical pathology

1) Symptomatic Irreversible pulpitis.
2) Asymptomatic irreversible pulpitis.
3) Asymptomatic pulp necrosis.
4) Chronic hyperplastic pulpitis.
5) Internal resorption.
6) Cracked tooth syndrome.
7) Medically compromised patients who have to make an effort visit to for treatment.
8) Physically compromised patients who have to make an effort visit to for treatment examples paralysis, handicap.
9) Apprehensive patients who require sedation.
10) Anterior teeth where esthetic is concern.

Two or three visit RCT

Diseases of the pulp with periapical pathology

1) Acute alveolar abscess.

2) Chronic alveolar abscess.

3) Periapical granuloma.

4) Infected periapical cyst before doing apicectomy.

5) External resorption.

6) Poor accessibility examples mesially angulated second and third molars.

7) Patient with limited mouth opening examples trismus.

8) Patient with temporomandibular disorders.

9) Presence of extra root or canals.

10) Canal calcifications.

11) Canal obstruction.

MULTIPLE VISITS ROOT CANAL TREATMENT (RE-RCT)

1) Post root canal acute periodontitis or post root canal Acute periodontal abscess caused due to anatomic discrepancy or procedural errors like:

Missed canals

- Mb2 in maxillary molars.
- Disto lingual or distobuccal canal in mandibular molars.
- Lingual canals in mandibular anterior.
- Extra canals in mandibular and maxillary second premolars.
- C shaped canals in lower posteriors.
- Extra canals in mandibular and maxillary canines.

Missed complex anatomy of tooth like

- Webs and fins
- Isthmus
- Lateral canals
- Accessory canals
- Furcal canals
- Multiple foramens
- Deltas

Procedural complication

1)   Perforation
2)   Instrument breakage
3)   Stripping
4)   Zipping
5)   Under obturation
6)   Over obturation
7)   Ledges
8)   Apical blockages
9)   Transportations

2)   Endodontic lesions of periodontal origin (perio-endo lesions)

Apicectomy

It is done in anterior teeth. 3 mm of apical 1/3rd. of root is removed.

Indications

1)   Non- resolved pyogenic granuloma.
2)   Peri radicular cyst.
3)   Instrument breakage beyond apex.
4)   Selected cases of horizontal root fractures.
5)   Over obturated severely infected necrotic tooth.
6)   Tooth with wide open apex.
7)   Complex anatomy of tooth.

Hemi-section

Re infected either mesial or distal root is removed which cannot be retreated with re-root canal treatment.

Root resection (maxillary molars)

Re infected either distobuccal or mesio buccal root is removed which cannot be treated with re-root canal treatment.

Bi-cuspidation

Surgical division of mandibular molars in two halves when there is furcation involvement.

Example

Root furcation caries.

Trephination

Drainage of pus through bone.
It is done in Mandibular & maxillary premolars.

4
Magnification & Illumination

We can only treat what we can see. Human eyes have the ability to resolve two lines or two discrete entities that are 0.2mm apart. Clinically, most dental practitioners will not be able to see an open margin smaller than 0.2mm. Traditional endodontics has been based on feel not sight. Together with radiographs and electronic apex locators this blind approach has produced surprising success. There is, however significant failure rates, especially in long terms. Magnification helps the user, not only to see more, but to see well. High levels of magnification increases aggregate amount of visual information available to endodontists for diagnosing and treating dental pathology. Improved ergonomics and zero defect endodontics. The film thickness of most crown and bridges cement is 0.025mm, well beyond the resolving power of the naked eye.

Human mouth is a small space to work in, especially considering the size of available instruments, and comparatively large size of the operator hands.

Few procedures that demand tolerance well beyond the 0.2mm limit

➤ Caries removal
➤ Root canal orifice location
➤ Furcation and perforation repair
➤ Post placement or removal
➤ Crown margins
➤ Scaling procedures
➤ Incisions
➤ Bone and soft tissue grafting

Human eyes and age!!

A baby can clearly see objects that are 7cm away from 25 to 30 years old person at 30cm, on reaching the age of 40 most people become presbyopic, the distance between object and the eye becomes increasingly bigger.

Traditional endodontics have been based on feel not sight, together with radiographs and electronic apex locators this blind approach has produced surprising success. There is however a significant failure rate especially in long-term magnification helps the user not only to see more but to see well. Significant advances in the use of magnification and illumination and supportive armamentarium in recent years have benefited treatment protocols in non-surgical and surgical endodontics such that teeth which might otherwise have been extracted now have a predictable chance for retention.

Magnification	Resolution
Unaided human eye	200u
2.5x loupes	100u
4x loupes	50u
Sharp explorer	40u
8x microscope	25u
10x microscope	20u
14x microscope	14.3u
20x microscope	10u

Several elements are important for consideration in improving clinical visualization.

➢ Stereopsis

➢ Magnification range

➢ Depth of field

➢ Resolving power

➢ Working distance

➢ Spherical and chromatic distortion

➢ Ergonomics

➢ Eyestrain

➢ Head and neck fatigue

➢ Cost

The need for better visualization in the field of endodontics has been an ongoing challenge the unaided vision is inadequate. The combination of improved lighting and magnification has been provided by several means like

■ Loupes

■ Fiber optic headlamps

■ Surgical operating microscopes

■ Ora-scope

Loupes

Historically, dental loupes have been the most common form of magnification used in apical surgery.

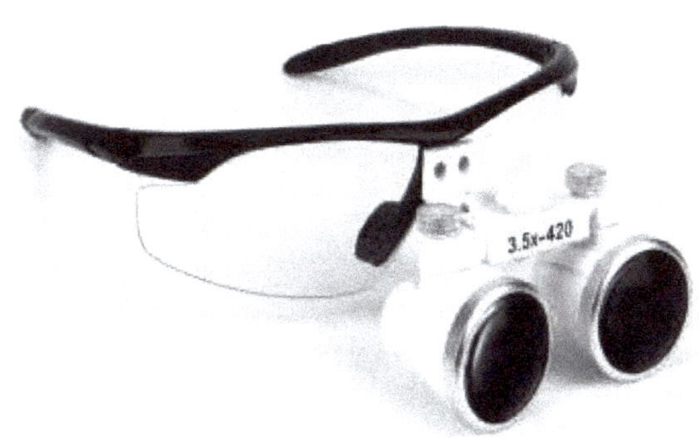

Fig. 4.1: Loupe

Dental loupes are small magnification devices attached to frames that allow the user to see a magnified view of an object. Loupes are kind of telescope. The telescope has two lenses the

I.   Ocular or eye piece that the dentist looks in to

II.   The objective lens or the lens closest to the object

Loupes are essentially two mono ocular microscopes with lenses mounted side by side and angled inward to focus on an object. The disadvantage of this arrangement is that the eyes must converge to view an image. The convergence over time will create eyestrain and fatigue and, as such loupes were never intended for lengthy procedures most dental loupes used today are compound in design and contain multiple lenses.

Principle

The refraction of light through a series of lenses.

Types

Flip-up loupes

- We can adjust the interpupillary distance
- Can be flipped out of sight when not in use
- Interpupillary distance, convergence angle and declination angle can be changed
- Relatively cheaper
- Sharing among operators permitted
- May be worn with the loupes or incorporated in to the frame

TTL loupes (through the lens loupes)

- Actual magnification put through the lenses_fixed barrels may hinder eye contact during communication
- Interpupillary distance, convergence angle and declination angle is fixed change not needed
- Sharing among operators not possible
- Lighter in weight
- More expensive

Galilean system

The Galilean system utilizes two or three lenses provides a magnification range from 2x up to 4.5x and is small, light and very compact system.

Prism loupes (Keplerian system)

Prism loupes are actually low power telescopes that use refractive prisms. Prism loupes utilize multiple lenses and   provide magnification up to 6x and produce better magnification, larger field of view, wider depths of field and longer working distance.

These loupes have sophisticated optics, which rely on internal prisms to bend the light. The disadvantage of this arrangement is that eyes must converge to view an image. These convergence over time will create eyestrain and fatigue. Only the dental operating microscopes provides better magnification and optical characteristics than prism loupes.

Magnification with loupes

- With Single lens 2x
- With Dual lens 3x
- With Multiple lenses 4 to 5x

Advantages

Economical

Easy to use

Disadvantages

Gives vision which is converging

Eye strain

Fatigue

Pathologic vision changes especially after prolonged use

Limitation

Maximum convenient range of magnification is 4 to 5x that is not sufficient some times

Microscopes

Endodontists have frequently boasted that they can do much of their work blindfolded simply because there is nothing to see. But, the truth of the matter is that there is great deal to see if only we had the right tools. Before the introduction of the operating microscopes, we could feel the presence of a problem a ledge, perforation, blockage, broken instrument and the clinical management of that problem was never predictable and depended on happenstance but now with the help of microscope we can deal with such complicated cases and the whole procedure becomes more predictable.

Most microscopes can be configured to magnifications up to *40 and beyond but limitations in depth of field and field of view make it impractical.

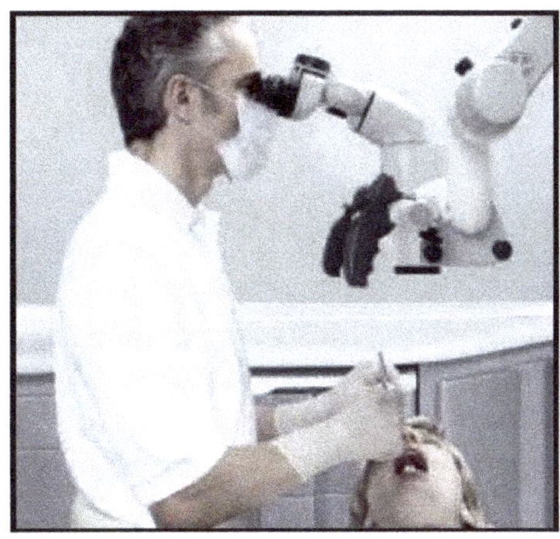

Fig. 4.2: Surgical microscope

Definition

Microscope is an instrument used to see objects that are too small for the naked eye.

Micro means= Small

Scope means= To look

A microscope is a tool that produces an accurately enlarged image of small objects.

Classification of microscopes

Based on use

- Surgical microscope
- Examination microscope

Based on installation
- Ceiling mounted
- Floor mounted
- Wall mounted

Based on magnification
- Lower magnification
- Midrange magnification
- High range magnification

Principles

- Working distance
- The distance measured from the dentist eye to the treatment filed being viewed
- Working range
- Interpupillary distance
- Field of view
- The area that is visible through optical magnification
- Depth of field
- Refers to the ability of the lens system to focus on objects that are both near and far without having to change the loupe position.

How surgical operating microscopes works?

- Magnification
- Illumination
- Instrumentation
- Documentation
- Magnification

Parts of microscope

Eyepiece

- Eyepieces which are available in powers of 6.3x,10x,12.5x,16x ,20x
- Just like a magnifying glass the two eyepieces magnify the intermediate image produced in the tube.
- Eye piece consists of
- A viewing side with rubber cup
- Adjustable diopter settings (-5 to +5)
- Binoculars which are used to hold eye piece which may be straight, inclined or inclinable and again of shorter and longer focal length

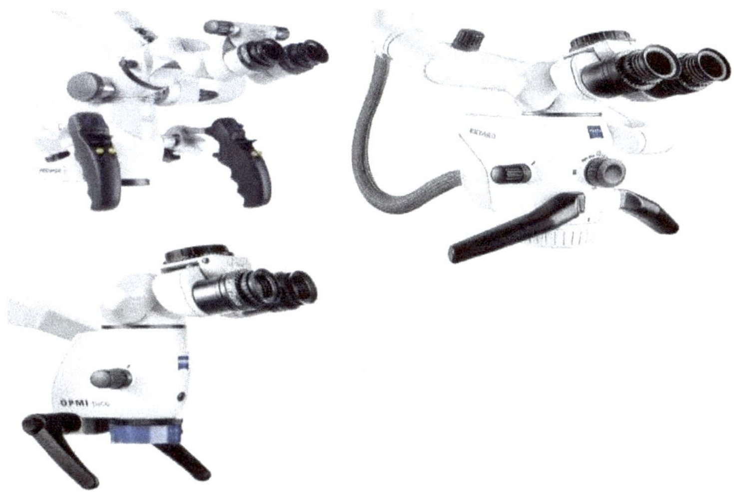

Fig. 4.3: Parts of microscope

Tube head

- Straight
- The tubes are parallel to the head of the microscope
- Inclined
- A -inclined tube head is fixed angle of 45 degree offers limited ergonomics
- Inclinable tubes
- B-inclinable tube head 0 to 180 degree allows the dentist to alter the angle of the eyepiece holder

Magnification changer

- A 3,5,6 step manual changer or a power zoom changer located within the head of the microscope permits the smooth transition between magnifications
- A 3,5,6 step manual changer 3 steps or 5 steps
- 3.5x ,5.1x,8.5x,13.6x,21.25x
- 6x,10x,16x,20x,25x

Objective lens

The objective lens is the first optical component that the image information crosses on its path from the object to the eye. Whose focal length (which ranges from 100 to 400mm) determines the operating distance between lens and surgical field.

The lenses vary in their focal distance (=focal length

The most common working distance are 200,250 and 300mm

Light

- Halogen=yellow picture
- LED
- Xenon=brighter, color true picture
- Components of microscopic for documentation
- Camera
- Beam splitter
- Supplies light to direct the image to a camera or an axillary observation tube and also supplies light to accessories
- Essential for documentation
- Camera adapter

Uses of microscopes in endodontics

The dental operating microscope has become an integral part of endodontic practice for both non-surgical and surgical endodontic therapy. Treatment rendered using the dental operating microscope results in superior care for patients, and modern endodontic therapy is more effective because of its use.

Diagnosis

- Examination of the external surface of the tooth.
- To detect caries
- To prepare conservative access cavity designs and preservation of tooth structure.
- To detect cracks and micro fractures (methylene blue staining). The dentist should always look for internal vertical coronal and radicular cracks and fractures when using the microscope. These would be difficult to detect without the high magnification and illumination.

Locate canals

- Make canal location easier by magnifying and illuminating the grooves in the pulpal floor and differentiating the color differences between the dentin of the floor and the walls. What was considered a rare exception in the past has become a routine finding when using the microscope
- 50% of all molars have a 4th canal
- 30% of all premolars have a 3rd canal
- 25% of all anterior teeth have 2 canals

Locating hidden canals

With proper assessment of the radiographs and with the aid of microscopic magnification and ultrasonic we can locate the hidden missed canals. Microscope make easy visualization of the MB2 canal in maxillary first and second molars. Studies confirm that this root canal exist in percentage very close to 100%. If we compare these results with previous studies published years ago, we conclude that the increased percentage is not due to change of the root canal anatomy but to the better skills of the clinicians who use the operating microscope.

i.   Atypical position or form of a root canal orifice
ii. Isthmuses and accessory root canals
iii. Calcified canals
iv. Missed canals
v.   Aberrant canals
vi. Dilacerated canals
vii. Canals blocked by restorative materials

Management of calcified canals

Changes in color, translucency, and refractive indexes

Perforation repair

Under microscopic magnification we can accurately identify and evaluate the damaged site, determine the granulation that invade the perforation site. After removing that tissue, the exact dimensions of the perforation are clearly visible. Then a precise application MTA to the perforation area is more accurate with the help of magnification.

Removal of fractured instrument

Precise and short strokes under complete visualization, magnification and illumination with ultrasonic tips can minimize the damage to the surrounding dentin and allow us to disengage the instrument from the surrounding dentine and become loose to retrieve.

Identify and evaluate subtle changes in dentin

Removal of residual obturating material from the canal

Final examination of the canal preparation

A small amount of sodium hypochlorite is deposited in to the canal and observed carefully at high magnification, if there are bubbles coming from the prepared canal then there is still remnant pulp tissue in the canal.

Surgical endodontics

Moderate bevel of the root resection, retrograde root canal filling

Patient education

Ergonomics

Ergonomics is a scientific discipline concerned with the understanding of interaction between humans and other elements of a system simply ergonomics means working correctly.

Over load: -If the settings of the system operator are not correct an adverse effect in terms of back and neck discomfort can appear so work ergonomically to reduce the overload. The following basic position should be used to reduce overload.

1. Dentist should assume an adequate seated position.
2. Patient should be placed in the correct position.
3. Microscope should be positioned comfortably.

Dentist position

The 12 o'clock position relaxing straight back and neck behind the head of the supine patient is the ergonomical position for most dental procedures.

Patient position

For the patient, a comfortable supine position should be found this can be improved through special padding and head and neck support. head rest positioned for indirect view of the maxillary teeth with maxillary occlusal plane vertical. Head rest adjusted for indirect mirror view of mandible where the mandibular occlusal plane is vertical. For better view of treatment field, it is enough to simply have the patients head to the left or right. In many cases this provides a direct view of the treatment field.

Microscope position

90 degree to the floor, focal distance should be correct

1. Microscope must be poisoned at 90 degree to the floor
2. Microscope must be set, the right working distance

Assistant ergonomics

To enable the work to be carried out ergonomically, assistance tailored specifically to the needs of micro dentistry is essential. This aspect must not be underestimated because it contributes to efficient work flow during procedure.

Instrument change

Documentation always on

The laws of ergonomics

Class1 motion: -moving only the fingers

Class2 motion: -moving only the fingers and wrists

Class3 motion: -movements originating from the elbow

Class4 motion: - movements originating from the shoulder

Class5 motion: -movements that involves twisting and bending at the waist.

Micro endodontic instruments

Because of the level of precision that can be achieved when using the microscope special instruments are required. These include instruments that help to identify structures and allow the more accurate removal of tooth tissues by improving visual access.

Mirrors

There are three different mirror surfaces

- Standard
- Rhodium
- HR mirrors

standard mirrors result in double images and a loss in definition. We need at least rhodium mirrors these reflect 75% of the light. HR mirror have the highest reflectivity on the market today 99.9%.

Micro-instrument files with a handle

Micro-opener: -used to look for the entrances of the canal it may also be useful in the identification of a bifurcation or a ledge.

Micro-debrider: -which is based on a head storm file used to remove tissue from the wall of the canal or root canal filling material.

Regular hand instruments can also be used by attaching them to locking tweezers.

Stropkov syringe

This instrument is really useful for drying the canals at a precise point. It is used in micro-apical surgery for drying the canal before obturation and in separated instrument cases.

Burs

It is important to use long shank burs so that the tip of the bur can be controlled precisely and not impaired by the head of the hand piece.

Ultrasonics

It is a vital part of the armamentarium needed in primary and re-treatment cases, both surgical and non-surgical

IRRISAFE Tip: -used for activating irrigating solutions.

ET25 Tip: -used for instrument retrievel.

ET18 D Diamond coated Tip: -used for removal of calcification

Uses of ultrasonics

- ➢ Removal of fractured instruments
- ➢ Canal location especially where canals are sclerosed
- ➢ To refine access cavities
- ➢ Post removal
- ➢ Root end preparation in endodontic surgery

Advantages

- ✓ Improved visualization, magnification, and illumination of the root and tooth structures
- ✓ Improved diagnosis
- ✓ Broader therapy treatment spectrum
- ✓ Reduced trauma
- ✓ Increased precision and predictability in procedures
- ✓ Increased manipulation of tissues
- ✓ More thorough cleansing of root canal systems
- ✓ Increases the patient comfort, reduces tissue trauma, post-operative pain and inflammation healing is faster.
- ✓ Patient education marketing benefits to the clinician's professional practice.

Disadvantages

- Need for specific training
- As a dental microscope has a restricted working field 11mm -55mm
- An operator using a dental operating microscope can see only the tip of the instrument and they are used in delicate movements of small amplitude.
- Relatively high initial cost of the equipment and instruments
- The need for retraining of the auxiliary staffs
- Adjustment period for the new treatment paradigms and operator postures

- May increase treatment costs and reduce initial productivity besides the need for rescheduling
- Its size which is difficult to fit in a small operatories.
- It takes the operator some time to get used to the equipment
- Adaption to indirect vision
- Narrow field
- Movement of the patient

Illumination

The physical stress of clinical dental hygiene practice is an occupational risk factor for developing musculoskeletal disorders (MSDs). Coaxial illumination, combined with magnification, can improve visual accuracy, ergonomics, and diagnostic capabilities for oral health professionals. A 1-3 quality light source and magnification will reduce strain on the eyes and the need to lean in closer to the oral cavity, improving posture.

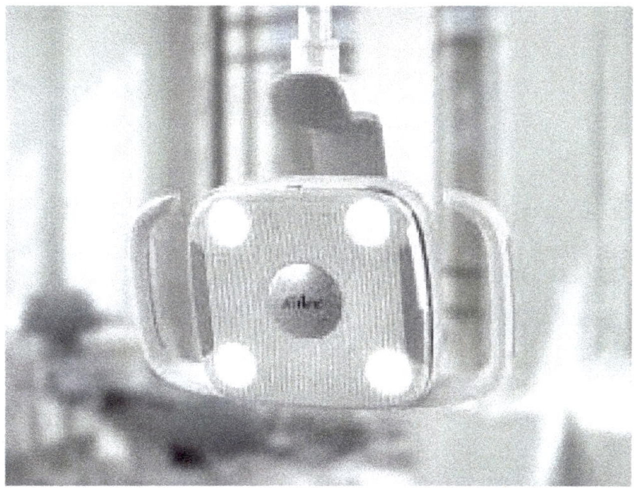

Fig. 4.4:

Need of illumination

- Dental hygienists work in the small dark area of the oral cavity, limiting visual acuity. A good lighting system can help improve practitioners' ergonomics, reduce fatigue, and is essential for optimizing visual performance and comfort. A study related to nursing and medication dispensing errors found that adequate lighting was one of the top environmental solutions for avoiding mistakes. The clinical dental hygienist needs to detect slight tissue changes and pathology even more intricate and tiny than medication labels. The purpose of clinical illumination is to help oral health professionals see the oral cavity and anatomical features clearly while in a comfortable working posture. Good clinical illumination should provide the following.

- Prevent the clinician from being forced into poor working postures
- Help to see the detail and color of the point of interest
- Enable control of light intensity
- Reduce eye strain and pain

Downsides of overhead lighting

- Traditionally, the light used to illuminate the oral cavity during treatment has been an overhead light on a track or a chair-mounted light, neither of which provides significant benefit to visual acuity. Studies have found that overhead lighting is often out of reach causing the clinician to use awkward postures to reach it, and it frequently cannot be adjusted with one hand. Results also showed that overhead lighting provided inadequate luminance levels for the operating field. Studies analyzed the effects of overhead lighting on dental hygienists. They found that this type of lighting created overhead glare, illuminance (brightness) and uminance (distribution) levels that were too high or too low, and luminance (distribution) uniformities that were too high or too low. While overhead lights are typically adequate for illuminating flat objects, they are less effective at illuminating deeper body cavities, like the oral cavity.

- The increased interest in enhancing visual acuity and desire to reduce MSD risk have increased the popularity of coaxial illumination.

Coaxial illumination is a type of lighting that provides a parallel source of light, reducing the incidence of shadows in the field of vision. During clinical practice, dental hygienists easily block their source lighting, compromising neck and back ergonomics. This problem is eliminated because coaxial illumination provides a target source of light.

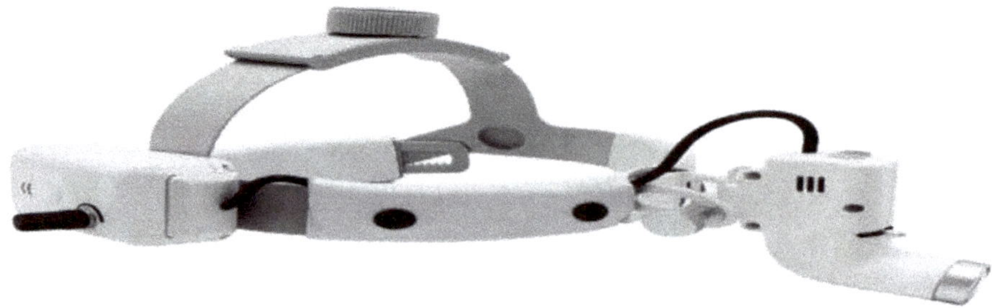

Fig. 4.5: Overhead lighting

Technology

- LED lighting has become an excellent source of illumination in the dental field. LED lights are extremely small, lightweight, and provide a high-quality light source with greater output than traditional light sources and better color rendering. These are desired qualities in a mounted light as correct brightness and true color allow for more clear vision and may even make tissue and anatomic changes more discernible during dental hygiene diagnosis and treatment. However, the greatest output is not necessarily the safest. Some studies demonstrated that LED lighting provided the best visual acuity as measured on symbol identification and color recognition compared with fluorescent lighting.

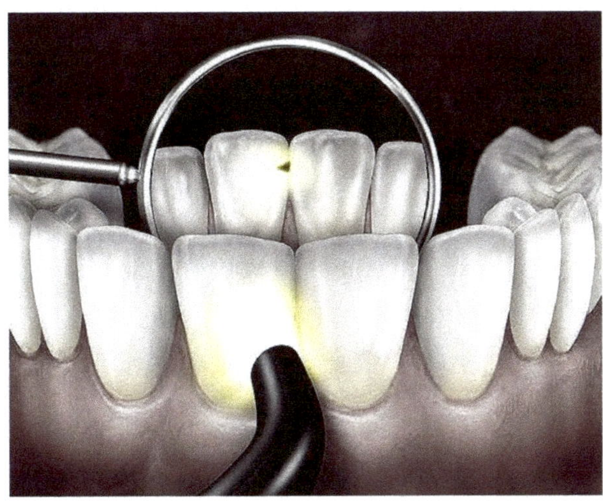

Fig. 4.6: LED lighting

Clinical considerations:

Finding the light that best supports ergonomic practice is important. LED headlights are classified into four types according to how the light beam is generated single lens optic, reflective optic, single lens/reflective optic, and achromatic multi-lens optic. Single lens optics are not uniform, contain blue light around the main beam, and their beam patterns and color uniformity fluctuate with changes in working distance. Achromatic multi-lens optics offer uniformity in beam patterns and color-LED lights come in varying colors: neutral white, cool white, and extreme cool white. It is important to evaluate the beam uniformity and color rendering before choosing a light. Shine the light on a white piece of paper to check for uniformity. The edges of the beam should not appear ragged or fading. Check the color rendering by illuminating anatomical objects to make sure they are true to color. In order to see accurate colors, consider an LED light with a neutral white color, or a color that accurately portrays the anatomical structure. The intensity of the beam should also be considered, as too high an intensity could cause a glare, which is potentially harmful to the clinician and patient. Too low of an intensity may lead the clinician to hunch or lean forward, or even strain the eyes to see more clearly. A light with an adjustable beam intensity may eliminate many of these issues. The light's weight and size should be considered, as a light that is too heavy or cumbersome may force the clinician into unhealthy postures or even harm vision.

5
Medicines in Endodontics

ANTIBIOTICS

Antibiotics require blood supply to reach and kill bacteria. Teeth lack collateral circulation because pulp is enclosed in a closed chamber. Abscess are devoid of blood supply, thus antibiotics cannot reach bacteria present in the abscess. so antibiotics merely have any role to play in endodontic infections It's of no use to prescribe antibiotics in endodontic infections. Address the cause and eliminate the source of infection, The best drug in endodontic, is root canal treatment.

Antibiotics are not needed in endodontics unless there is systemic manifestation of bacteremia present.

Antibiotics are not needed unless patient has immunocompromised disorders. Sensible and wise use is recommended to avoid bacterial mutation and its consequences.

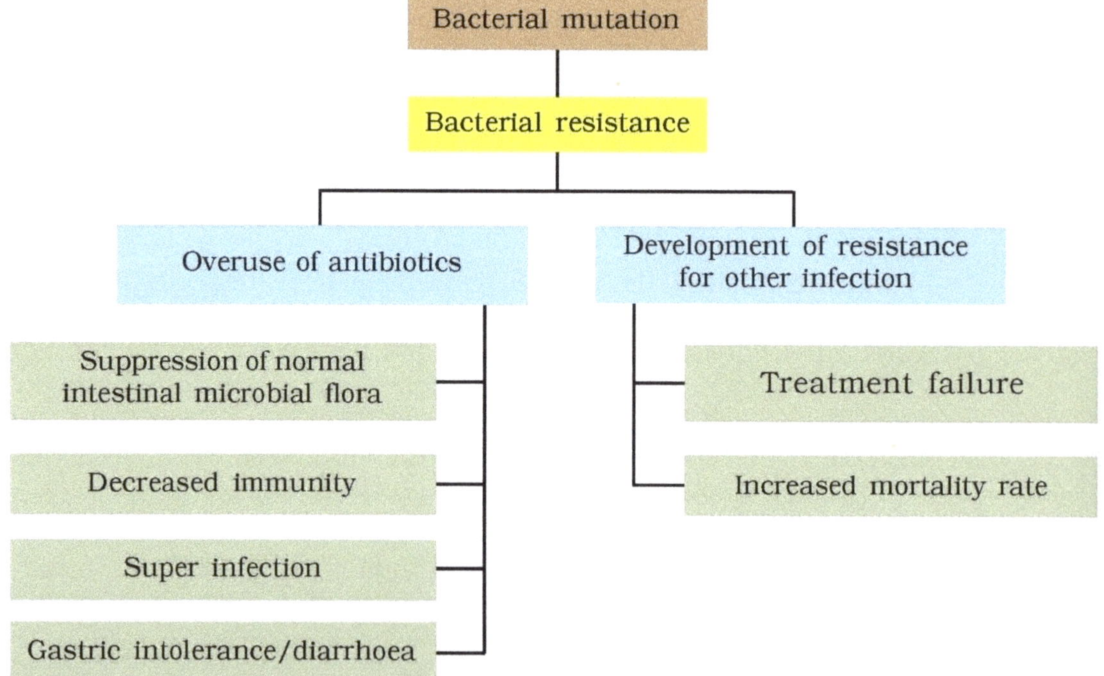

Indications

1) Acute periapical abscess with Signs and symptoms of systemic involvement such as

Fever

Malaise

Lymphadenopathy

Swelling

Trismus

2) Acute periapical abscess in immune compromised patients like

Diabetes mellitus.

Patient on prolonged corticosteroid therapy

Adrenal insufficiency

Bone marrow suppression

Leukaemia's

Patient on immunosuppressant like in organ transplants

Hiv and Aids

Radiation therapy

3) Prophylaxis to prevent subacute bacterial endocarditis or infective endocarditis in medically compromised patients like

Congenital valvular defects

Prosthetic valves

Patients with recent heart surgeries

4) Progressive space infections like

Osteomyelitis of jaw

Canin space infection

Buccal space infection

Ludwig's angina

Submandibular space infection

5) Persistent infections

6) Endodontic flareups

7) Phoenix abscess

8) Prophylaxis prior to reimplanting avulsed tooth;

Contra indications

- ➤ Reversible pulpitis
- ➤ Symptomatic irreversible pulpitis
- ➤ Asymptomatic irreversible pulpits
- ➤ Pulp necrosis
- ➤ Chronic hyperplastic pulpitis
- ➤ Acute periapical periodontitis associated with vital tooth
- ➤ Acute periapical periodontitis with non-vital tooth without the signs & symptoms of systemic involvement
- ➤ Acute periapical abscess without the signs and symptoms of systemic involvement
- ➤ Chronic periapical abscess
- ➤ Periapical granuloma
- ➤ Periapical cyst unless infected.

PENICILLIN'S

Amoxycillin

Mode of action - Bacteriostatic

Mechanism of action-

- Inhibits the growth and multiplication of bacteria by interfering with cell wall synthesis
- These are narrow spectrum & effective against gram +ve bacteria.
- Amoxycillin is used in combination with Clavulanic acid, which enhances the spectrum of activity of amoxycillin. Clavulanic acid acts on bacterial wall by inhibiting â lactam enzyme synthesis.

Uses (prophylactic uses)

In patient with acquired/congenital Heart disease to prevent Bacterial endo-carditis.

In patient with compromised or impaired immunity to prevent primary & secondary infections associated with bacteraemia. Dose/Drug (trade names).

- Novomox 125/250/500 mg
- Bluemox DT 250/500 mg.
- Augmentin 375 mg/625 mg
- Clavam 375/625 mg (amoxycillin 300/500 & clavulanic acid 75/125 mg).
- Moxikind CV 225/375/625
- Dosage and duration is dependent on age & weight of patient & severity of infection

FLUOROQUINOLONES

Ciprofloxacin and ofloxacin

- Acts by inhibiting bacterial DNA gyrase.
- Bactericidal.
- Broad spectrum of action.

Prophylactic use

- If patient is allergic to penicillin.
- If patient is non responsive to penicillin.
- Used as an intracanal medicament in combination with ornidazole and metronidazole.

Dosage

- Ciprofloxacin 250/500 mg.
- Ofloxacin used in combination with Tinidazole.

LINCOSAMIDE ANTIBIOTICS

Act by inhibiting bacterial protein synthesis

Mode of action

- Bacteriostatic
- Effective against gram positive microorganisms possess narrow spectrum activity.

Prophylactic use

- Second drug of choice when patient allergic or non-responsive to penicillins.
- Also used in severe soft tissue and hard tissue infections when patient allergic or non-responsive to fluoroquinolones.
- Lincomycin used in osteomyelitis because of its effective deep penetration in bone.
- Clindamycin used in soft tissue serious infections because of its soft tissue penetration.
- Clindamycin very effective in actinomyces of jaw.

Adverse effects

Pseudomembranous colitis

Diarrhoea

Inj clindamycin 150 mg/ml

Inj lincomycin 300 mg/ml

MACROLIDE ANTIBIOTICS

Act by inhibiting bacterial protein synthesis, possess narrow spectrum of activity.

Mode of action

Primarily bacteriostatic attains bactericidal activity at higher concentration against susceptible microorganisms.

Prophylactic use

Effective against penicillin resistant strains. Last choice of drug when patient allergic or non-responsive to penicillin.

Commonly used drug in sinusitis and cellulitis.

Adverse effects

Gastric intolerance Hepatotoxicity

Stevens-Johnson syndrome

Cap Azithromycin 250 mg, 500 mg

NITROIMIDAZOLES

Effective against anaerobic microorganisms. Acts by inhibiting bacterial nucleic acid synthesis. Drugs included in this group are metronidazole and tinidazole. Metronidazole should be used with other antibiotics.

Uses

In mixed infections

Acute alveolar abscess with systemic manifestations

In endodontic lesions of periodontal origin.

Contra indications

should not be used in alcoholic patients and epileptics

E.g.: Tab MO2, Tab O2, Ofloxacin 200 mg + Ornidazole 200 mg.

Side effect - Metallic taste

Adverse effect – Great bacterial resistance

AMINOGLYCOSIDES

Acts by inhibiting bacterial protein synthesis. It is Bactericidal in nature. Effective against gram negative Bacteria.

Uses

Severe serious infections like acute alveolar abscess progressing towards cellulitis and space infection. It is also given intramuscularly. Example Inj. Gentamicin 40 mg/ml Twice daily

TETRACYCLINE

Broad spectrum effective against gram positive and gram-negative Bacteria and atypical microorganisms like chlamydia, micro plasma and rickettsia. It is bacteriostatic in nature.

Mechanism of action

It acts by inhibiting bacterial protein synthesis.

Uses

- Used as an intracanal irrigant in necrotic non vital tooth.
- Used as intracanal medicament in severe serious infections and re root canal cases.
- Used in triple antibiotic paste
- Used in perio-endo lesions

Inj.: Doxol

ANALGESICS

NON-OPIOIDS

Acts by inhibiting the synthesis and release of mediators of inflammation.

Uses

Used in mild to moderate pain

Drugs

- Salicylates – Aspirin,
- Para aminophenol derivative – Acetophenone.
- Aryl acetic acid derivative–Diclofenac. Propionic acid derivative – Ibuprofen.
- Indole derivative – Indomethacin.
- Pyrrole derivative – Ketorolac.

Side effects

- Nausea and vomiting
- Constipation
- Gastric intolerance
- Precipitation of asthmatic attacks
- Ulcers
- Increased BP
- Liver and kidney disorders

Contraindications

Asthma, known Hypersensitivity, Bleeding disorders, Hypertension, Pregnancy, Peptic ulcer, Liver and kidney disease

PARACETAMOL OR ACETAMINOPHEN

- Potent analgesic but poor anti-inflammatory
- Higher and safer pain killer
- Best pain killer in older and aged patient
- Plain paracetamol used in pregnancy

IBUPROFEN

- Preferred pain killer in endo-perio lesions because of its osteogenic potential
- Better tolerated than aspirin
- Side effects are milder compared to aspirin
- Preferred in acute musculoskeletal pain along with other analgesics.
- Like aspirin ibuprofen is contraindicated in pregnancy, asthma, bleeding disorders, ulcers

KETOROL DT

- For short duration intense pain
- For instant and immediate relief of acute pain

Side effects

- High BP Dyspnea
- Vision disturbances

Contraindications

- Alcoholics
- Dehydration
- Known allergy

Commonly used drugs

- Tab diclomol (diclofenac 50 mg + paracetamol 500 mg)
- If patient not responding to diclomol
- Tab ketorolac or tab tramadol is used
- If swelling is present triple combination drugs such as
- Tab Enzoflam (paracetamol + diclofenac + serratiopeptidase) Tab Lysoflam (paracetamol + diclofenac + hyaluronic acid)

OPIOIDS

- Act by inhibiting synthesis and release of neurotoxins. Act by Inhibiting the formation of synapsis.
- Act by inhibition of transmission of pain path way.

Uses

- Severe pain not subsided by NSAIDs.
- Chronic recurrent pain.
- Prior to treatment to relieve anxiety.
- Recommended painkillers in pregnancy especially in first trimester.
- Recommended drugs in patients who are under anticoagulant therapy.

Note: Used in low dose for short period.

Side effects

- Constipation.
- Blurring of vision.
- Sedation.
- Fall in BP.
- Respiratory depression.

Adverse effect

Drug dependence and drug addiction.

E.g.: Morphine 10 mg, codeine 15 mg, propoxyphene 5 mg.

ANTI-ANXIETY DRUGS

Tranquilizers

- Act by depressing the central nervous system.
- Make the patient tranquil, calm, cool and tension free by reducing the anxiety and agitation.
- Diazepam – 10 mg previous night.
- 5 mg 1 hour before appointment.

Sedatives

- Act by depressing central nervous system.
- In higher doses produces general anaesthesia.
- Flurazepam 20 mg previous night.

Note: Dose and duration depends upon general health and age of the patient

STEROIDS

Used to treat the post-operative pain & discomfort caused due to the irritating effects of

a. Over extended obturated materials.

b. Accidental extrusion of sealers in the periodontal space.

Mechanism of action
Acts by immunosuppressive, anti-inflammatory, antiallergic

Indication

1. Severe Infections (acute/chronic abscess, phoenix abscess) pain not subsided by opioids and non-opioids.

2. Atypical mixed bacterial infections.

3. Used as intra canal medicament in root canal procedure.

4. Allergy and hypersensitivity reactions

Prednisolone 5 mg/10 mg.

Used in low dose for shorter duration.

Hydrocortisone = 5 mg IM.

ANTI-HISTAMINE

Acts by inhibiting the synthesis and release of histamine

Indication

- In allergic reactions caused due to analgesics, antibiotics, chemicals, As a premedication to avoid nausea and vomiting.
- As a premedication to produce mild sedation and xerostomia in medically compromised patients.
- Tab cetirizine 10 mg
- Tab avil.

6
Preventive Endodontics
Vital Pulp Therapy

A) INTRODUCTION

Significant importance is given to maintain the vitality of the tooth because vital tooth shows better defence against any pathologic assault and survive more in the oral cavity compared to the endodontically treated tooth. The root canal treated tooth after losing its innervation and vascular supply becomes more prone to any lesion. The basis to vital pulp therapy is inherent ability of vascular living tissues to heal and repair in the absence of microbial contamination. It is done in both deciduous and permanent dentition and particularly done in immature young permanent tooth for the continual uninterrupted development of root (root length growth and maturation) and closure of apical foramina (apexogenesis).

TERMINOLOGY

Immature teeth

- Recently erupted developing teeth in the oral cavity whose rootformation has not yet completed.
- It takes 3 years to complete the full formation of the root apex after eruption of the tooth into the oral cavity.

Mature teeth

Whose physiologic root formation has been completed.

Young permanent teeth

Immature or mature permanent teeth present in people whose age is between 6 years and mid teen (17 to 18 years).

Example

6, 7, 8, 9 years molars are called immature young permanent molars because their physiologic root formation has not been completed. From 10 years to 17 years are called mature young permanent molars because their physiologic root formation has been completed.

Definition

It is the procedure initiated to preserve and protect the pulp that has been compromised due to caries, trauma and restorative procedures.

Aim

Preservation of vitality of tooth to maintain the functional and structural integrity of tooth and its supporting tissues.

Objective

Dental health has direct influence on physical and mental development of children and young adults.

To have pain free healthy growing children and young adults by

- Early prevention of pain and inflammation
- Elimination of sensitivity and discomfort
- Elimination of pain
- Elimination of infection
- Avoiding root canal treatment
- Avoiding extractions

Rationale

Inflamed pulp repair and recover in the absence of microbial contamination. Healing ability of pulp is the basis to vital pulp therapy. The following factors influence the healing ability of pulp and should be considered before initiating vital pulp therapy.

1) Vascularity or blood supply (volume of healthy normal pulp)
2) Health and integrity of supporting tissues
3) Immunological status of tooth (diabetic, steroid therapy or any other immune compromised disorders)
4) Age and General health of patient (size of roots and pulp chamber, number of roots, volume of vascularity)
5) Genetic make up
6) Patient's inner drive and self-motivation to get healed naturally
7) Type of technique employed
8) Type of medicament and bioactive material used
9) Regular follow ups and monitoring
10) Patient on any medication.

Mechanism

- Odontoblasts are the structural and functional units of teeth

- Preserving and maintaining existing odontoblasts and inducing the formation of new odontoblasts is the key.

1) Removing caries completely eliminates the bacteria and their by-products which eventually avoids further damage to existing odontoblasts.

2) Constant mild irritation of calcium hydroxide or bioactive materials stimulate the undifferentiated mesenchymal cells of pulp to form odontoblast like cells and fibroblasts. The odontoblast like cell secretes reparative dentin and fibroblast secretes fibrinogen.

3) Moderate to severe irritation of calcium hydroxide or bioactive materials stimulate the primary odontoblast to secrete reactionary dentin.

4) Finally, tertiary dentin calcific bridge is formed with the help of reparative dentin and reactionary dentin.

Recovery and repair more readily occur in a young permanent tooth with normal pulp or minimally inflamed pulp or compromised pulp.

- Due to high cellular activity and high vascularity immature young permanent tooth exhibits significant potential to recover and repair.

- Due to the presence of pluripotent stem cells in pulp and multipotent undifferentiated mesenchymal cells in periapical area, repair more readily occurs in young permanent tooth.

- Revascularization more readily occurs through wide open apex due to the presence of rich vascular supply in peri apical area of immature young permanent tooth.

Benefits

By bringing back the tooth to its natural state, the tooth's natural immune system will be brought back to its normal function.

Preservation, protection and maintenance of vitality of tooth have following benefits:

- Maintenance of normal function
- Maintenance of natural aesthetics
- Maintenance of arch length
- Prevention of displacement of tooth
- Prevention of malocclusion

GENERAL GUIDE LINES FOR CASE SELECTION

- Tooth has to be normal - Normally responsive.
- Tooth has to be vital - Healing ability.
- Periodontal status has to be normal and healthy without any pathosis and lesions.
- The inflammation should be minimal - Recoverable.
- The inflammation should be reversible - Repairable.

Diagnosis

Correct diagnosis, employing appropriate technique, following right protocols using suitable materials is the key to success of vital pulp therapy.

Clinical and radiographic examination

Pulpal inflammation must be confined to coronal portion of the pulp without the signs and symptoms of periapical pathosis.

Pain

There should be no history of spontaneous pain, continuous pain, postural pain, referring pain and sleep disturbed due to pain.

Nature of pain should be inductive, transient, intermittent, short, momentary.

Palpation test

Soft tissue should be normal with no swelling, abscess or fistula, sinus tract

Percussion test

Should be negative.

PERIODONTAL PROBING

There should be no evidence of any pockets, vertical cracks or any defective morphology.

Mobility

Should be firm and stable in socket without any pathologic mobility.

Cold test

Sharp, Transitory pain, localized pain disappears immediately after removal of cold stimulus.

Hot test

Pain should not aggravate after taking hot and should not continue even after the removal of hot stimulus.

Electric pulp test

Should respond to low currents

Requirements of medicaments and bioactive materials

- Antimicrobial – should completely eliminate bacteria and neutralize existing infection.
- Formative – should induce and promote the formation of tertiary dentin calcific bridge.
- Should exhibit good sealing properties to prevent microleakage. Long term coronal seal is the key to the success of vital therapy.
- Should be biocompatible.
- Should be nontoxic, non-mutagenic and non-carcinogenic.
- Should be inexpensive and easily available.

Material and medicament used

- Calcium hydroxide
- Tricalcium silicates
- MTA
- Bio dentin
- Formocresol
- Ferric sulphate

Parameters to assess the success of vital pulp therapy

- Tooth should be normal (normally responsive to all tests).
- Patient should be asymptomatic without sensitivity and pain.
- There should be no signs and symptoms of irreversible pulp damage.
- There should be no signs and symptoms of periapical or para-apical pathology like sinus, fistula, abscess and tenderness on percussion.
- There must be radiographic evidence of root end closure in young immature permanent tooth.
- There must be radiographic evidence of root length development in immature permanent tooth.
- There must be radiographic evidence of calcific barrier formation beneath the restoration.

B) INDIRECT PULP CAPPING

It is successfully done in both deciduous and permanent dentition. It is the most appropriate treatment in primary teeth to manage deep dentinal caries approaching the pulp without involving the pulp. If done in an appropriate case following proper protocols, it has high success rate compared to other vital therapies.

Definition

It is a clinical procedure to treat the deep carious lesions of the tooth where the status of pulp is judged to be normal or minimally inflamed.

Aim

1) Arresting of caries process by completely excavating aggressive caries.

2) Neutralization of existing infection by sealing the cavity with bioactive materials.

3) Remineralization of affected dentin by achieving a sterile bacteria free environment.

4) Induction and promotion of formation of tertiary dentin calcific bridge adjacent to the affected dentin which in turn protects the pulp from further injury.

Advantages

- Saving the vitality of the tooth. Preserve the immunological status of the tooth which thereby maintains normal function and integrity of the tooth.

- Early prevention of pain

- Elimination of sensitivity and immediate comfort to the patient

- Avoid more complex pulp therapies

- Has high success rate compared to pulpotomy

- Less expensive.

Indications

1) Tooth with hard, non-progressive sterile caries close to the pulp

2) Deep dentinal caries close to the pulp without involving the pulp

3) Gross caries lesions may or may not be associated with sensitivity

4) Traumatic fracture involving enamel and dentin near pulp exposure but not exposing the pulp

5) Deep dentinal exposure close to the pulp not exposing the pulp

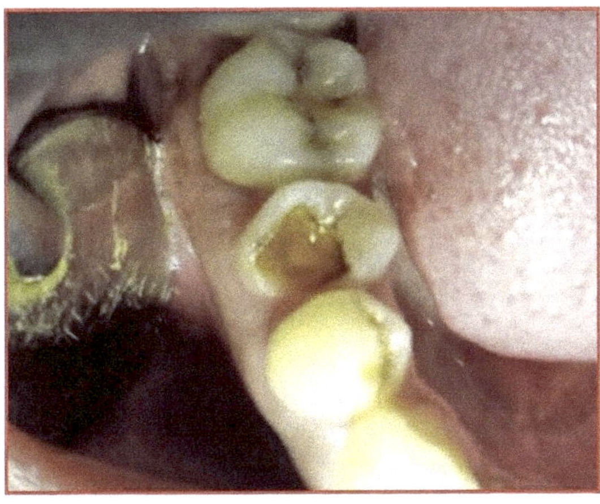

Fig. 6.1: Deep Dentinal cariers

Mode of actions

1) Removing infected caries and sealing the cavity with bioactive materials cuts off the nutrient supply to the bacteria. Due to starvation bacteria cannot grow and multiply and eventually bacterial count is reduced.

2) Due to high alkaline pH of bioactive materials the surveillance of bacteria become difficult. No bacteria can survive at 12.5 pH. of calcium hydroxide.

3) Direct bactericidal action of bioactive materials reduces the bacterial count.

4) Finally, in a bacteria free environment the progressive caries slowly shifts in to arrested caries and affected dentin slowly gets Re-minerali.

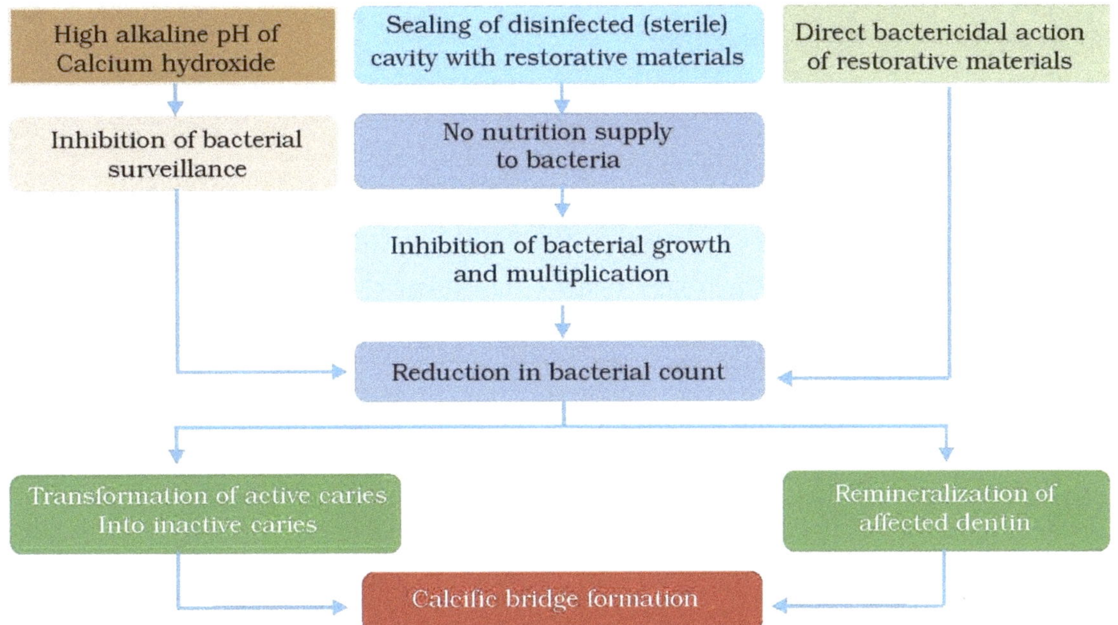

To Understand and manage indirect pule capping effectively deep carious lesions of the tooth are divided into two types.

1) Arrested caries

The carious process becomes stagnant. It does not have tendency to progress, hence the removal of deep caries layer adjacent to the pulp is not necessary and so adequate thick layer of dentin adjacent to the pulp is left behind. If this thick layer of dentin is removed, it would lead to pulp exposure.

Rationale

Overtime, in the absence of microbial contamination, the left behind adequate thick layer of arrested caries, dentin gets remineralized and converted in to normal dentin.

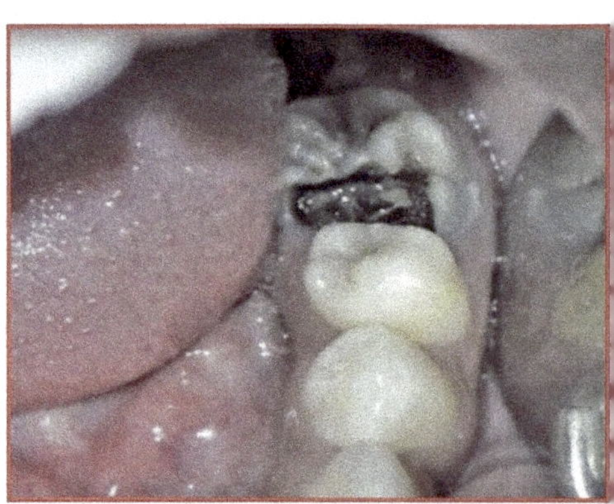

Fig. 6.2 : Arrested Caries

Features

- Color – Dark brown or black
- Consistency – Hard, difficult to remove
- Texture – Smooth and shiny
- Bacterial activity – Absent
- Pain on probing – Absent
- Sensitivity – Absent

2) Non arrested caries

The carious process is active and has tendency to progress, its complete removal is must.

Rationale

Disinfection of residual affected dentin is more readily accomplished in primary and young permanent tooth through following mechanisms.

Young enamel acts like a semipermeable membrane.

Flushing out of interstitial fluid of the dentin flushes out the microorganisms clogged in dentinal tubules coronally.

Sweating of dentin during cutting flushes out the microorganisms clogged in dentinal tubules out of dentin.

Features

- Color – Light yellow, light red, light brown or deep red
- Consistency – Soft and easy to remove
- Texture – Rough and dull
- Bacterial activity – Present
- Pain on probing – Present

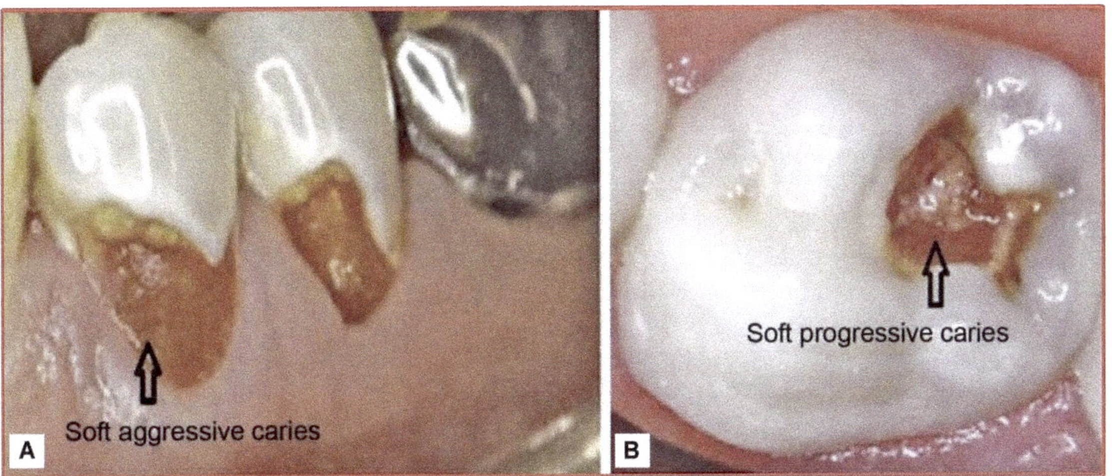

Fig. 6.3 : (A) Soft aggressive caries: (B) Soft progressive caries

Contraindications

1) Non restorable tooth
2) Soft leathery dentin
3) Spontaneous pain

Case selection

Rely upon accurate assessment of pulp status. Pulpal status should be normal with no or reversible pulp damage.

Material used

1) Calcium hydroxide
2) Tricalcium silicates
3) MTA
4) Bio dentin
5) Full coverage stainless steel or zirconia crowns

Procedure

Single appointment indirect pulp capping

It is done in arrested type of caries where whole caries removal is not required. And done by applying medicament over a thick layer of caries dentin.

STEPS

Isolation

complete isolation of tooth from oral cavity by using rubber dam is done to prevent the contamination with microorganisms present in oral fluids.

Excavation of caries

A large round bur at high speed with adequate water spray is used to remove gross caries. Care must be taken to remove all the peripheral caries from axial and lateral walls which is critical to achieve good marginal seal of the restorative materials. Marginal seal prevents microleakage and ingress of microorganisms, thus enhances the prognosis. Adequate thickness of carious dentin adjacent to the pulp left behind to avoid pulp exposure and further damage to the pulp.

Placement of bioactive material lining

After caries excavation, cavity is rinsed with normal saline or diluted sodium hypochlorite and air dried.

A layer of tricalcium silicate (MTA or bio dentin) or hard setting calcium hydroxide is placed over a thick layer of left behind dentin by applying mild pressure.

Final restoration

Once the bioactive material sets, the cavity is filled with direct bonding resin modified high strength glass ionomer cement as sub base and finally permanent restoration done with crowns or composite restorations.

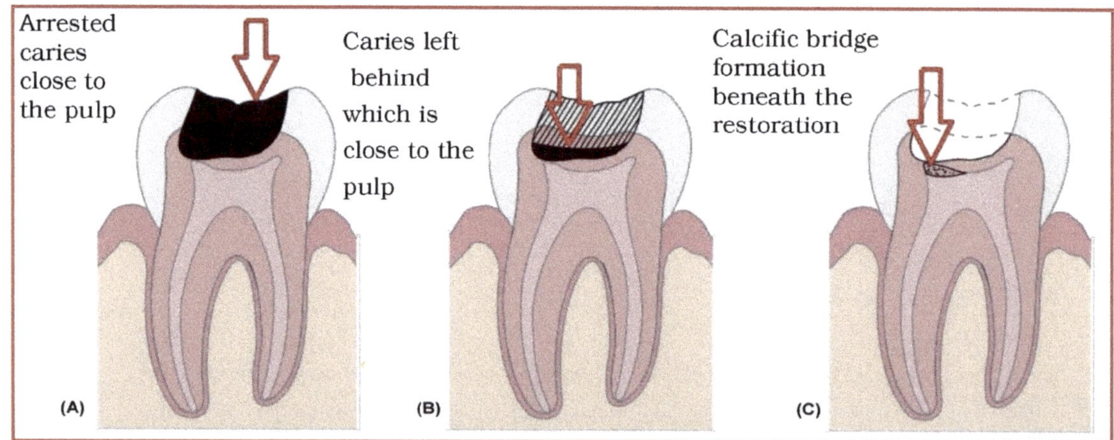

Fig. 6.4: Single visit indirect pulp capping

Two or multiple appointment indirect pulp capping

It is done in progressive non arrested type of caries. Caries excavation carried out in stepwise incremental manner in multiple visits.

First visit

It is a judgmental procedure. It involves complete removal of soft active caries as much as possible from deep dentinal caries lesion without exposing the pulp followed by leaving behind very thin caries immediately adjacent to the pulp which if removed would lead to pulp exposure.

The thin layer of infected dentin remaining over a nearly exposing pulp is covered with medicament. Temporary dressing is given and patient is recalled for second visit two months later. The Idea is shifting the progressive carious lesion into non progressive lesion or completely removing all caries before doing final restoration.

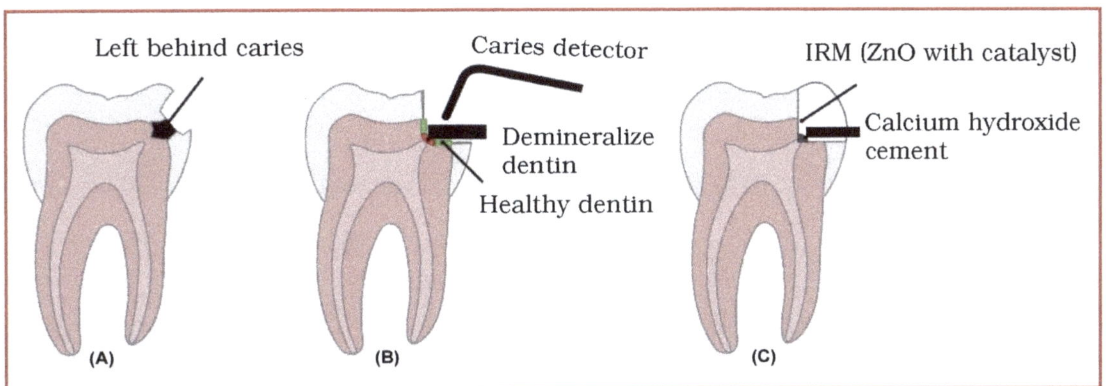

Fig. 6.5: First visit

Second visit

Cavity is re-entered, the caries which was left behind adjacent to the pulp is removed. Care must be taken not to expose the pulp. Its success depends upon managing to completely remove soft active caries lesion without exposing the pulp.

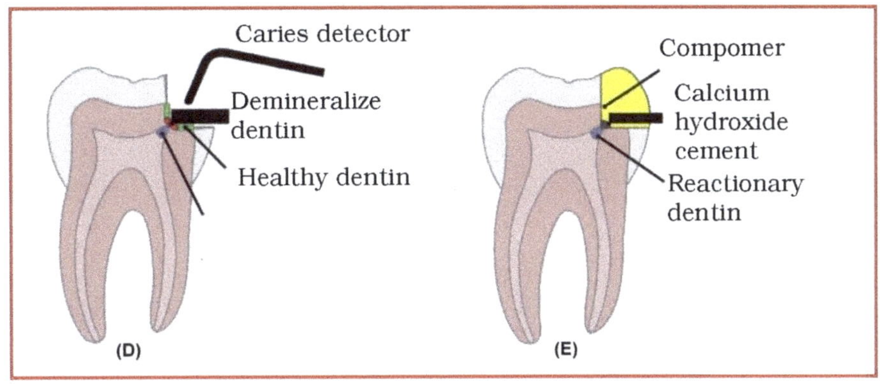

Fig. 6.6: Second visit (after 2 months)

Prognosis of indirect pulp capping

Prognosis depends upon the following factors

1) Removal of all active carious lesion without exposing the pulp,
2) The amount of remaining sound dentin underneath the restoration
3) Type of medicament used.
4) Type of restorative material used for coronal seal which determines the seal against microleakage
5) Complete disinfection and remaining sound margins below the restoration is more important compared to type of materials used to the final outcome.

C) DIRECT PULP CAPPING

This procedure is primarily performed to manage a pin point iatrogenic exposure of the pulp in asymptomatic teeth. Pulp exposed unintentionally in asymptomatic teeth during routine restorative procedures serve better compared to inflamed pulp infected from caries or trauma. Case selection is the key to final out-come.

Direct pulp capping in primary dentition is done only if optimal outcome is anticipated.

Definition

It is an attempt to treat and save the exposed dental pulp with materials which induce and promote the formation of tertiary dentin calcific bridge which in turn covers and protects the pulp from further injury.

Aims

To protect and preserve the exposed pulp in order to maintain the vitality of tooth.

Case selection

Case selection is extremely important for success. The following factors should be considered especially inflamed pulp infected from caries or trauma.

Type of exposure

Non carious exposures have more potential for healing and recovery compared to carious exposure of pulp.

Location

More coronal the exposure better would be the prognosis

Time

fresh exposure without contamination with oral fluids, better would be the prognosis.

Size of exposure

No break in the continuity or slight break in the continuity of dentinal wall (classic pin point exposure) covering the pulp better would be the prognosis, depth of exposure influences more compared to width of exposure.

Age

In children and young adults due to high healing capacity and faster recovery, prognosis is better.

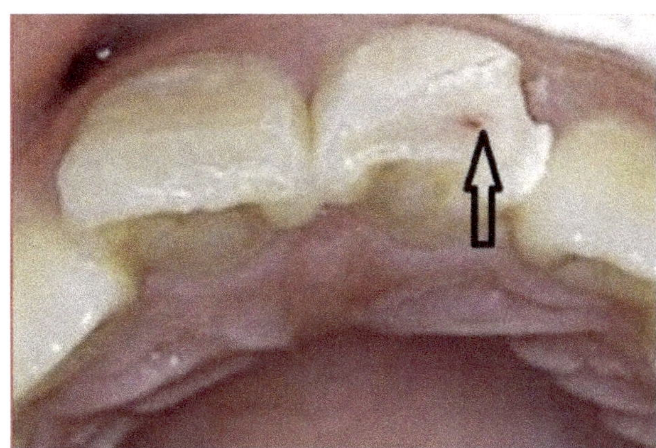

Fig. 6.7: Pin point traumatic exposure

Size and volume of pulp cavity

More the size and volume of pulp tissue, more the vascularity and more would be the healing capacity.

E.g.: Multi rooted molars and maxillary anterior.

Status of pulp

In cases of severe pulp calcifications and fibrosis prognosis is poor.

E.g.: Old and aged pulps.

Indications

Pin point accidental or mechanical exposure during crown cutting, restorative procedures.

Pin point caries exposure of pulp less than 0.5 mm in immature young permanent tooth where there is high chance for favorable response.

Pin point caries exposure of pulp less than 0.1 mm in young permanent tooth where there is high chance for favorable response.

Note

Caries exposure through affected dentin not infected dentin. If caries exposure occurs through infected dentin pulpotomy or root canal treatment should be considered.

Pin point traumatic pulp exposure due to deep dentinal fractures reported within 12 hours in aseptic state that is in dry condition without contamination.

Few chosen cases of deciduous teeth nearing their exfoliation. exfoliation period is within 6 months.

Contraindications

Carious pulp exposure in deciduous tooth due to high cellularity in deciduous dentition there may be diffuse inflammation and internal resorption.

1) Pulpal exposure along the axial wall. *E.g.:* Class 2 cavity
2) Non restorable tooth.
3) Pulp calcifications and pulp fibrosis.
4) Mentally compromised patient where isolation of tooth is difficult.
5) Immunocompromised patients where healing and recovery is poor.
6) Aged and older patients with atrophied and calcified pulp.

Prerequisites

- Asymptomatic permanent tooth
- No bleeding or already controlled bleeding
- Normal pulp or reversibly inflamed pulp

Prognosis

- High failure rate is observed in deciduous tooth due to internal resorption so case selection in deciduous tooth must be done very cautiously.

- In permanent dentition bacterial contamination plays key role, so it should be performed immediately after the exposure and coronal seal must be air tight to resist any microleakage.

Material used

1) Calcium hydroxide
2) Tricalcium silicates
3) MTA
4) Bio dentin

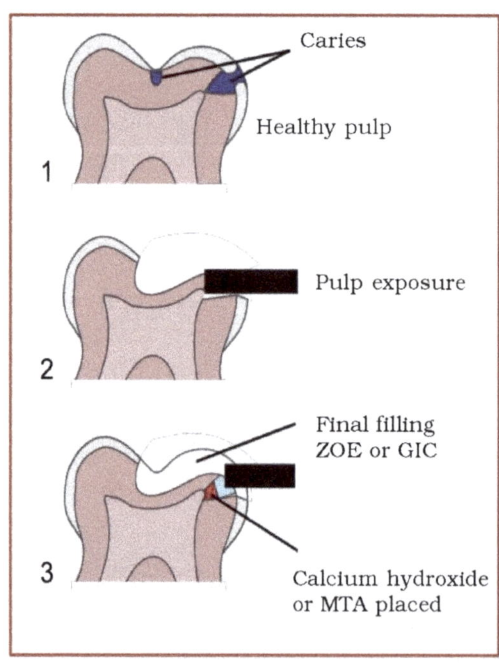

Fig. 6.8: Direct pulp capping

Procedure

Isolation

Complete isolation of tooth from oral cavity is done with help of rubber dam or cotton rolls to avoid contamination of pulp with oral fluids, prognosis is better with rubber dam isolation.

Hemostasis

Stop bleeding by applying gentle pressure with sterile moist cotton wool pellet

Disinfection

Clean and disinfect the exposed site by rinsing with normal saline or highly diluted sodium hypochlorite or chlorhexidine depending upon type of exposure- carious or traumatic.

Application of medicament

A layer of calcium hydroxide or tricalcium silicate is applied over clean and dry exposed site with no pressure.

Achieving hermetic marginal seal

This is an extremely important step which has direct impact on outcome. Thick layer of direct bonding glass ionomer cement is filled over medicament followed by final filling with mechanically bonding composite resins.

Preventing long term marginal leakage and contamination by achieving air tight seal is crucial for success of direct pulp capping.

D) PULPOTOMY

It is routinely done in primary tooth and immature young permanent tooth with good success rate.

Definition

- It is a surgical procedure which involves partial or complete removal of compromised coronal pulp followed by covering the remaining larger portion of healthy pulp or amputated root stumps or remaining vital radicular pulp with medicaments or bioactive materials.

Aims

Preserving, protecting and maintaining remaining vital healthy pulp in order to save the vitality of tooth.

Rationale

- Recovery and Repair of remaining healthy pulp of primary teeth and young permanent tooth occurs due to high cellular activity and high vascularity.
- Recovery and repair more readily occur in immature young permanent teeth due to the presence of pluripotent stem cells in pulp and multipotent undifferentiated mesenchymal cells in periapical area.
- Revascularization more readily occurs through wide open apex due to the presence of rich vascular supply in the peri apical area of immature tooth.

Benefits

Structural and functional integrity of tooth is maintained by preserving the vitality of tooth.

Uninterrupted physiologic root development in immature young permanent tooth.

Case selection

- Tooth has to be vital
- Tooth has to be restorable
- At least 2/3 root length must be present
- Isolation of tooth must be feasible

Prerequisites

- Inflammation must be confined to the coronal portion of tooth
- Inflammation has to be reversible
- Inflammation has to be minimal (mild to moderate)
- Periodontal status of tooth has to be normal

Classification

1) *Depending upon type of material used*
   a) Formo-cresol pulpotomy
   b) Calcium hydroxide pulpotomy
   c) Trisilicate pulpotomy
   d) Ferric sulphate pulpotomy

2) *Depending upon extent of removal of coronal pulp*
   a) Superficial or partial or subtotal or Cvek pulpotomy or shallow pulpotomy
   b) Cervical pulpotomy or Total coronal pulpotomy

3) *Depending upon method*
   a) Conventional pulpotomy
   b) Laser pulpotomy
   c) Electrosurgical pulpotomy

1. PARTIAL PULPOTOMY OR SHALLOW PULPOTOMY

Definition

- Surgical removal of superficially compromised pulp followed by covering the remaining healthy coronal and radicular pulp with medicament or bioactive materials.

- It is mainly done in traumatic exposures of pulp of immature young permanent tooth with high success rate.

Indications

- Mechanical exposure less than 1 mm
- Traumatic exposure less than 1 mm if reported immediately in dry condition
- Caries exposure lees than 0.5 mm in immature permanent tooth

Advantages

- Wound management and hemostasis is easy.

- Only pulp horns or superficial chamber tissue is removed conserving more healthy coronal pulp.

- Complete deroofing is not required.

- Slight or partial portion of the roof is removed which saves more tooth structure and strengthens the tooth.

- Provides seat for medicament placement which enhances the marginal seal and prevents microleakage.

Procedure

- It is done by removing small portion of compromised coronal pulp 1 to 2 mm or more to the depth of healthy tissue.

- Small round bur corresponding to the size of exposure and highspeed hand piece with good supply of coolant are used.

- Cutting is performed intermittently without applying unwanted pressure.

- Bleeding is controlled by applying mild pressure with cotton wool pellet against the wound or continuous rinsing with normal saline. Clinician should achieve hemostasis without blood clot formation and bleeding should stop within 2 to 3 minutes, if not cervical pulpotomy or root canal treatment should be considered.

- Disinfection is carried out by rinsing with sodium hypochlorite or chlorhexidine. Dry the area with cotton wool pellet. Place calcium hydroxide or MTA over the operating area. At least 1.5 to 2 mm thick layer of MTA should cover the exposure and surrounding entire dentin.

Note: In anterior tooth white MTA is used to avoid discoloration of tooth and in posterior tooth grey MTA is used to get more predictable results.

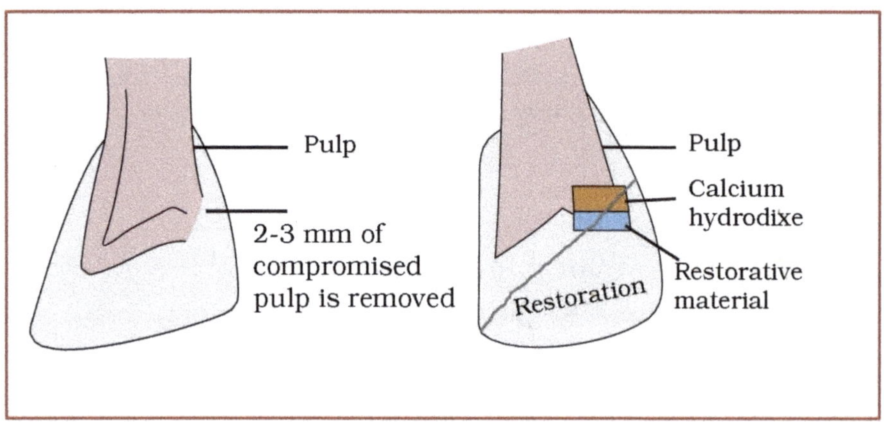

Fig. 6.9: Partial pulpotomy

2. CERVICAL PULPOTOMY

Indication

- Reversible pulpitis and a very few selected cases of early irreversible pulpitis in immature young permanent tooth.
- Carious exposure of pulp in primary tooth.
- Carious exposure of pulp less than 2 mm in immature young permanent tooth.
- Mechanical exposure of pulp greater than 2 mm in young permanent tooth.
- Traumatic exposure of pulp in young permanent tooth due to enamel dentin fractures reported within 24 hours of injury.

Contraindication

- Irreversible pulpitis
- Spontaneous pain
- Calcification of pulp chamber
- Internal resorption

Contraindication during the procedure

- Uncontrolled bleeding after amputation of coronal pulp
- Thick viscous sluggish bleeding
- Dull dark bleeding

Procedure
Premedication

If necessary, premedication with anti salivary drugs like propantheline and scopolamine is given to inhibit salivary secretion and promote dry working environment.

Local anesthesia without vasoconstrictor (plain 2% lignocaine hydrochloride). Adrenaline is a vasoconstrictor; it decreases the blood flow to assess the exact degree of bleeding. After amputation plain local anesthesia is recommended.

Isolation with rubber dam

Completely isolate the tooth from oral cavity to prevent the contamination from oral fluids. This is the key to the success of the procedure.

Occlusal clearance

A clearance of 1.5 to 2 mm is given, it aids in removal of superficial Bacteria and healing of tooth.

Excavation of caries

Complete removal of caries is done by using large round burs at high speed. Care must be taken to remove all the peripheral and core caries before deroofing the pulp.

Deroofing the pulp chamber

After rinsing the cavity with sodium hypochlorite or chlorhexidine, complete deroofing is done with small no. 6 sterile round bur at low speed. Safe ended bur is used in primary teeth to avoid furcation perforation because the distance between pulp chamber and floor is less.

Surgical pulpotomy

Make a clean cut at the level of pulpal floor or at the level of orifice of canals with the help of sterile abrasive bur at high speed with adequate coolant to resect coronal pulp tissue. The purpose of using high speed and coolant is to avoid further damage to the pulp tissue. The size of the bur should correspond to the size of pulp chamber. Small sharp spoon excavator can also be used for the same purpose. The residual tissue tags should be removed as they interfere with hemostasis.

Hemostasis

Bleeding is controlled by applying mild pressure with moist cotton wool pellet soaked in normal saline. Rinsing continuously with sterile water helps to achieve hemostasis without the formation of clot. If bleeding is not controlled within 3 to 5 minutes it indicates hyperemic irreversibly inflamed pulp. Pulpotomy is no more indicated.

Antisepsis

If needed antisepsis is done with highly diluted sodium hypochlorite or chlorhexidine depending upon the status of pulp.

Applying therapeutic agents

Apply the medicament or bioactive material to the amputated site and finally restore with interim or permanent fillings depending upon type of pulpotomy.

Formo-cresol pulpotomy:

- Most commonly and widely done method with high success rate in carious exposure of primary tooth
- Solution ! Composition of Formo-cresol solution
- 19% formaldehyde
- 35% cresol
- 15% glycerin
- Buckley's formo-cresol—1:5 concentration of formo-cresol solution

Mechanism of action

- Formaldehyde is a potent bactericidal agent.
- It acts by fixation. It prevents the autolysis of cells by reversibly bonding proteins, basic overall structure of cells remains same.
- Fixation occurs in Coronal 1/3.
- Middle 1/3 presents loss of cellular integrity.
- Apical 1/3 shows granulation tissue growth.

Advantages
- Bactericidal
- Germicidal
- Cheap and commonly available
- Long shelf life

Disadvantages
- Controversial material
- Highly caustic
- In high doses toxic
- Exhibits mutagenic and carcinogenic potential

Procedure

One appointment formocresol pulpotomy

A sterile cotton pellet soaked in 1:5 concentration of Buckley's formocresol is placed over the amputated root stumps for 3 to 5 minutes and check for signs of fixation. The root stumps become darkish brown and the cotton pellet turns to brownish color. Dry the area with new cotton pellet, fill the cavity with zinc oxide eugenol cement in direct contact with the root stumps and finally cover the tooth with stainless steel crown.

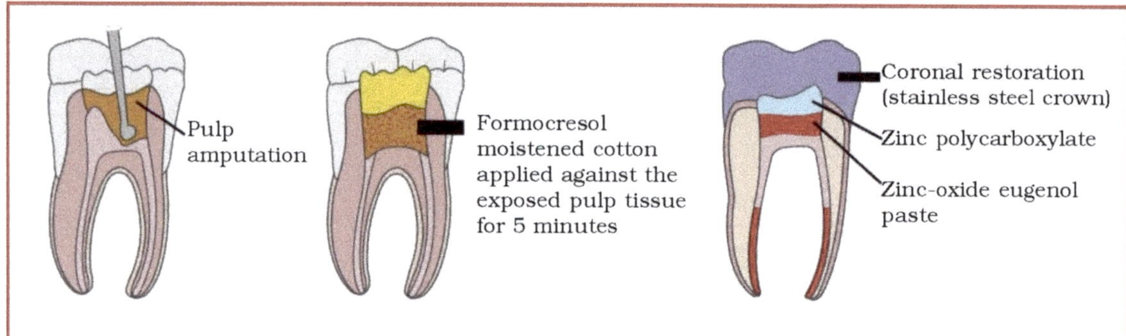

Fig. 6.10: One appointment formocresol pulpotomy

Two appointment formocresol pulpotomy

A sterile cotton pellet soaked in diluted formocresol is sealed in the chamber for 4 days with temporary cement. At second appointment temporary cement and cotton is removed, chamber is irrigated with highly diluted sodium hypochlorite or chlorhexidine. After thoroughly air drying the area, completely fill the cavity with fast setting high strength zinc oxide eugenol cement and finally cover the tooth with stainless steel crowns.

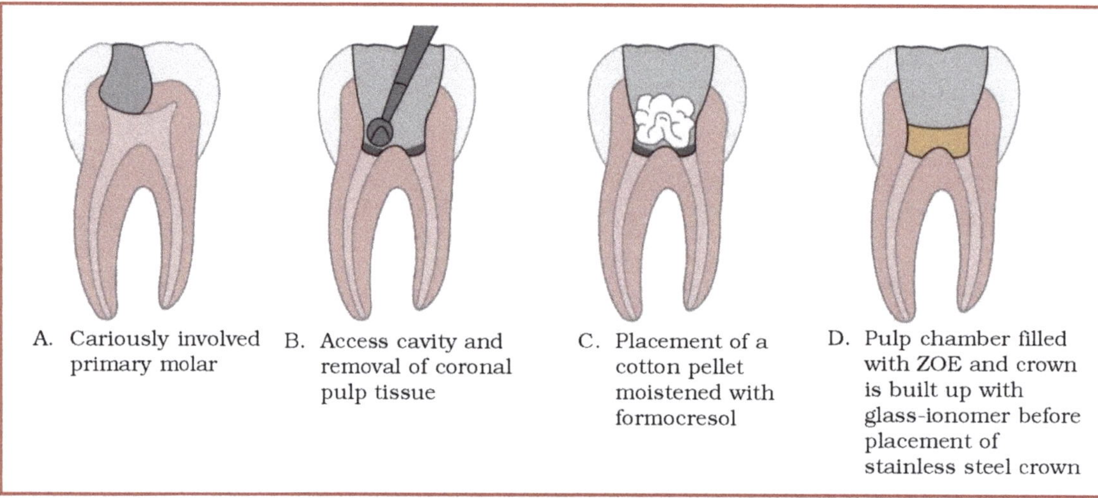

Fig. 6.11: Two appointment formocresol pulpotomy

Calcium hydroxide pulpotomy

It is contra indicated in primary tooth because it causes diffuse chronic inflammation and internal resorption.

It is more frequently done in immature young permanent tooth with incomplete root formation and less frequently done in mature young permanent tooth.

It is done by gently covering the amputated root stumps with calcium hydroxide paste by applying very mild pressure with a plastic condenser and drying with cotton pellet. Place a modified glass ionomer cement as sub base. Finally restore the tooth with composite resins.

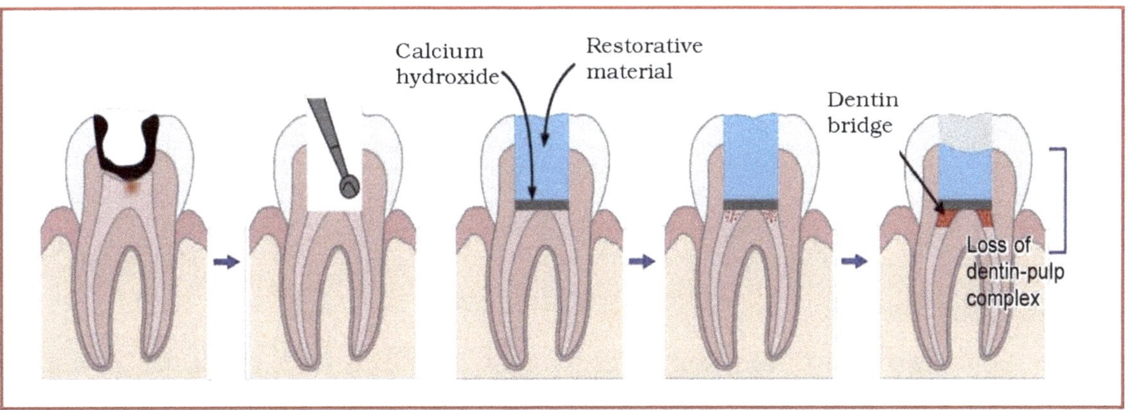

Fig. 6.12: Calcium hydroxide pulpotomy

Note: Care must be taken not to place calcium hydroxide over blood clot in order to avoid internal resorption because high alkaline pH of calcium hydroxide induces metaplasia in blood clot which leads to formation of odontoclasts which in turn increases odontoclastic activity and causes internal resorptions.

Advantages

- Excellent antimicrobial property
- Less expensive and commonly available.
- Easy to handle

Disadvantages

Calcific barrier is of poor quality with multiple tunnel defects and porosities. Lacks adhesive property.

More soluble in oral fluids and dissolves over time. Inability to provide long term seal against microleakage.

Ferric sulphate pulpotomy

It is done by applying 15% ferric sulphate solution over the amputated root. Stumps for 15 seconds.

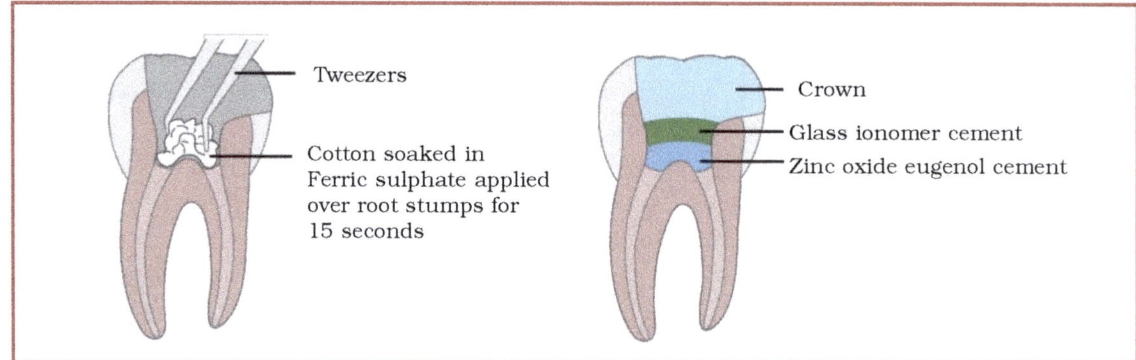

Fig. 6.13: Ferric sulphate pulpotomy

Mechanism

It acts as an astringent and hemostatic agent. The iron in ferric sulphate reacts with proteins to form metal protein complex which mechanically occludes the lumens of blood capillaries to cease blood flow and avoid clot formation.

Advantages

- Economical and easily available

- Non-toxic and non-carcinogenic

- Ferric sulphate also used in calcium hydroxide pulpotomy as a hemostatic agent.

Disadvantages

Internal resorption

Mineral trioxide pulpotomy

It is done in both deciduous and permanent tooth.

Procedure

Mix the MTA with sterile water on a sterile glass slab. The final mix should have a wet sand like consistency.

Safely carry and place the mix over the amputated root stumps, gentle pressure with a moist cotton wool pellet is applied to spread and condense the material all over the root orifice and floor.

The thickness of compacted material should be 4 to 5 mm, care must be taken to condense it properly without voids. The moist cotton wool pellet is left in the pulp chamber and cavity is filled with temporary cement to allow the MTA to set.

In the following appointment temporary cement and cotton pellet is removed and the tooth is restored with permanent restoration.

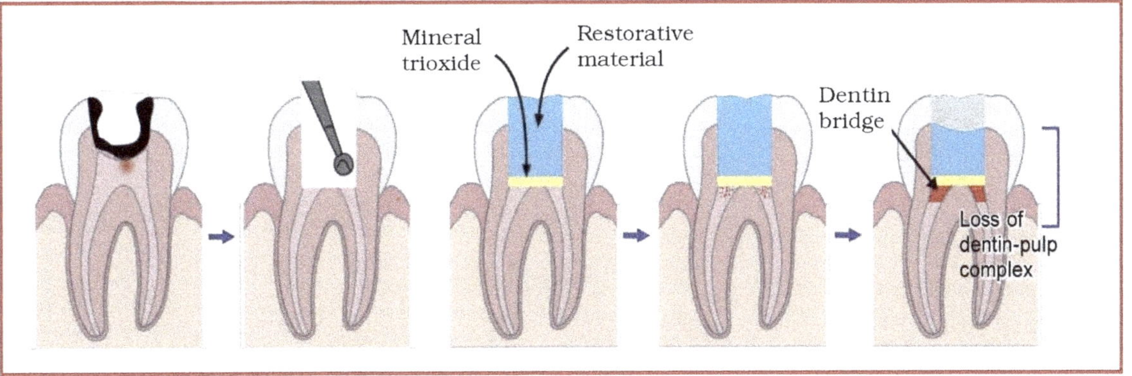

Fig. 6.14: Mineral trioxide pulpotomy

Advantages

- Exhibits broad spectrum antimicrobial activity. MTA has antibacterial and antifungal properties.
- Calcific barrier is of good quality with less tunnel defects and porosities.
- Better biocompatibility, non-mutagenic and less cytotoxic.
- Less solvable in oral fluids and non-permeable. Better resistance against microleakage.
- Expands during setting, marginal adaption and sealing ability is better.
- Radio-opaque.

Disadvantages:

- Requires two appointments because of long setting time
- More expensive
- Poor handling features
- High solubility before final setting
- Discoloration of tooth.

e) APEXOGENESIS

Apexo means root end or root apex. Genesis means formation

The physiologic formation of root apex is called apexogenesis.

IMMATURE TEETH

- Recently erupted developing teeth in the oral cavity whose root formation is not yet completed.
- It takes 3 years to complete the full formation of root apex after eruption of the tooth into the oral cavity.

MATURE TEETH

Whose physiologic root formation has been completed.

YOUNG PERMANENT TEETH

Immature or mature permanent teeth present in people aged from 6 years to mid teen.

Example

6, 7, 8, 9 years molars are immature young permanent molars because their physiologic root formation has not been completed.

From 10 years to 17 years Mature young permanent molars because their physiologic root formation has been completed.

IMMATURE YOUNG PERMANENT TOOTH

Injury to immature young permanent tooth due to trauma or caries results in cessation of blood supply which halts the formation and deposition of minerals which in turn eventually leads to incomplete or underdevelopment of root of the tooth with following features

1) Short roots

2) Thin and fragile root walls

3) Parallel or diverging root walls

4) Wide open apex

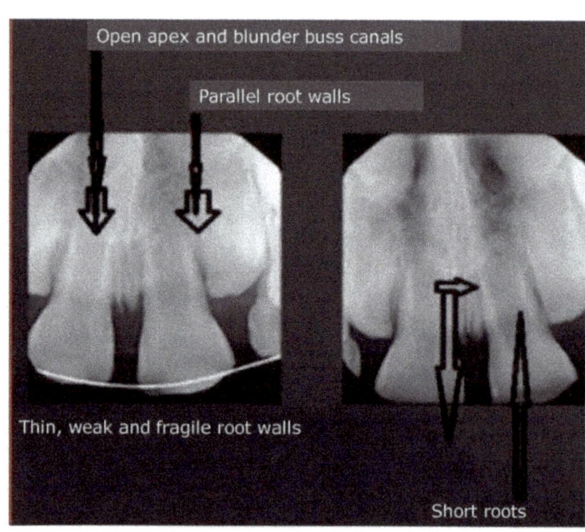

Fig. 6.15:

DIFFICULTIES ASSOCIATED WITH IMMATURE TOOTH

Conventional root canal treatment and apical surgery - ortho grade filling in immature young permanent tooth is contraindicated due to following reasons:

1) Lack of apical stop.

   Due to wide open apex, it is impossible to achieve three-dimensional air tight apical seal which is critical for endodontic success.

2) Lack of taper, due to divergent or parallel root walls.

   Difficult to achieve compact obturation of root canal filling materials.

3) Thin and fragile dentinal walls prone to fracture. Weak and fragile walls do not resist lateral and vertical forces during obturation or apical surgery and orthograde filling.

Definition

It is a procedure to treat vital normally inflamed or compromised pulp of immature young permanent tooth in order to allow continual root development and closure of open apex.

Methods

Depending upon extent of injury and pulpal status following methods are used to induce apexogenesis.

1) Indirect pulp capping when the status of pulp is normal or minimally inflamed.

2) Direct pulp capping when the pulp is minimally inflamed.

3) Partial pulpotomy when the pulp is slightly compromised and the inflammation is confined to the pulp horns or superficial layer of coronal pulp.

4) Cervical pulpotomy when the pulp is compromised and inflammation is confined to the coronal pulp.

Objectives

- Elimination of infection.
- Neutralization of existing infection.
- Preservation of vitality of pulp.
- Permitting the continual physiologic process of root end development (root growth, maturation and root end closure).
- To attain favorable crown root ratio.
- Inducing and promoting the tertiary dentin calcific barrier formation beneath the medicaments or restorations.

Rationale

- Recovery and repair more readily occur in an immature young permanent tooth with normal pulp or minimally inflamed pulp or compromised pulp.
- Due to high cellular activity and high vascularity immature young permanent tooth exhibits significant potential to recover and repair.
- Due to the presence of pluripotent stem cells in pulp and multipotent undifferentiated mesenchymal cells in periapical area repair more readily occur in young permanent tooth.
- Revascularization more readily occur through wide open apex due the presence of rich vascular supply in peri apical area.

Indication

- Traumatically exposed immature young permanent vital tooth.
- Caries exposure of immature young permanent vital tooth.
- Luxation of immature young permanent vital tooth.
- Iatrogenic injuries of immature young permanent vital tooth.

Contraindication

- Non vital immature young permanent tooth.
- Longitudinal crown root fractures require interradicular retention for restoration.
- Grossly destructed non restorable tooth.
- Crown fracture at the level of CEJ or horizontal cervical 1/3 root fracture.

Diagnosis and Case selection

Thorough clinical and radiographic investigation carried out before selecting the case.

Pulpal inflammation must be confined to coronal portion of the pulp without the sign and symptoms of periapical pathosis.

Pain

There should be no history of spontaneous pain, continuous pain, postural pain, referring pain and sleep disturbances due to pain.

Nature of pain should be inductive, transient, intermittent, short, momentary.

Palpation test

Soft tissue should be normal with no swelling, abscess or fistula, sinus tract.

Percussion test

Should be negative.

Periodontal probing

There should be no evidence of any pockets, vertical cracks or any defective morphology.

Mobility

Should be firm and stable in socket without any pathologic mobility.

Cold test

Sharp, intermittent, transitory pain, short, localized, momentary pain, induced pain disappears immediately after removal of cold stimulus.

Hot test

Pain should not aggravate after taking hot and should not continue even after the removal of hot stimulus.

Electric pulp test

Should respond to low currents.

Radiographic examinations

- There should be no evidence of periapical radiolucency.
- There should be no evidence of intra-radicular radiolucency.
- No widening of periodontal ligament space.
- No break in the continuity of lamina dura.
- No root caries and furcation involvement.

Material used

1) Calcium hydroxide.
2) Tricalcium silicates.
3) MTA.
4) Bio dentin.
5) Full coverage stainless steel or zirconia crowns.

7
Morphology of Tooth

WHEN WE KNOW BETTER, WE CAN DO BETTER.

KNOWING BOOSTS CONFIDENCE.

CONFIDENCE BREEDS POWER.

POWER LEADS TO PERSONA.

PERSONA DEFINES SUCCESS.

PERSONA IS EVERYTHING IN CLINICAL PRACTICE.

Starting from access opening to obturation, the techniques, type of instrumentation and materials used are all based on the anatomy of tooth. In other words, morphology of the tooth is the basis to endodontics. So, thorough knowledge of the anatomy of the tooth is essential and is the paramount ingredient

KEY POINTS

The average length of a tooth is 22 mm. Except maxillary and mandibular canine which is 27 mm and 26 mm respectively. An average crown length is 10 mm. An average root length is 13 ± 1 mm. Average height of the pulp is 4 mm. The average distance between occlusal surface of the tooth and roof of the pulp chamber is 6 mm.

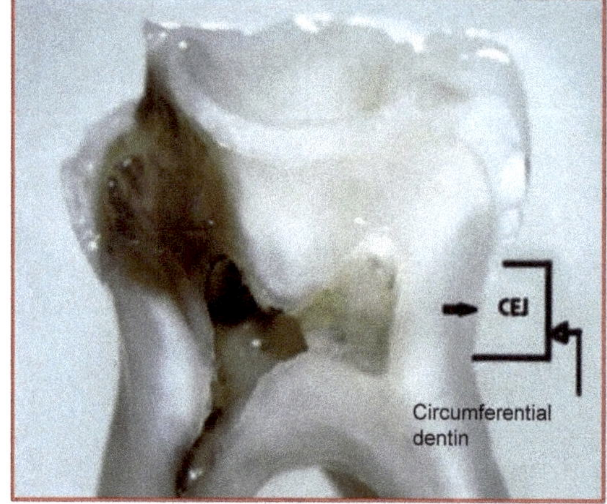

Fig. 7.1: Cementoenamel junction

Cementoenamel junction

It is the most constant anatomic landmark. It determines the floor of the pulp chamber. The area 6 mm above and 6 mm below CEJ is called peri cervical dentin. Preservation of peri cervical dentin is crucial as it empowers the tooth against various occlusal stresses. Peri cervical dentin (circumferential dentin) gets more removed during pre-coronal widening with large Gates-Glidden drills.

Cementodentinal junction

It is the point where cementum meets the dentin. It's the point where the pulp ends and peri-radicular tissue starts. Location of CDJ ranges from 0.3-3 mm short of the anatomical apex. It is a histologic land mark, it cannot be seen radiologically, but it can be felt with finger tactile sense with experience.

Apex locater is used to determine its exact location.

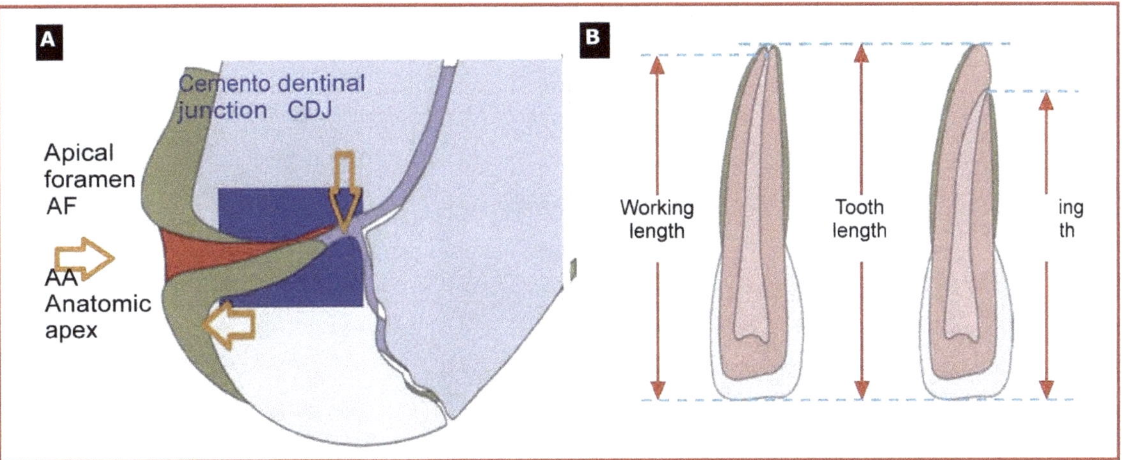

Fig. 7.2: (A) Cemento-dentinal junction; (B) Variation in location of CDJ.

Roots

All roots are straight from the cervical to middle one third except:

1) Mesio-buccal root and distobuccal root of maxillary molars
2) Maxillary lateral incisors and
3) Mesial root of mandibular molar

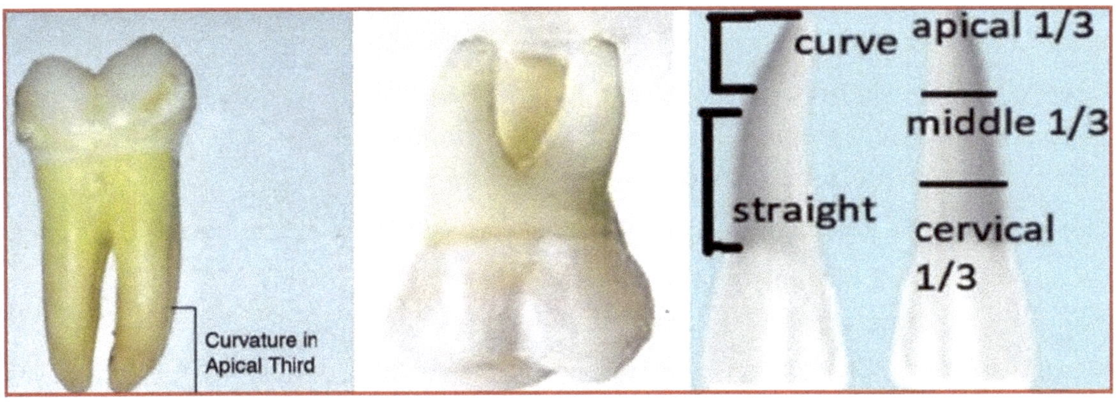

Fig. 7.3. Root's Curvature Roots

- Curvatures starts from apical 1/3 and apices curve distally. Maxillary centrals and canine curve disto-labially

- Maxillary laterals curve distolingually

- Upper anterior and lower anterior teeth are conical in shape, broader buccolingually and narrower mesiodistally.

- In anterior teeth, number of roots and root canal is one except mandibular lateral incisors.

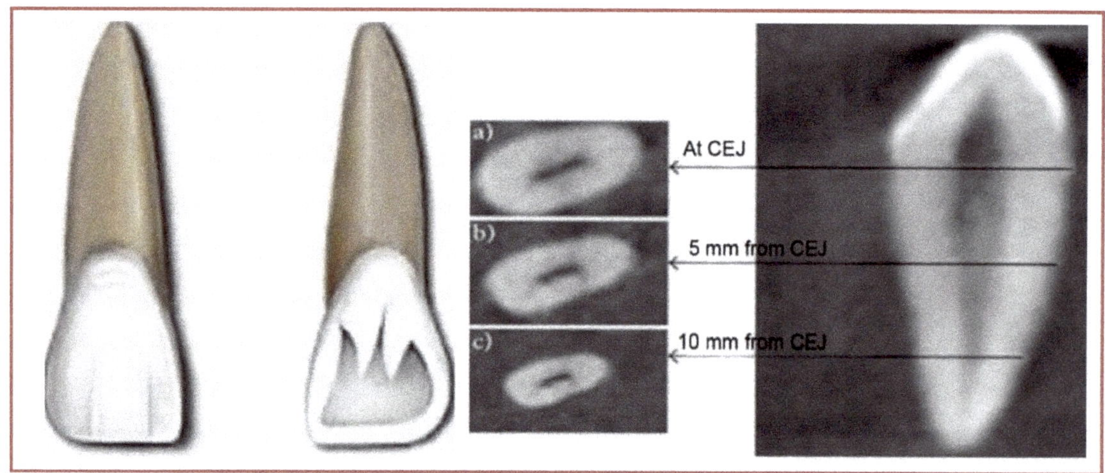

Fig. 7.4. Cross Section of Anteriors

Cross section:

In cross section, cervical and middle one third of almost all roots is roughly oval or elliptical and apical one third is round.

In cross section, roots that are flattened mesio-distally may have two canals or more than two canals.

Example –   Mesio buccal root of maxillary first molars

Mesial roots of mandibular first molars

Mandibular incisors

The roots which are round or oval in cross section have single canal.

Example –   Maxillary anterior

Disto-buccal roots of maxillary molars

Maxillary posteriors have three roots and three canals except maxillary first premolar which has two roots and two canals and mandibular second premolar which has one root and one canal.

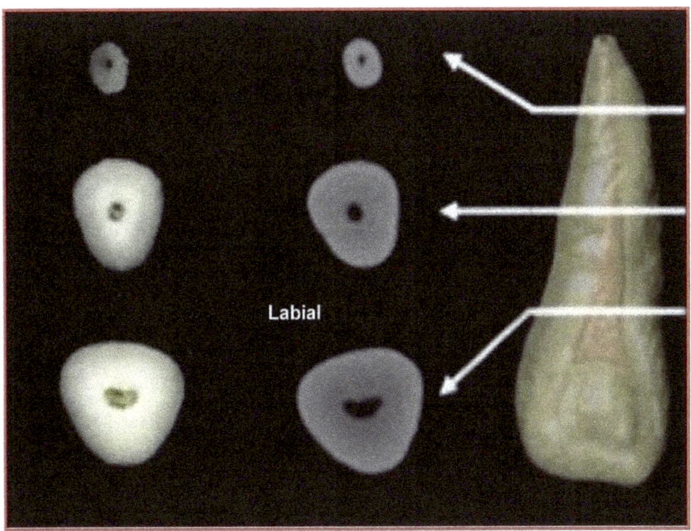

Fig. 7.5 : Cross section posteriors

- The palatal roots of maxillary molars and distal root of mandibular molars are straight and apices curve buccolingually.

- The buccal and palatal roots of maxillary 1st. premolars and roots of mandibular 2nd premolars are straight and apices curve buccolingually.

- Roots of mandibular 1st premolar are conical, short and straight.

- Mandibular molars have two roots and three canals and apices curve distally.

- Mandibular premolars have one root and one root canal except mandibular second premolars which may sometimes have two canals.

- Mandibular first premolars rarely surprise with three canals or complex internal anatomy.

- In maxillary molars the shape of access cavity is trapezoidal whereas in lower molars it is triangular in shape.

- The pulp chamber of all posteriors is directed mesially.

- Roots of all teeth inclined distally except maxillary and mandibular central incisors which may sometimes are straight or curved mesially.

- Roots of lower third molars and upper third molars show great variations in internal anatomy and morphology of teeth with respect to   number and inclinations of roots.

Mandibular anterior teeth

Central incisors

- Eruption = 6 to 7 years
- Root completion =9 years

- Smallest tooth in the arch
- Average tooth length tooth length 20.8mm
- Average crown length 9mm
- Average root length 12.5mm

Pulp chamber

- The pulp chamber is wide Labiolingually
- Small and flat mesiodistally and tapers –incisally

Cross section

- Coronal one third - slightly ovoid
- Middle one third –round
- Apical one third –round

Roots

Mandibular central incisors have a single root which is broader labiolingually but narrow and flat mesiodistally comprise developmental depression present in mesial and distal root surfaces.

- Straight – 60%
- Distally curved -24%
- Labially curved -15%

Canals

When two canals are present the labial canal was the straighter the point of division for divided canals was in the cervical third of the root.

Vertucci configuration

- Type 1 - 70%
- Type 2 - 5%
- Type 3 - 22%

Occurrence of Lateral canal – 6%

The apical foramen is situated centrally in the root in 25%

Lateral incisors

- Eruption = 7 to 8 years
- Root completion =10 years
- Average tooth length tooth length 22.6mm
- Average crown length 9.5mm
- Average root length 14 mm

Pulp chamber

Similar to central incisor but slightly larger dimensions the pulp chamber is wide Labiolingually.

Small and flat mesiodistally and tapers –incisally

Cross section

- Coronal one third - slightly ovoid
- Middle one third - round
- Apical one third - round

Roots

Mandibular lateral incisors have a single root which is broader labiolingually but narrow and flat mesiodistally comprise developmental depression present in mesial and distal root surfaces.

- Straight - 60%
- Distally curved - 23%
- Labially curved -13%

Canals

When two canals are present the labial canal was the straighter the point of division for divided canals was in the cervical third of the root

Vertucci configuration

- Type 1 - 75%
- Type 2 - 5%
- Type 3 - 18%

Occurrence of Lateral canal –13.3%

The apical foramen is situated centrally in the root in 20%

Mandibular canines

- Eruption = 9 to10 years
- Root completion =12 to 14 years
- Average tooth length tooth length 25.6mm
- Average crown length 11mm
- Average root length 16mm

Cross section

- Coronal one third - ovoid
- Middle one third - ovoid
- Apical one third - round

Roots

Tooth usually has a slight labial axial inclination of the crown. although the tooth usually has a single root. It may have two in 2.3%of cases.

- Straight – 68%
- Distally curved -20%
- Labially curved -7%
- Canals

Vertucci configuration

- Type 1 - 94%
- Type 2 - 14%
- Type 3 - 18%

Occurrence of two canals –6%

Mandibular first premolar

- Eruption = 10 to12 years
- Root completion =12 to 13 years
- Average tooth length tooth length 21.9mm
- Average crown length 8.5mm
- Average root length 14mm

Transitional tooth between anterior and posterior teeth anatomic structures it resembles both types of teeth. The prominent buccal cusp and smaller lingual cusp give the crown of mandibular first premolar about a 30degree lingual tilt.

Roots

Usually has a single short conical root which is broader buccolingually and narrower mesiodistally.

Comprise developmental depression on distal surface which is deeper than mesial surface.

Ovoid or hourglass shape in cross section.

- Are straight - 48%
- Distally curved -35%
- Mesially curved -0%
- Lingually curved -7%
- Buccally curved -2%
- Bayonet 7%

Pulp chamber

No distinct demarcation exists between the pulp chamber and the root canals

Bucco lingually –wider with prominent buccal pulp horn.

Mesiodistally –narrow

Prominent buccal cusp and small lingual cusp

Cross section

- Coronal one third— very narrow and ovoid
- Middle one third –round
- Apical one third –round

Canals

If one canal is present it will be cone shaped and simple in outline. mesiodistally such a root canal narrow, buccolingually it is broad and tapers towards the apical one third.

Wein's configuration

- Type 1 - 73.5%
- Type 2 - 6.5%
- Type 3 - 19.5%

Occurrence of three canals 0.5%

Second premolar

- Eruption = 11 to 12 years
- Root completion =13 to 14 years
- Average tooth length tooth length 22.3mm
- Average crown length 8mm
- Average root length 14.5mm

Roots

Usually has single root which is broader buccolingually and narrower mesiodistally

Comprise developmental depression on distal surface but mesial surface of root is flat or convex, the root is slightly larger than first premolar.

Ovoid in cross section.

- Straight –39%
- Distally curved -40%
- Mesially curved -0%
- Lingually curved -3%

- Buccally curved -10%
- Bayonet 7%
- Trification curves 1%

Pulp chamber

- Bucco lingually –wider with prominent lingual pulp horn
- Mesiodistally - narrow
- Prominent buccal cusp and small lingual cusp

Cross section

- Coronal one third - very narrow and ovoid
- Middle one third - less ovoid
- Apical one third - round

Canals

Wein's configuration

- Type 1- 85%
- Type 2 - 1.5%
- Type 3 - 11.5%

Occurrence of three canals 0.5%

First molar

- Eruption = 6 to7 years
- Root completion =9 to 10 years
- Average tooth length tooth length 21.9mm
- Average crown length 7.5mm
- Average root length 14mm

Roots

Typically, two well differentiated roots are present in the mandibular first molar one mesial and one distal both roots are broad and flat buccolingually which are widely separated mesial and distal roots separated with a furcation level buccally 3mm and lingually 4mm.

Both mesial and distal root surfaces of roots are concave with a depression in the middle of the roots. The concave depression on the distal surface of mesial root is more prone striping compare to convex mesial surface which is thick and away from furcation.

Distal root ovoid in cross section.

Mesial root	Distal root
Straight –16%	74%
Distally curved -84%	21%
Mesially curved -0%	5%
Lingually curved -0%	0%
Buccally curved -0%	0%

Pulp chamber

The roof of the pulp chamber in the mandibular first molar is often rectangular in shape the mesial wall is straight the distal wall is round, the buccal and lingual walls converge to meet the mesillay inclined mesial and distal walls to form a rhomboidal form floor. The roof of the pulp chamber has four pulp horns mesiobuccal, mesiolingual, distobuccal and distolingual. The roof the pulp chamber is located in the cervical one third of the crown and the floor is located in the coronal one third of the root. Three distinct orifice are present in the pulpal floor mesiobuccal, mesilingual and distal. The mesiobuccal orifice is under the mesiobuccal cusp. The mesiobuccal and mesiolingual orifice may be close together under mesiobuccal cusp Distal orifice is oval in shape with widest diameter present buccolingually can be explored by stating from a mesial direction if the orifice is penetrated in marked distobuccal or distolingual direction there are more chances of presence of distolingual or distobuccal canal.

Canals

Wein's configuration

Mesial root	Distal root
Type 1- 0	71.1%
Type 2 - 40.3%	61.5%
Type 3 - 59.5%	38.5%
Occurrence of three canals 0.1%	Occurrence of two canals 28.9%

Second molars

- Eruption = 11 to 13 years

- Root completion =14 to 15 years

- Average tooth length tooth length 21.4mm

- Average crown length 7mm

- Average root length 13.5mm

Roots

Majority of the mandibular second molars have two roots mesial and distal which are close together and more frequently fused together.

Majority of the mandibular second molar has two roots 71% but teeth with one root 27% and teeth with three roots 2%.

Mesial root	Distal root
Straight – 27%	58%
Distally curved - 61%	18%
Mesially curved - 0%	10%
Lingually curved - 0%	0%
Buccally curved - 4%	4%
Bayonet - 7%	6%

Tooth with single root

Straight	-	53%
Distally curved	-	26%
Mesially curved	-	0%
Lingually curved	-	0%
Buccally curved	-	2%
Bayonet	-	19%

Pulp chamber

The pulp chamber is smaller than that of mandibular first molar and root canal orifices are smaller and closer together. all three canals are small.

Canals

Three root canals are usually present the most frequent variation is the presence of two canals.

Wein's configuration

Mesial root	Distal root
Type 1 - 13%	92%
Type 2 - 49%	5%
Type 3 - 38%	3%

Maxillary anterior teeth

Maxillary central incisors

- Eruption = 7 to 8 years
- Root completion =10 years
- Average tooth length tooth length 23.5mm
- Average crown length 10.5mm
- Average root length 13mm

Pulp chamber

- Pulp located in the center of crown equidistant from dentinal walls
- Broad ovoid mesiodistally broadest part located incisally
- Follows contours of crowns and has three pulp horns which corresponds to mamelons

Roots

- Single rooted straight trunk
- Triangular or void in cross section tapers towards lingual
- Single root canal system
- Majority are straight - 75%
- Distally curved - 8%
- Mesially curved - 4%
- Palatally curved - 4%
- Labially curved - 9%
- Lateral canals - 23%
- Apical ramifications- 9%

Single root canal system

Maxillary central incisor usually has one canal there are many case reports of two root canals in maxillary central incisors. The canals follow the direction of curved roots. The canal is large, simple in outline and conical in shape. Canal is centrally located.

Mid root and apical lateral canals are common

Root apex and apical foramina disto-labially

Vertucci configuration

Type1 - 100%

Cross section
- Coronal one third— ovoid
- Middle one third – ovoid to round
- Apical one third –round

Maxillary lateral incisor
- Eruption = 8 to 9 years
- Root completion =11 years
- Average tooth length tooth length 22.5mm
- Average crown length 9mm
- Average root length 13mm

Pulp chamber

Shape is similar to that of maxillary central incisors but smaller in size the division between pulp chamber and root canal is indistinct.

Two pulp horns corresponding to developmental mamelons.

Roots

Single slender root which is wider labiolingually than mesiodistally. Root trunk smaller than central incisor .the root apex is sharper than that of central incisor displaying a common deflection to distal and palatal side (sickle shape apex) Circular or ovoid in cross section tapers towards lingual.
- Distally curved -53%
- Others are straight - 30%
- Lateral canals - 26%
- Apical ramifications - 12%

Single root canal system

Vertucci configuration

Type1 - 100%

Root apex and apical foramen are displaced distolingual

Cross section

Coronal one third - slightly ovoid becomes progressively round

Middle one third - slightly ovoid to round

Apical one third - round

Maxillary canine

- Eruption = 11 to 12 years
- Root completion =13 to 15 years
- Average tooth length tooth length 26mm
- Average crown length 10mm
- Average root length 17mm

Single rooted largest tooth in dentition typically straight and symmetrical labiolingually tapers to sharp apex. Root is wider labiolingually Developmental depression present in mesial and distal surfaces.

- Ovoid in cross section
- Usually single root canal system
- Root apex and apical foramen are displaced distolabially

Pulp chamber

Triangular in shape with apex towards single cusp and broad base in cervical third of crown. mesiodistally.

Narrow resembling a flame. Has only one pulp horn.in cross section the chamber is ovoid in shape with greater diameter labiopalatally.

Cross section

- Coronal one third - slightly ovoid
- Middle one third - canal is smaller and remains ovoid
- Apical one third - round

Roots

- Are straight –39%
- Distally curved -32%
- Mesially curved -0%
- Palatally curved -7%
- Labially curved -13%
- Lateral canals—24%
- Apical ramifications- 8%

Maxillary first premolar

- Eruption = 10 to 11 years
- Root completion =12 to 13 years
- Average tooth length tooth length 21.5mm

- Average crown length 8.5mm
- Average root length 14 mm
- Prominent developmental depression on mesial and distal root surfaces, mesial root concavity more prominent.
- Broader buccolingually and narrow mesiodistally
- Kidney shaped cross section at CEJ

Pulp chamber

- Narrow mesiodistally, wider buccopalatally
- Pulp horn under each cusp ,buccal pulp horn more prominent
- Floor is convex
- Two canal orifice lie deep in coronal third of root below cervical line

Cross section

- Coronal one third - ovoid
- Middle one third - round
- Apical one third *round
- Canal system

Two roots When fused roots ,a groove running in occlusso-apical direction divides the root in to buccal and palatal portions each containing a single root canal.

Maxillary second premolar

- Eruption = 10 to12 years
- Root completion =12 to 14 years
- Average tooth length tooth length 21.6mm
- Average crown length 8.5mm
- Average root length 14 mm
- Single rooted form-most common
- Broader buccolingually and narrow mesiodistally
- Prominent developmental depression on mesial and distal surfaces
- Single canal system –50.3%
- Pulp chamber
- Narrow mesiodistally, wider buccopalatally than maxillary first premolar
- Pulp horn under each cusp buccal pulp horn more prominent

Cross section

- Coronal one third - ovoid
- Middle one third - round
- Apical one third -round

Canal system

- Single root –90.3%
- 2 well developed roots -2%
- 2 roots partially fused -77%
- When two canals are present, they will be distinct and separated along the entire length of root

Maxillary first molar

- Eruption = 6 to 7years
- Root completion =9 to 10 years
- Average tooth length tooth length 21.3mm
- Average crown length 7.5mm
- Average root length 13mm
- Mesio-buccal root
- Broad buccolingually
- Developmental depressions in both distal and mesial root surface
- Distobuccal root
- Round or ovoid in cross section
- Palatal root
- Broad mesiodistally
- Ovoid in cross section
- Buccal curvature at the apical one third

Pulp chamber

- Largest in the arch. four pulp hors mesiobuccal ,mesiopalatl, distobuccal distopalatal.
- Roof-rhomboidal in shape, roof converges palatal wall disappears and farms triangle .anatomic dark lines in the floor connect the orifices, orifices are located in the three point angles of the floor mesobuccal orifice under mesiobuccal cusp tip, distobuccal orifice under distobuccal cusp tip and palatal orifice under palatal cusp tip. May have depression in the palatal end of mesiobuccal orifice where the fourth canal may be present. MB2 canal is located mesial to or directly on a line between the MB and palatal orifice.

Roots

- Mesiobuccal root
- Have distal curvature 78%, straight 21% and bayonet 1%
- Narrowest of three canals. Apical foramen centrally located
- Distobuccal root
- Distal curvature 17%, straight 54% and bayonet 10%
- Apical foramen centrally located
- Palatal root
- Largest root and diameter, ovoid mesiodistally, tapers apically
- Buccal curvature at the apical one third
- Locating MB2
- Locating MB2 difficult as it is buried under dentine bridge formed as result of aging.
- Reparative dentin formation as a result of caries and trauma.
- Canal located mesial to or directly on a line between the MB1 and palatal orifice, within 3.5mm palatally and 2mm mesially of MB1 orifice

Maxillary second molar

- Eruption = 12 to 13 years
- Root completion =14 to 16 years
- Average tooth length tooth length 17.1mm
- Average crown length 7mm
- Average root length 12mm

Similar to maxillary first molar

- Roots have a distal inclination
- Normally has three roots
- Roots tend to close together, higher tendency toward fusion of two or three roots

Pulp chamber

Similar to maxillary first molar except narrower mesiodistally

Roof - rhomboidal

Floor obtuse triangle

Mesiobuccal and distobuccal canals closer together

Canal system

- Mesiobuccal root
- Broad buccolingually
- Prominent depression in mesial and distal surface
- One or two canals
- Distobuccal root
- Rounded or ovoid single
- Orifice appears on same line joining mesiobuccal and palatal canals
- Palatal root
- Broad mesodistally
- Ovoid single

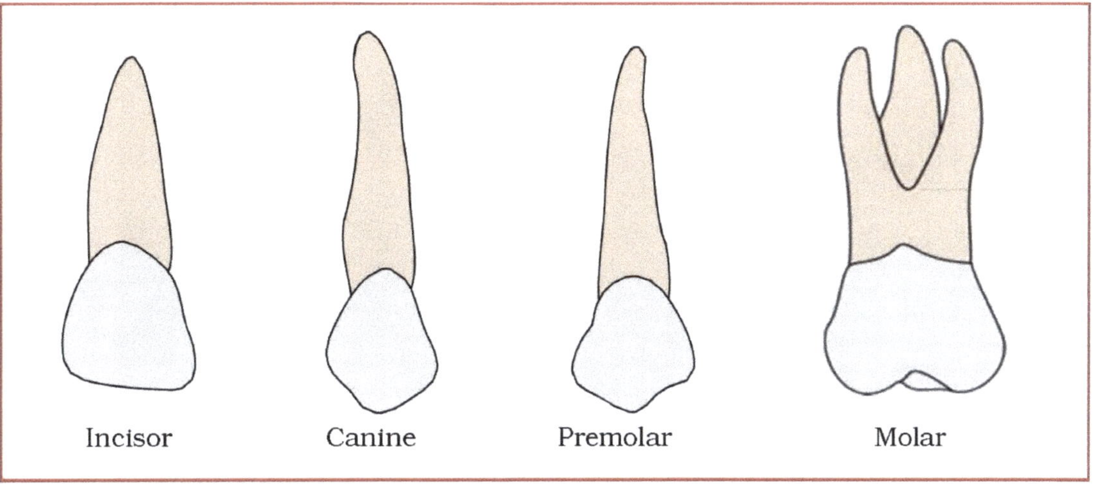

Fig 7.6: Root's curature

Note

Distal roots of mandibular first molar, occasionally have two canals *i.e.* distolingual, distobuccal.

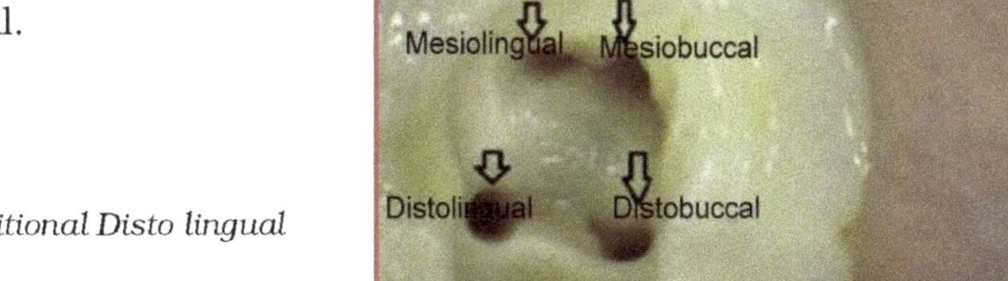

Fig. 7.7. Additional Disto lingual

Mesiobuccal root of maxillary first molar may have two canals: MB2 which is located 2 to 3 mm palatal to MB1.

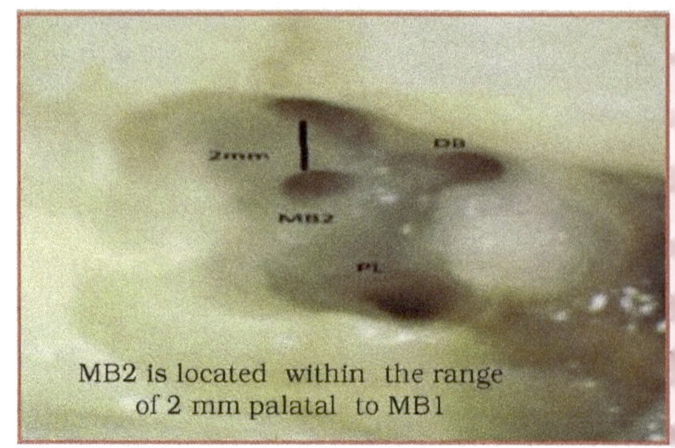

Fig 7.8: Additional Mesiobuccal canal

Cavity of mandibular lateral incisors and premolar may be bifurcated to present two canals.

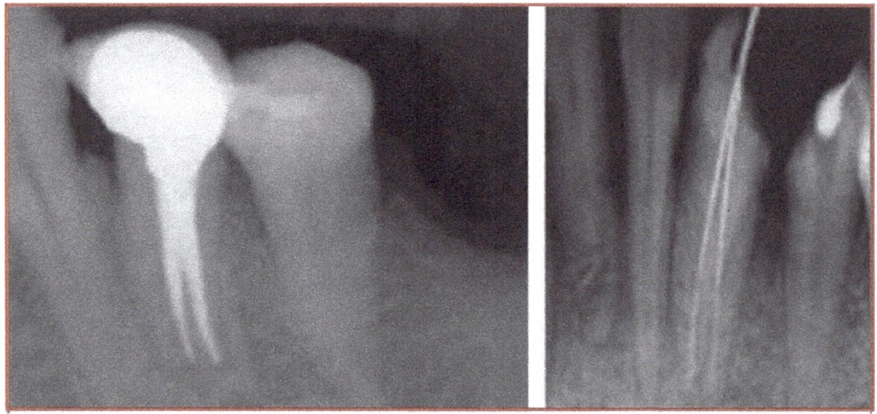

Fig. 7.9 : Lower lateral incisier with additional Lingul canal

Isthmus and C shaped canals are common with mandibular second molars and rarely with mandibular premolars.

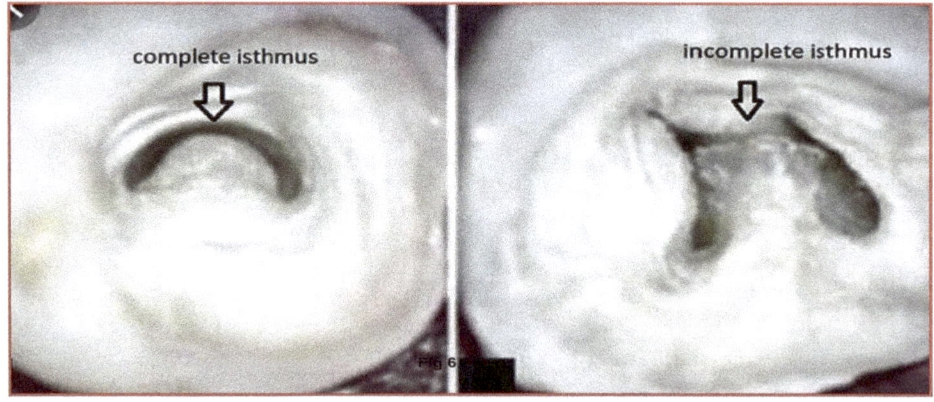

Fig 7.10 : Isthmus

Maxillary second molar surprises sometimes with 2 canals or with 4 canals rarely with one canal.

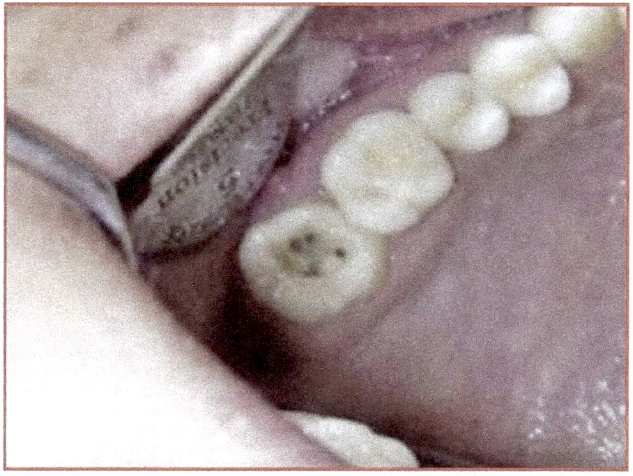

Fig. 7.11 : Upper IInd molar with additional palatal canal

RADIX ENTOMOLARIS TOOTH

Commonly mandibular first molars have two roots rarely mandibular first molar has mid mesial root which is present between mesial root and distal root. The tooth with this extra root is known as radix entomolaris.

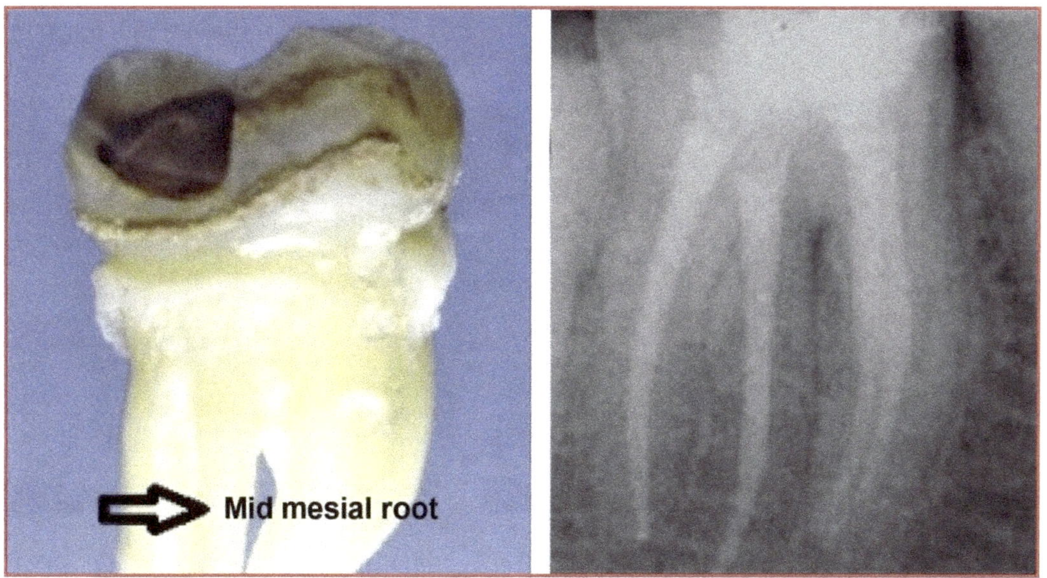

Fig 7.12.: Radix entomolaris root

RADIX ENTOMOLARIS CANAL

Rarely midmesial canal is present in the groove between mesiobuccal canal and mesiolingual canal this extra midmesial canal is called radix entomoloris canal.

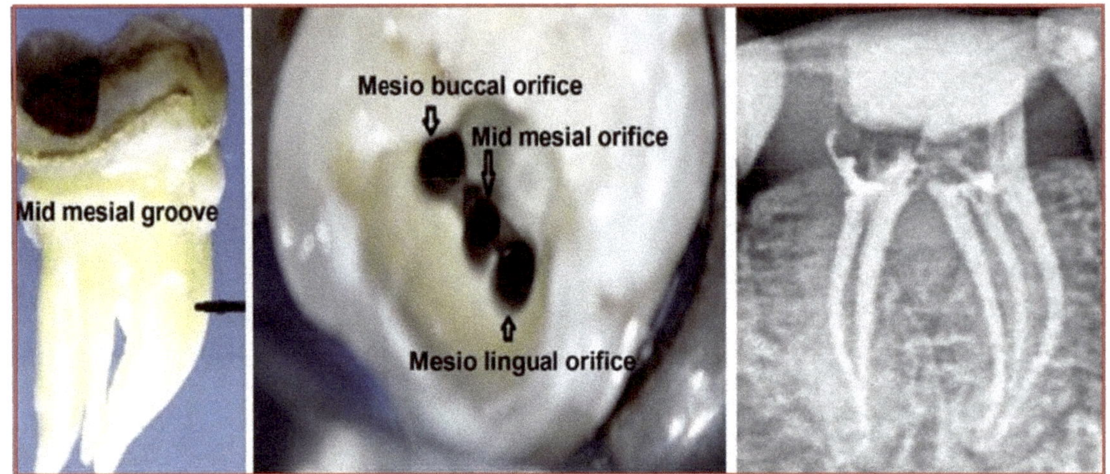

Fig 7.13.: Radix entomolaris canal

8

Internal Anatomy of Tooth

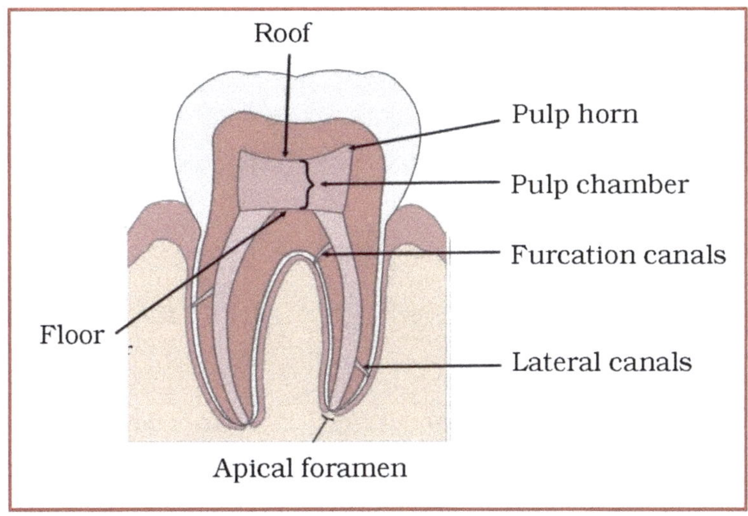

Fig. 8.1: Anatomy of the pulp chamber

Internal anatomy of tooth is a complex system of finely tuned small tributaries running through the entire length and breadth of tooth. Since during root canal treatment we cannot see much inside the area we work, meticulous understanding and knowledge of various complexities of the spaces we are expected to clean and fill is crucial to perform a successful endodontic treatment.

Problems encountered during the treatment occur because of inadequate understanding of the pulp space anatomy knowledge of internal anatomy help us to provide exact working length and width of canal which guide us to effective debridement, disinfection and three dimensional obturation.

Pulp cavity

- Core cavity within the tooth entirely enclosed by dentin contains pulp. Extends from tip of pulp horns to the Cemento-dentinal junction.

- It is divided into two portions-coronal and radicular pulp. Coronal portion is called pulp chamber.

- Radicular portion is called root canals.

PULP CHAMBER

In anterior teeth pulp chamber gradually merges in the root canal with no clear distinction between pulp chamber and root canal, where as in multi rooted teeth there is clear distinction between pulp chamber and root canals.

Roof

Coronal or incisal wall of pulp chamber covered by dentin parallel to the occlusal surface of the tooth. An average distance between the occlusal surface of the tooth and roof of the pulp chamber is 6 mm.

Pulp horns

Extension of pulp directly under cusps or developmental lobes. More prominent and highly placed in young tooth. Recedes and becomes less prominent with advancing age.

Floor

Apical wall of pulp chamber runs parallel to roof. Always darker than the walls.

Canal orifice

Small opening in the floor leading or guiding into the root canals.

Root canal

Extends from orifice to the apical foramina. May be single, straight or curved. Runs in Bucco-lingual direction.

Apical foramina

The most apical wider portion of canal which opens on the root surface to communicate with the apical periodontium.

It's a cemental portion of canal, funnel shaped. Wider portion of the funnel contains periodontal tissue with the base of funnel faces toward PDL and apex of funnel faces at CDJ giving it callalily flower like appearance. The anatomy changes with age.

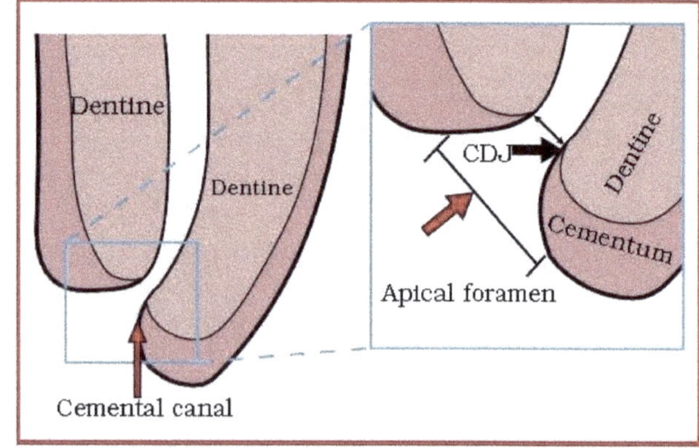

Fig. 8.2:

ISTHMUS

Narrow wedge-shaped communication between two root canals. Contains pulp tissue.

It is a danger zone. Harbours micro-organisms. Should be cleaned with ultrasonic files and obturated. Commonly seen in Molars. It presents between two canals with in the same root as ribbon shaped intracanal connection or corridor or transverse anastomosis. Whenever two or more root canals are present an isthmus should be suspected and all attempts should be made in detecting and debriding it.

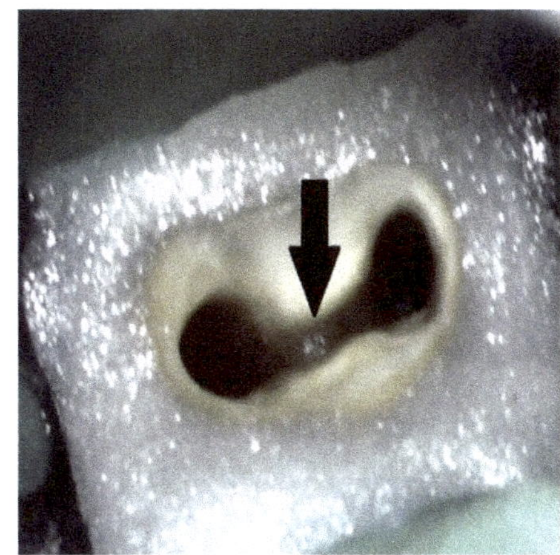

Fig. 8.3:

Classification of isthmuses

Type 1

It is an incomplete isthmus characterized by no notable communication or faint communication between the two or three canals.

Type 2

It is a complete isthmus characterized by a definite connection between the two main canals.

Type 3

Very short complete isthmus between two or three canals.

Type 4

When canals extend in to isthmus area.

Type 5

The true connection or corridor throughout the section

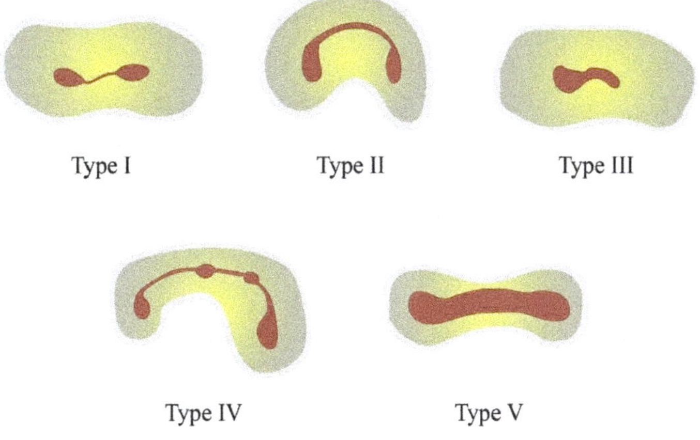

Fig. 8.4:

Furcal canals

- Seen in trifurcation and bifurcation of multirooted tooth. Extends from floor to furcation area
- Harbours micro-organisms.
- Should be cleaned and obturated.
- Commonly seen in first molars

'C' Shaped canals

- Common cause of failure of root canal treatment in posterior teeth is the occurrence of C shaped canals and its improper negotiation.
- There are two patterns of c shaped canals.
- A single ribbon like C -shaped canal from orifice to apex –less common.
- Three distinct canals below the C shaped orifice - more common.
- C shaped canals prevents effective cleaning, shaping and obturation during a root canal treatment.

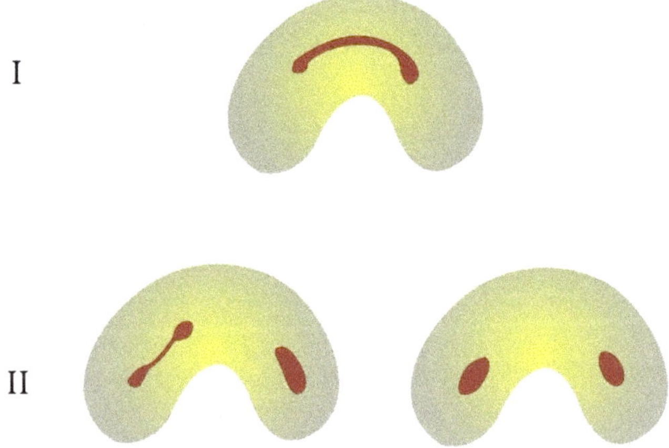

Fig. 8.5:

Lateral canals

lateral canals are accessory canals and integral part of normal pulp cavity rather than an anomaly or an exception branches off at right angles to the main canals.

A lateral canal can be found anywhere along the length of the root but commonly seen in the body of canals (cervical and middle third).In posterior teeth molars. the presence of lateral canals in the furcation areas of molars teeth is well documented and their incidence is high.

Seen in mandibular premolars and maxillary central incisors. Size of lateral canals ranges from 1mm to size of blood vessels.

Accessory canals

Accessory canals are formed by the entrapment of periodontal vessels in hertwigs epithelial root sheath during calcification hence considered as integral part of normal pulp cavity rather than an anomaly or an exception.

Accessory canals contains connective tissue and blood vessels do not supply the pulp with collateral circulation.

Branches off from the main canals in the apical one third of canal commonly seen in mandibular premolars and maxillary central incisors.

Size of accessory canals ranges from 1mm to size of blood vessels and the mean diameter of accessory foramina 6 to 60nm.

Frequently Large number of accessory canals are fan out towards the apex of the tooth in a canoe shaped arrangement or y shaped arrangement to form **apical deltas** commonly found in distal roots of lower molars and palatal roots of upper molars.

Apical deltas describe the primary or secondary canal that terminates short of the apex with lateral canals fanning out from this point to the end of root surface.

Following endodontic treatment, the necrotic pulp tissue in the uninstrumented branches may become source of reinfection and cause for failure of root canal treatment.

These ramifications and accessory canals were increasingly eliminated by.

1mm root end resection -52%

2mm root end resection -78%

3mm root end resection -98 %

Apical 1/3 of root

A detailed knowledge of the apical 1/3 root anatomy is vital as it is common area for procedural errors during instrumentation inadequate knowledge and mismanagement of apical one third may affect long term and short term prognosis of endodontic treatment.

Apical 1/3 of root exhibits great variations in internal anatomy, presence of fins, deltas, accessory canals, multiple foraminas, resorptions and dentinal aberrations makes the shaping and cleaning of canals difficult.

Apical 1/3 exhibits great variations in morphology occurrence of different canal curvatures, different location of apical constriction, shape, size and position of apical foramina makes the obturation difficult.

Hence it is morphologically complex, therapeutically challenging, radiographically most obscure and prognostically most important region.

Note

Generally apical 3 mm of root is resected during apicectomy in order to eliminate canal aberrations.

Vertucci Types of canals

Type 1	:	Single canal extends from the pulp chamber, to meet at the apex.
Type 2, 2-1	:	Two separate canals extend from the pulp chamber, join short of the apex forming a single canal.
Type 3, 1-2-1	:	Single canal leaves the pulp chamber divides into two canals then joins to form a single canal.
Type 4, 2-2	:	Two separate canals leaving the pulp chamber joining two separate foramens.
Type 5, 1-2	:	One single canal divides into two separate canals.
Type 6, 2-1-2	:	Two separate canals leave the pulp chamber, merge in the body of the root and redivide short of the apex to exit as two distinct canals.
Type 7, 1-2-1-2	:	One canal leaves the pulp chamber, divides and then rejoins in the body of the root, and finally redivides into two distinct canals short of the apex.
Type 8, 3-3	:	Three separate distinct canals extends from the pulp chamber to the apex.

Type 1 1-1	Type 2 2-1	Type 3 1-2-1	Type 4 2-2	Type 5 1-2	Type6 2-1-2	Type 7 1-2-1-2	Type8 3-3

Fig. 8.6 : Types of canals

Wein's classification

Type 1

Single canal with single orifice and single apical foramen.

Type 2

A canal with a single orifice that divided into two canals and exist with a single foramen.

Type 3

Two canals with two orifice and two separate single foramina.

Type 4

Single canal with two orifices and two separate apical foramens.

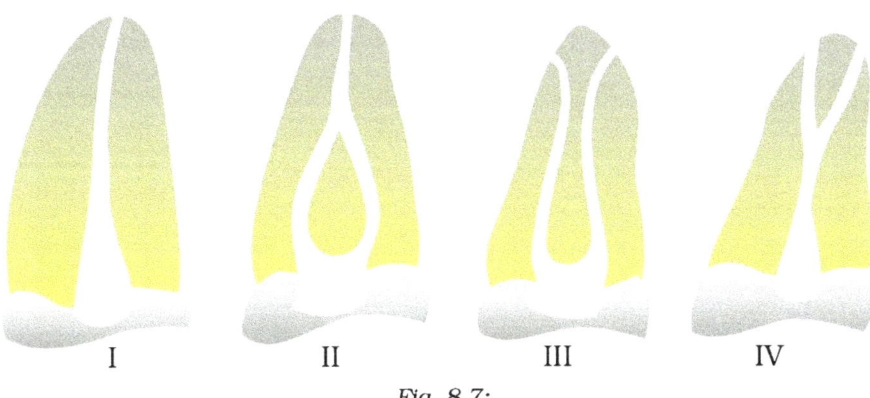

Fig. 8.7:

Apical foramina

From apical constriction the canal widens as it approaches the apical foramina The location and shape of apical foramina may undergo changes as a result of functional influence on tooth, mesial drift and occlusal pressure. the principal apical foramina might be in the center of the root. Originally the foramina gradually shifts with aging due to continuous cementum deposition. It is frequently eccentrically located away from the anatomic or radiographic apex . The shape of the space between minor and major diameter has been described as, hyperbolic or morning glory. The location of apical foramen is not necessarily always at the center of root apex, located laterally away from the anatomic apex average distance is 0.4 to 0.7mm.

Types of root canals

Type 1 : Curved root canals with apical foramen distant from apex

Type 2: Curved root canals with apical foramen near the apex

Type 3: Straight constricted canals with apical foramen at the apex

Type4 : Double curvature of root canals with the foramen at a distance from apex

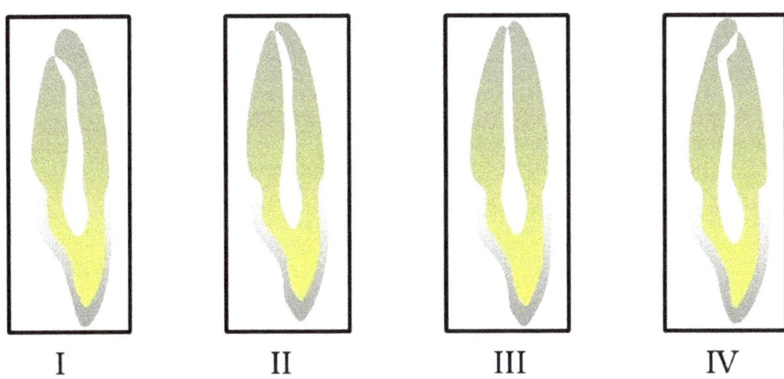

Fig. 8.8:

Mandibular anterior teeth

Central incisors
Pulp chamber

- The pulp chamber is wide Labiolingually
- Small and flat mesiodistally and tapers – incisally

Cross section

- Coronal one third - slightly ovoid
- Middle one third - round
- Apical one third - round

Canals

When two canals are present the labial canal was the straighter the point of division for divided canals was in the cervical third of the root.

Vertucici configuration

Type 1 – 70%

Type2 – 5%

Type 3 – 22%

Occurrence of Lateral canal – 6%

The apical foramen is situated centrally in the root in 25%

Lateral incisors

Pulp chamber

- Similar to central incisor but slightly larger dimensions the pulp chamber is wide Labiolingually.
- Small and flat mesiodistally and tapers – incisally

Cross section

- Coronal one third – slightly ovoid
- Middle one third – round
- Apical one third – round

Canals

When two canals are present the labial canal was the straighter the point of division for divided canals was in the cervical third of the root.

Vertucici configuration

Type 1 – 75%

Type2 – 5%
Type 3 – 18%
Occurrence of Lateral canal – 13.3%
The apical foramen is situated centrally in the root in 20%

Mandibular canines

Cross section
- Coronal one third – ovoid
- Middle one third – ovoid
- Apical one third – round

Vertucici configuration
- Type 1 – 94%
- Type 2 – 14%
- Type 3 –18%
- Occurrence of two canals – 6%

Mandibular first premolar

Pulp chamber
No distinct demarcation exists between the pulp chamber and the root canals
Bucco lingually –wider with prominent buccal pulp horn.
Mesiodistally –narrow.
Prominent buccal cusp and small lingual cusp.

Cross section
- Coronal one third— very narrow and ovoid
- Middle one third –round
- Apical one third –round

Canals

If one canal is present it will be cone shaped and simple in outline. mesiodistally such a root canal narrow, buccolingually it is broad and tapers towards the apical one third.

Wein's configuration
- Type 1 – 73.5%
- Type 2 – 6.5%
-    Type 3 – 19.5%
- Occurrence of three canals 0.5%

Second premolar

Pulp chamber

- Bucco lingually –wider with prominent lingual pulp horn
- Mesiodistally –narrow
- Prominent buccal cusp and small lingual cusp

Cross section

- Coronal one third - very narrow and ovoid
- Middle one third – less ovoid
- Apical one third –round

Canals

Wein's configuration

- Type 1 – 85%
- Type 2 – 1.5%
- Type 3 – 11.5%
- Occurrence of three canals 0.5%

First molar

Pulp chamber

The roof of the pulp chamber in the mandibular first molar is often rectangular in shape the mesial wall is straight the distal wall is round, the buccal and lingual walls converge to meet the mesillay inclined mesial and distal walls to form a rhomboidal form floor. The roof of the pulp chamber has four pulp horns mesiobuccal, mesiolingual, distobuccal and distolingual. The roof the pulp chamber is located in the cervical one third of the crown and the floor is located in the coronal one third of the root. Three distinct orifice are present in the pulpal floor mesiobuccal, mesilingual and distal. The mesiobuccal orifice is under the mesiobuccal cusp. The mesiobuccal and mesiolingual orifice may be close together under mesiobuccal cusp.

Distal orifice is oval in shape with widest diameter present buccolingually, can be explored by starting from a mesial direction if the orifice is penetrated in marked distobuccal or distolingual direction, there are more chances of presence of distolingual or distobuccal canal.

Canals

Wein's configuration

Mesial root	Distal root
Type 1 – 0	71.1%
Type 2 – 40.3%	61.5%
Type 3 – 59.5%	38.5%
Occurrence of three canals 0.1%	Occurrence of two canals 28.9%

Second molars
Pulp chamber
The pulp chamber is smaller than that of mandibular first molar and root canal orifices are smaller and closer together. All three canals are small.

Canals
Three root canals are usually present the most frequent variation is the presence of two canals.

Wein's configuration

Mesial root	Distal root
Type 1 – 13%	92%
Type 2 – 49%	5%
Type 3 – 38%	3%

Third molar
Pulp chamber

The pulp chamber of the mandibular third molar anatomically resembles the pulp chamber of mandibular first and second molars. It is large and possesses many anomalous configurations such as C shaped canal orifice.

Canals
Number of canals ranged from

1to 3 in teeth with one root

2 to 6 in teeth with two roots

3 to 5 in teeth with three roots

4 to 5 in teeth with four roots

The anatomy of a mandibular third molar can not be predicted on the basis of number of roots.

Maxillary anterior teeth
Maxillary central incisors

Pulp chamber

- Pulp located in the center of crown equidistant from dentinal walls.

- Broad ovoid mesiodistally broadest part located incisally.

- Follows contours of crowns and has three pulp horns which corresponds to mamelons.

Single root canal system

Maxillary central incisor usually has one canal. There are many case reports of two root canals in maxillary central incisors. The canals follow the direction of curved roots. The canal is large, simple in outline and conical in shape. Canal is centrally located.

Mid root and apical lateral canals are common.

Root apex and apical foramina disto-labially.

Vertucci configuration

Type 1 - 100%

Cross section

- Coronal one third - ovoid
- Middle one third - ovoid to round
- Apical one third - round

Maxillary lateral incisor

Pulp chamber

- Shape is similar to that of maxillary central incisors but smaller in size the division between pulp chamber and root canal is indistinct.
- Two pulp horns corresponding to developmental mamelons.

Single root canal system

Vertucci configuration

- Type 1 - 100%
- Root apex and apical foramen are displaced distolingual.

Cross section

- Coronal one third - slightly ovoid becomes progressively round.
- Middle one third - slightly ovoid to round.
- Apical one third - round.

Maxillary canine

Pulp chamber

- Triangular in shape with apex towards single cusp and broad base in cervical third of crown, mesiodistally.
- Narrow resembling a flame. Has only one pulp horn. In cross section the chamber is ovoid in shape with greater diameter labiopalatally.

Canal system

Usually single root canal system wider labiopalatal than mesiodistal in the middle it tapers gradually to an apical constriction.

Vertucci configuration

- Type 1 - 100%
- Root apex and apical foramen are displaced distolabially.
- The apical foramina centrally located in the anatomic apex in 14% cases. The mean distance of apical foramina from the root apex ranges from 0.30mm to 0.62mm.

Cross section

- Coronal one third - slightly ovoid
- Middle one third - canal is smaller and remains ovoid
- Apical one third - round

Maxillary first premolar

Pulp chamber

- Narrow mesiodistally, wider Bucco palatal.
- Pulp horn under each cusp, buccal pulp horn more prominent. The roof of the pulp chamber coronal to the cervical line.
- The floor of the pulp chamber is convex usually with two canal orifices one buccal and the other palatal and it lies deep in the coronal third of the root below the cervical line.
- Two canal orifices lie deep in coronal third of root below cervical line.

Root canal system

In a tooth with a single canal through the length of the root, the canal is ovoid in shape, wider buccolingually than mesiodistally in the cervical and middle third and round in apical one third when two canals are present the palatal canal is generally the larger of the two canals, it is directly under palatal cusp and its orifice can be penetrated by following the palatal wall of the pulp chamber. The buccal canal is directly under the buccal cusp and its orifice can be penetrated by following the buccal wall of the pulp camber. The cervical thirds are ovoid in shape at mid-root they are almost round and in the apical third they are round and small.

Wein's configuration

Type 1 - 9%

Type 2 - 13%

Type 3 - 72%

Three canals three foramina's - 6%.

Transverse channels between the canals are common.

Cross section

- Coronal one third - ovoid
- Middle one third - round
- Apical one third - round

Maxillary second premolar

Pulp chamber

Narrow mesiodistally, wider Bucco-palatally than maxillary first premolar.

Pulp horn under each cusp buccal pulp horn more prominent. The roof of pulp chamber coronal to cervical line. The pulpal floor is deeper if two canals are present. If one canal is present the root canal orifice will be indistinct but if two canals are present two distinct orifice will be visible .in cross section the pulp chamber has a narrow ovoid shape.

Canal system

- Single root single canal – 90.3%
- 2 well developed roots two separate canals -2%
- 2 roots partially fused -77%
- When two canals are present, they will be distinct and separated along the entire length of root.

Wein's configuration

- Type 1 - 75%
- Type 3 - 24%
- Three canals three foramina's - 1%
- Apical foramina centrally located in 12% of cases
- Laterally located 78% of cases

Cross section

Coronal one third - ovoid and narrow.

Middle one third – When one canal is present it is ovoid and when two canals are present, they are round.

Apical one third – canal is round regardless of whether one or two canals are present.

Maxillary first molar
Pulp chamber

Largest in the arch. Four pulp horns mesiobuccal, mesiopalatl, distobuccal, distopalatal.

Roof-rhomboidal in shape, roof converges palatal wall disappears and farms triangle. Anatomic dark lines in the floor connect the orifices, orifices are located in the three point angles of the floor mesobuccal orifice under mesiobuccal cusp tip, distobuccal orifice under distobuccal cusp tip and palatal orifice under palatal cusp tip.

Palatal orifice

It is the largest, round or oval in shape and easily accessible for exploration.

Distobuccal orifice

Is located slightly distal and palatal to the mesiobuccal orifice is accessible from the mesial for exploration.

Mesiobuccal orifice

Mesiobuccal orifice is located under mesiobuccal cusp point angle created by the buccal wall, mesial wall and subpulpal floor.

Long buccopalatlly may have depression in the palatal end of mesiobuccal orifice where the fourth canal may be present.MB2 canal is located mesial to or directly on a line between the MB and palatal orifice.

Root canals

Mesiobuccal canal have distal curvature 78%, straight 21% and bayonet 1%.

Narrowest of three canals. Apical foramen centrally located.

Locating MB2.

Locating MB2 difficult as it is buried under dentine bridge formed as result of aging and Reparative dentin formation as a result of caries and trauma.

Canal located mesial to or directly on a line between the MB1 and palatal orifice, within 3.5mm palatally and 2mm mesially of MB1 orifice.

Distobuccal canal is narrow tapering canal generally cone shaped ending in a small, round canal in apical one third. Distal curvature 17%, straight 54% and bayonet 10%.

Apical foramen centrally located in 19% of cases and canal exist to lateral surface 81% of the times.

Palatal canal is largest of three canals, it is ovoid mesiodistally, tapers apically where it becomes a small round canal with buccal curvature at the apical one third. Apical foramina located centrally in 18% of cases. The canal exists to a lateral surface 88.5% of the cases.

Wein's configuration

Mesiobuccal root

Type 1 - 41.1%

Type 2 - 40%

Type 3 - 18.9%

Maxillary second molar

Pulp chamber

Similar to maxillary first molar except narrower mesiodistally.

Roof of the pulp chamber is more rhomboidal.

Floor of the pulp chamber is an obtuse triangle.

And the mesiobuccal and distobuccal canals closer together and may appear to have a common opening but they are readily distinguishable from each other.

Some times all three canal orifices may be in a straight line occasionally canal curve into the chamber at a more horizontal angle, making it necessary to remove a lip of dentin so that the canal can be entered more in a direct line with the canal axis.

Canal system

- Mesiobuccal root
- Broad buccolingually
- Prominent depression in mesial and distal surface
- One or two canals
- Distobuccal root
- Rounded or ovoid single
- Orifice appears on same line joining mesiobuccal and palatal canals
- Palatal root
- Broad mesodistally
- Ovoid single

Wein's configuration
Mesiobuccal root
Type 1 - 63%

Type 2 - 13%

Type 3 - 24%

Maxillary third molar
Pulp chamber
The pulp chamber of maxillary third molar similar to that of second molar with three canal orifices but it may also have an odd shaped chamber with four or five root canal orifice or a conical chamber with only one root canal.

Root and root canals
The maxillary third molar has three well developed roots that are closely grouped. It may also have fused roots, one conical root or four or more independent roots. The roots may be straight, curved or dilacerated and they may be fully or partially developed.

Maxillary third molars with root presented an extremely unpredictable internal anatomy ranging from one to six canals.

Variations in internal anatomy of tooth
a)   Variations due to congenital defects

    Germinations

    Fusions

    Dense evaginatus

    Dense invaginatus

    Dilacerations

    Dentogenesis imperfecta

    Concrescence

    Talon cusp

    Taurodontism

    Lingual groove

b)   Variations in shape of pulp cavity due to developmental defects

    Gradual curves

    Apical curves

    C shaped

    Sickle shape

    Bayonet shape

c) Variations due to aging
   Pulp calcifications
   Pulp stones

d) Variations due to pathology
   Internal resorption
   External resorption

e) Variations in size of tooth
   Microdontia
   Macrodontia

f) Variations in apical 1/3 of root
   Different locations of apex
   Status of apex (open or closed apex)

AGE CHANGES

Size of pulp decreases with age

Shape of the access cavity is not constant it changes with the age of the patient. During cavity preparation, the intensity of feeling the drop decreases due to decrease in pulpal height and there is less demarcation between pulpal roof and pulpal floor.

Width of the canals decreases with the age

The initial file size decreases with advance in age

a) Young age   —   15 k
b) Middle age   —   10 k
c) Old age   —   8 k and 6 k

Size of the apical foramen and apical constriction becomes smaller with the age

Chances of apical blockage, ledge formation and file separation are more with advance in age

The number of lateral canals, accessory canals, multiple foramens decreases with age

Long term prognosis is good with advancing age. It is all due to continuous deposition of secondary/tertiary/reparative dentin.

Frequency of diffuse pulp calcification and pulp stones are more with advancing age.

Due to calcification and fibrosis dentinal map is less evident and location of orifice becomes difficult.

Due to continued deposition of cementum with advancing age the Cemento dentinal junction moves more coronally from the radiographic apex.

Due to gingival recession, there is exposure of dentin and cementum and thus older patients are more prone to root caries. Negotiation of canals in root caries is difficult.

Intra pulpal anaesthesia is difficult as the volume of pulp chamber is reduced with advancing age.

Intra ligamentary injections are difficult as the width of periodontal ligament.

is reduced with advancing age.

Due to increased bone density infiltration is slow and ineffective with advancing.

Note :

The shape of the access opening is determined by the shape and size of pulp chamber.

In anterior teeth and premolars: In children it is triangular in shape, in young adults it is round/ovoid in shape, in old patients it is round.

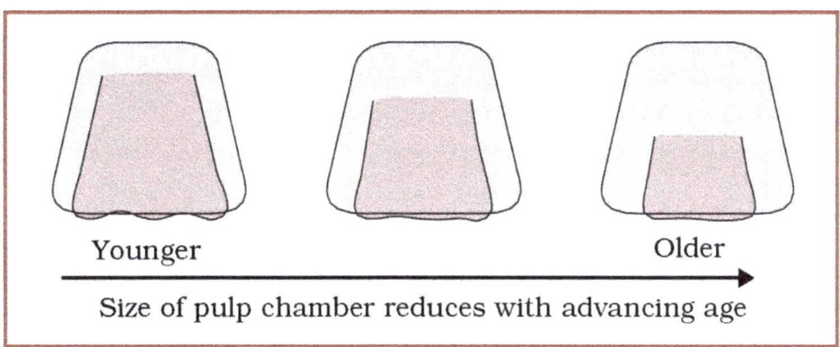

Fig. 8.9: Age changes of pulp chamber

9

Root Canal Treatment

A) ACCESS OPENING

ACCESS DETERMINES ENDODONTIC ACTIVITY. WHERE THERE IS ENDODONTIC ACTIVITY THERE IS DECOMPRESSION, DRAINAGE AND ALLEVIATION.

IT IS THE ACCESS WHICH DESIGNS AND SHAPES THE ENDODONTIC SUCCESS.

IT IS THE ACCESS WHICH SAVES AND MAINTAINS THE TOOTH. NO ACCESS – NO ENDO – NO TOOTH.

Introduction

The main goal of performing root canal treatment is to remove all infection from root canal system that has been infected and obliterate the empty root canal system space with three-dimensional stable filling material to prevent further infection in order to accomplish this entrance to the canal system is essential, gaining entrance to the canal system is called access cavity preparation. Access cavity preparation is a preliminary step that opens the door to augment cleaning, debridement, shaping, irrigation, obturation and post endodontic restoration. The effectiveness of these steps relies on optimal access cavity preparation design, any error in this step would compromise subsequent steps hence access preparation is referred as 'Access to success', must be performed with attention, patience and right attitude.

Definition

Creating a designed opening in coronal portion of crown derived by internal anatomy of the tooth to gain entrance to the root canal system for the purpose of performing root canal treatment.

Types of access cavity designs or Different approaches

As access opening is the most crucial step and influences the long-term prognosis of endodontically treated tooth. It requires strategy, patience and attention to conserve as much as crucial dentin possible by meeting the needs of modern instrumentation techniques and filling materials. There should be fine balance between operator needs, instrumentation needs, restoration needs and tooth demands.

1) Traditional or Conventional approach
2) Conservative approach
   a. Contracted access cavity - Clark and Khademi
   b. Truss cavity - Auswin and Ramesh
   c. Ninja access cavity - Belogard M
   d. Guided access cavity - Zehnder and Connert

Clinician should consider the following factors before selecting the type of access opening design

Age of the patient

The size of pulp decreases with age, in old patient pulp chamber is smaller and canals are narrower the access cavity design will be smaller and conservative, where as in young patient pulp chamber is larger and canals are wider though getting in to chamber and canals are easier may require larger design.

Status of pulp

Tooth with diffused calcified pulp chamber and large pulp stones may require complete deroofing.

Severity of pulpal and periapical infection.

Vital inflamed tooth may require less extensive preparation while Non vital tooth with purulent discharging canals may requires complete deroofing and larger access cavity design. Example draining acute and chronic periapical abscess.

Anatomy of tooth in question

The access cavity must not assume a predetermined design rather anatomy of pulpal floor, position of orifice, internal canal anatomy and occurrence of additional root or canals should dictate the design. Tooth with simple anatomy may require smaller conservative designs while tooth complex internal anatomy may require larger extensive design.

Developmental anomalies tooth

Developmental anomalies of tooth like fusion, gemination, taurodontism, bifurcation and trifurcation of canals at mid root with occurrence of additional root or canals level may require larger extensive preparation

Strategic position of tooth in the arch

Molars are close to temporomandibular joint thus to the hinge axis hence experience higher force and canines positioned in strategic areas of dental arches demands less removal of healthy tooth structure and more preservation of strategic dentin to withstand occlusal stress in order to prevent vertical root fracture which is the second most cause of failure of endodontically treated tooth.

Type of occlusion

Deep bite and decreased overjet cases demands less removal of healthy tooth structure and more preservation of strategic dentin to withstand occlusal stress.

Re-root canal treated tooth

Re-root canal treated tooth may require straight line access and extensive conventional design to scout missed canals, retrieve gutta percha, retrieve separated instruments and remove remnants of old filling materials.

Type of instrumentation technique and frequency of usage of rotary files

Recent technological advances in flexible rotary instrumentation systems and modern filling materials criticizes more destructive traditional access cavity designs. Heat treated high flex files automatically glide into the more curved portion of canals and gain straight line access, strategic more conservative cavity designs can be selected with single usage of these high flex files.

Availability of technological advances

The use of magnifying aids has provided endodontics with a significant improvement in vision of the operating filed, enhancing visualization and simplifies work. Operating microscopes, loupes, endoscopes enhance magnification and illumination of interest area and allows to perform very precise cavity's with minimal errors associated with any possibility's drilling bur reaching the canal orifices and also offers the possibility of visualizing before execution, the exact area where chamber opening should be performed. If magnification is not employed in the farm of loupes or microscopes perform blindly. The size of access becomes wider as it progresses deeper in to the tooth worsens when advance leading unnecessary removal of healthier tooth structure. phenomenon is called inverse funneling.

1) Employing illumination and magnification

   Employing magnification in the form of operating microscopes and loupes conservative and ultraconservative designs can be chosen.

2) Employing CBCT

   Employing advanced CBCT technology (small FOV's) more conservative and ultra conservative designs can be chosen.

Type of materials used for post-endodontic restoration

Use of flowable composites and thixotropic filling materials require larger conventional designs while use of modern filling materials like bio ceramic cements may require conservative preparations.

Type of obturation techniques

Cold and warm gutta percha condensation may require larger cavity preparation to accommodate placement of spreaders and pluggers while thermo plasticized condensation may require conservative cavity design and latest thermo hydraulic condensation may require ultraconservative design.

Shaping taper and working width

Smaller apical size preparation with 2% and 4% tapered single use high flex heat treated file may require conservative and ultraconservative cavity preparation while larger apical size preparation with 6% and 8% tapered may need larger access cavity design.

Experience and Good judgement

More modern designs require experience, proper judgement and excellent command over the anatomy of tooth being treated and its variations.

Complete deroofing approach or Conventional or Traditional approach

Conventional approach is an operator centric which primarily focuses on radicular aspect of cavity preparation while neglecting coronal aspect that is endo restorative-endo prosthetic aspect. This approach involves complete deroofing and direct straight-line axis to the apical foramina thus wider preparation and more removal of tooth structure.

Principle

Although technological advances have allowed better outcomes and made treatment more predictable endodontic success is not based exclusively on new techniques and devices it is grounded in the knowledge and application of basic biological and mechanical principles.

In traditional endodontic access cavity preparation, the tooth structure is removed in a controlled manner and access preparation extended adequately to prevent endodontic complications, it follows the principle of extension for prevention. Extension for prevention leads to complete deroofing of pulp chamber roof and facilitates the direct straight-line access to apical foramina thereby permit the complete direct vision of the pulpal floor and canal orifices without having to move the mouth mirror and allow the effective biomechanical removal of all the chamber contents and canal contents.

Objectives

- To remove all caries and existing faulty restoration.
- To penetrate through the occlusal surface of crowns.
- To discover the pulp chamber
- To completely unroof the dentin covers the pulp chamber
- To remove all the pulp horns
- To remove biomechanically all the infected tissue contents of pulp chamber vital or necrotic or both
- To find pulpal floor in order to uncover and locate all canals
- To disinfect the remaining tooth structure
- To obtain straight line access to the apical foramina
- To obtain uniform contact of the file with the access cavity walls
- To facilitate obturation and complete sealing of orifice of canals
- To establish restorative margins to minimize marginal leakage of restored tooth

Shape and Initial out line form

Traditional approach is an operator centric primarily focuses on the operator needs has a predetermined shape according to the type of tooth.

Tooth	Maxilla	Mandible
• Central incisors	Triangular	Ovoid or Elliptical
• Lateral incisors	Roughly ovoid	Oval
• Canine	Oval	Oval
• First premolar	Ovoid	Ovoid
• Second premolar	Ovoid	Ovoid
• First molar	Triangular	Rectangular or Trapezoidal
• Second molar	Triangular	Triangular

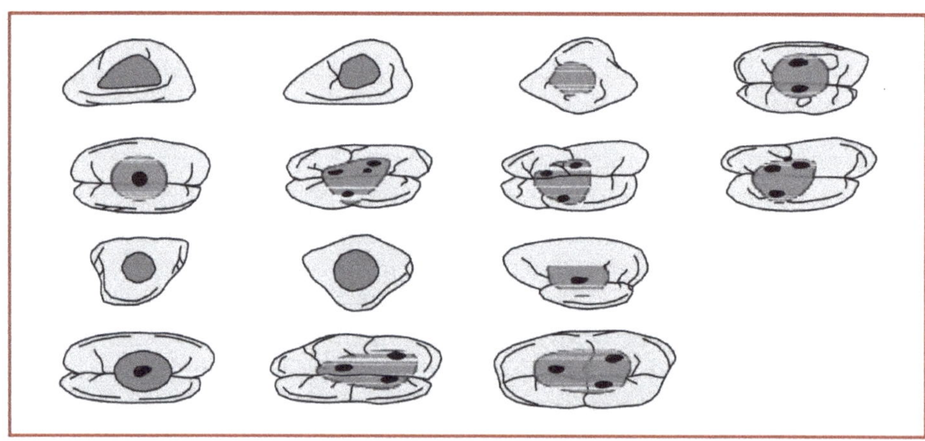

Fig. 9.1:

Anterior teeth

- The shape and outline are determined by age and status of pulp In children triangular in shape with the base of triangle facing incisally and tip of the triangle facing towards cingulum.

- In young adults rounded triangular in shape.

- In old adult's long oval in shape with greater diameter inciso gingivally

- In older patients it is rounded.

- Access opening of mandibular anterior teeth differ from maxillary anterior teeth in the following aspect.

- It is smaller in shape

- Shape is long oval with greater dimension inciso gingivally

- In mandibular anterior teeth when two canals are present facial canal is easy to locate. The lingual canal lies under lingual shoulder limited access will hinder the instrument getting into the canal hence access should extend well in to the cingulum gingivally.

Premolars

Maxillary first premolars

Oval in shape with greater dimensions buccolingually and lesser dimensions mesiodistally. If only one canal is present buccolingual extension is less when three canals are present outline becomes triangular with the base of triangle on the facial surface.

Maxillary second premolars

Similar to that of first maxillary premolar but does not have buccolingual extension as much as the first premolar unless it has two canals.

Mandibular premolars

- At the center of occlusal surface between buccal and lingual cusp.

- Due to lingual inclination of crowns and presence of nonfunctional lingual cusp the opening is buccolingual slightly towards the lingual surface of buccal cusp.

- Oval in shape with greater dimensions buccolingually and lesser dimensions mesiodistally.

- Slight variations exist between maxillary and mandibular premolars due to lingual tilt of mandibular premolars.

Molars

Maxillary first molars

Rounded triangular in shape with tip of the triangle pointing towards palatal cusp tip and base of the triangle pointing towards buccal surface. Trapezoidal when extended slightly mesial in case of presence of MB2. Transverse ridge and oblique ridge should be left intact without undermining.

Maxillary second molars

Similar to that of maxillary first molar three canals are present rounded triangle, Rhomboidal when four canals are present and oval when two canals are present widest in buccolingual direction. Transverse ridge and oblique ridge should be left intact without undermining.

Mandibular firs molars

Triangular in shape with tip of the triangle pointing towards central pit and base of the triangle pointing towards mesial surface. Rhomboidal when extended slightly distobuccally or distolingually in case of presence of distobuccal or distolingual canals.

Mandibular second molars

- Similar to that of mandibular first molars
- When two canals are present rectangular wide mesiodistally and narrow buccolingually. When single canal is present oval mesio-distally. because of Bucco axial inclination of crown, sometimes it necessitates the reduction of greater portion of mesio-buccal cusp to gain access in to mesio-buccal canal.

Initial penetration

The objective of penetration is to penetrate the pulp chamber by breaking through the roof with the bur. A drop in or falling in to vacuum effect of the bur may be felt if the chamber is large enough"-feel the drop and stop" The drop can be better felt by round bur the intensity of drop decreases with age as the height of pulp chamber decreases with advancing age and there is less demarcation between roof and floor. If the chamber is very narrow or completely absent because of development of diffuse calcification one should not expect sensation of felling the drop.

Anterior teeth

At the center of lingual surface just below the cingulum in upper anterior teeth and in case of lower anterior teeth just above the cingulum.

Premolars

Maxillary first premolars

At the center of occlusal surface between buccal and lingual cusps with one canal under buccal cusp tip and another under palatal cusp tip.

Maxillary second premolars

Similar to that of first maxillary premolar but does not have buccolingual extension as much as the first premolar unless it has two canals.

Mandibular premolars

At the center of occlusal surface between buccal and lingual cusp.

Molars

Maxillary first molars

At the center of mesial half of occlusal surface, the point of penetration is on central groove.

Maxillary second molars

Similar to that of maxillary first molar

Mandibular firs molars

At the center of mesial half of occlusal surface, the point of penetration is on central fossa.

Mandibular second molars

Similar to that of mandibular first molars

Complete deroofing

Complete deroofing involves complete removal of all the dentin overlying the roof and roof covering the pulp chamber in order to achieve the following objectives.

- To maximize visibility
- To locate additional canal orifices
- To find isthmuses
- To find hidden orifices
- To permit removal of pulpal remnants especially from the pulp horns
- To permit direct-the direct straight-line access to the apical foramina

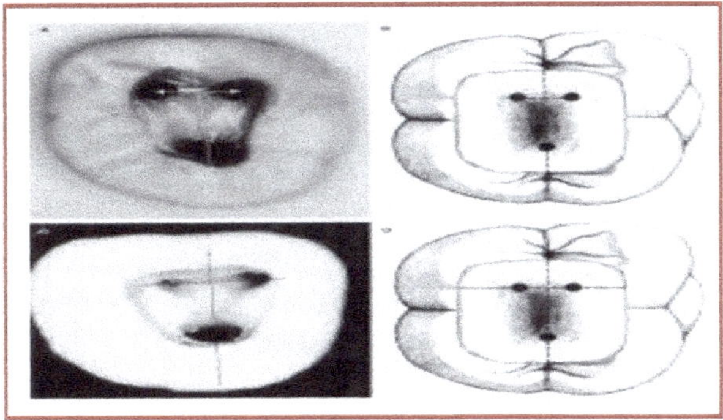

Fig. 9.2:

Straight line access

Straight line access decides the path of entry of instrumentation and materials for cleaning, debridement, shaping, irrigation, obturation and post endodontic restoration. It comprises coronal access and radicular access. Both coronal and radicular straight-line access is confirmed by observing the position of handle of initially placed file. If handle of initially placed file is upright parallel to the long axis of the tooth or skewed off long axis tooth. when handle of initially placed file is not upright parallel to the long axis of the tooth and it is skewed off long axis tooth then acknowledge that interferences must be removed to upright the file handle and position it on long axis.

Once access made it is important to remove the dentin lips or dentinal wedge overhangs on the access cavity walls.

Coronal access

Straight line axis to the orifice of the canal is achieved by considering the removal of :

1. All the dentin overlying the roof of the pulp chamber.
2. Prominences or triangles of dentin created after complete deroofing.

- In upper anteriors - palatal prominence of dentin formed by palatal roof and extends from cingulum 2mm apical to the canal orifice
- In lower anterior - lingual prominence of dentin formed by lingual roof and extends from cingulum 2mm apical to the canal orifice
- In Premolars- mesial and distal prominence of dentin
- In upper molars - buccal and mesial prominence of dentin
- In lower molars - mesial and distal prominence of dentin

Radicular axis

Straight line axis to the apical foramina is achieved by considering removal of triangles of dentin or wedges from the floor of the chamber this can be accomplished by :

I. Pre-flaring of orifice with Gate -Glidden burs or X- Gates
II. Pre-flaring of cervical one third of the canal with rotary files like Sx, Endoflare, one flare

Pre-flaring of orifice with Gate-Glidden burs or X- Gates

Gate Glidden burs can be safely used with brushing motion. The belly of GG serves to flare and blend the orifice in to the adjacent wall and helps to create smooth transition between coronal and radicular aspect of the root canal the size of the GG bur is selected according to the size of orifice largest GG bur is selected that can passively fit in to the given orifice.

Pre-flaring of cervical one third of the canal with rotary files like Sx-Endoflare, one flare

The objective of pre-flaring of cervical one third of canal is to produces a smooth flowing funnel to facilitate the subsequent placement of hand files pre-flaring of coronal one third is commonly performed in curved canals to intentionally relocate the coronal aspect of canal away from external root concavities and remove internal triangles of dentin. It also aids in accurate determination of working length and the apical diameter.

1) Pre-access analysis

A) Clinical analysis

Limited mouth opening and limited access

Limited mouth opening like in cases of trismus and /or an unfavorably positioned angulated tooth may result in the following.

- Difficulty to correctly align the bur along the long axis of crown
- Difficulty to correctly align the bur along the long axis of root

The difficulties can be overcome by employing /considering following

1. A well-positioned mouth prop.
2. A smaller head children's hand piece.
3. Standard size short length bur
4. Performing occlusal reduction by 2 to 3mm
5. Reducing the height of the buccal cusp tips by 2 to 3mm

Carious and defective fillings

First all caries and /or defective fillings removed completely then preparation gently extend to sound tooth structure towards the pulp chamber. All Caries must be completely removed irrespective of its location occlusal or buccal or proximal before proceeding to endodontic access opening. Caries and/or defective filling removal is different procedure and endodontic access cavity preparation is different procedure. After complete removal of caries and/or defective filling if prepared cavity is closer to the chamber it is better to enter the pulp chamber from same side itself. Let caries and defective fillings removal guide us to the pulp chamber. If proximal filling is extended sub-gingivally and is intact it should be retained to facilitate rubber dam placement and isolation. In some cases, teeth with intact crowns and stable occlusal contacts caries driven access is preferred.

Caries driven access preparation sometimes very useful in

a. Class V cavities in anterior teeth
b. Buccal pit or buccal surface caries in extremely tilted and angulated teeth
c. Root caries

Note: In root caries extreme caution is taken with respect isolation if necessary, crown lengthening and pre-endodontic buildup is considered.

Remaining caries dentin must remove for the following reasons

- To eliminate mechanically as many as bacteria as possible from the interior of tooth.
- To eliminate the discolored tooth structure that may ultimately lead to staining of the crown.
- To eliminate the possibility of any bacteria laden saliva leaking in the prepared cavity because caries dentin is leathery and highly permeable this is especially true in proximal or cervical caries and caries that extend into the prepared cavity.
- To increase entry of light and illuminate the cavity to improve vision as the caries is removed the prepared cavity turn from dark color to white color reflect light.

Restored and crowned teeth

Full coverage crowns, large defective restorations, inlays, onlays should be completely removed as it's difficult to asses the status of crown clinically and the status of pulp chamber radiographically this problem become even more worse in narrow pulp chamber with calcification.

If full coverage crowns are not removed without adequate magnification and illumination access cavity nothing more than a black hole and may present following difficulties.

- Crown masking the orientation of tooth
- The pulpal floor is difficult identifying
- The identification of orifice's is difficult
- The negotiation canals will be difficult
- There is always mesial drift or tilt in the crowns of abutment for bridges it is difficults asses to the angulation crown and root and long axis of root.
- Restorations impinging on straight access while instrumentation get lodged in to the pulp chamber thereby blocks orifices.

Benefits of Complete removal of crowns and restorations

- Allows the most favorable access
- Reduces the likelihood of removing sound dentin
- Confirm that there is sufficient tooth structure remaining
- Enhance accessibility and visibility
- Prevent coronal leakage through defective, fractured or leaky restorations

- Complete removal of existing restorations reveals hairline cracks on one or more axial walls which could influence the treatment plan and the endodontic prognosis root canal treated tooth.

Precautions

If restorations are done by you and is judged to be well bonding, esthetically pleasing and functionally designed then access through it. Proximal restorations extending sub gingivally must be spared to facilitate rubber dam placement and isolation.

Always remove restorations impinging on straight access even though it is judged to be well bonding, esthetically pleasing and functionally designed.

Seriously broken teeth

Sometimes due to gross carious destruction or trauma, rarely cervical resorption tooth left with no crown or minimal crown in such cases gingivectomy, crown lengthening and pre-endodontic build up should be considered.

Pre endodontic build up

A tooth that needs a root canal treatment rarely has an intact crown. It is always advisable to have all the four walls before access opening. Pre endodontic build up should mimic the natural anatomic tooth structures so they can use as a guide for the access cavity.

Commonly used materials are for pre-endodontic build up are

a.   Glass ionomer cements

b.   Flowable composite

c.   Composite resin plus glass ionomer cements using sandwich technique

Note:

If floor is located sub gingival glass ionomer cements are recommended or glass ionomer plus composite resin (sandwich technique) is recommended.

Objectives of pre-endodontic buildup

1.   To achieve stable rubber dam placement and isolation

2.   To provide reservoir for irrigating solutions after pre-endodontic buildup we can flood the pulp chamber with irrigating solutions

3.   To provide positive seat for interim restorations so that interim restorations do not fracture and get encroach in to interdental papillae between the appointments.

4.   To provide stable reference points for stoppers for consistent working length determination

5.   To prevent fracture of already weakened walls in between interappointment which can further complicate endodontic procedure

Note:

In cases where emergency drainage of pus through the canals required like acute periapical access first access opening and drainage is accomplished later pre endodontic build up is done.

In minimal or No crowns

Due to absence of guiding anatomy the long axis of root is difficult to trace so there is chance of misdirection of bur which leads to cervical perforation so it's imperative to take x-rays and evaluate distance between floor and remaining tooth structure of build tooth and angulation of root.

Tilted and angulated crown

Tilted and angulated crown mainly occur due to Loss of proximal contacts lead to mesial drifting.

Example

- Proximal caries
- Early loss of permanent tooth and creation of edentulous space.

In tilted and angulated tooth the long axis of the crown is not in alignment with long axis of root and may present following difficulties

- Difficulty to correctly align the bur along the long axis of crown
- Difficulty to correctly align the bur along the long axis of root
- The remaining tooth structure cover and mask the pulp chamber leading to poor visualization and poor accessibility.

Precautions

In tilted and angulated crowns access cavity should be prepared with great care to avoid procedural errors.

- Pre -operative radiographs are an absolute must to evaluate angulation of crown to the root.
- Visualization, illumination and magnification are primary requirements
- Long axis of the tooth is long axis of root not crown so always identify and determined long axis of root rather than long axis of crown to avoid procedural errors.

If care is not taken following errors may occur

- Failure to discover pulpal floor and identify dentinal map
- Failure to locate canal orifice
- Perforations
- Failure to discover pulpal floor and identifying of canals

- Excessive removal of tooth structure
- Improper debridement of pulp chamber
- Instrument separation
- Perforation
- Gauging of dentin

Crowded teeth

Crowding commonly occurs in lower and upper anterior region and rarely in posterior region. Due to misalignment and overlapping of teeth on each other there may be poor accessibility to center of crown conventional access cavity preparation approaches may be difficult.

Precautions

- Depending upon severity and direction of malalignment following precautions should be taken.
- Surface and site of access opening have to be altered, buccal or incisal approach may be taken in anteriors.
- Most recent guided access cavity approach, ultraconservative approach or orifice guided approach should be considered.
- Smaller canals have to be located in posteriors.
- Crowding in premolars region sometimes necessities pre-operative CBCT to assess relation of root tips to mental foramen.
- Never hesitate to refer.

Rotated teeth

If the tooth is rotated the outline form must follow the direction of rotation. suppose tooth is rooted in disto-palatal direction our access cavity preparation must also be in disto-palatal direction. Suppose tooth is rooted in mesiodistal direction our access cavity preparation must also be in mesiodistal direction.

Example

Mandibular premolars may rotate from their normal Bucco-lingual direction to mesiodistal direction. Access cavity preparation and extension must follow the direction of rotation that is mesiodistal.

If care is not taken following errors may occur

- Perforations
- Failure to discover pulpal floor and identifying of canals
- Excessive removal of tooth structure
- Failure to locate canal orifice

- Improper debridement of pulp chamber
- Instrument separation
- Perforation
- Gouging of dentin
- Instrument separation

B) Radiographic analysis

Preoperative radiographs are must and imperative requirement for selecting type of access opening design. Take IOPA's at two different angulations at least to evaluate 70 to 80 % tooth anatomy. Careful observation two or more angulated radiographs will give information of root morphology and curvature of number and curvature of roots or canals.

An ideal radiograph is one which provide maximum details, have desired density, covers adequate area of anatomic region of interest, radiograph should not be distorted, diffuse, darker, blurr, incomplete, shorten or elongated.

Preoperative radiographs define and determine the design of the access cavity by providing following information.

1) Morphology of tooth
    - Provides information about basic design or shape of tooth, whether straight or curved

2) Internal anatomy of tooth
    - Provides information about position, size and status of pulp chamber.
    - Provides information about different level of calcification of pulp chamber or resorptions if any.
    - Provide information about an angle of emergence of canals, number of canals, length of canals and branching of root canal system if any.
    - Provides information of about congenital anomalies of tooth like, Taurodontism, dense invaginatus.

3) Helps in measuring the distance between cusp tip to pulpal floor or from occlusal surface to roof of pulp chamber.

4) Helps to determine the position and status of apical foramina.

Calcified pulp chamber

In calcified teeth due to decrease in pulp volume there is less demarcation between roof and floor chance of feeling the droop is less, discovering pulp chamber by tactile sense is risky locating floor is difficult. It is not easy to remove pulp stones which are attached to the floor. Following precautions should be considered.

- Use of magnification in the form loupes and microscopes are of primary requirements for removing calcification and exploring pulpal floor.

- Complete removal of restorations and crowns if any is an absolute must.

- Use of long shank burs enhances the visualization.

- Complete deroofing approach is selected to remove large pulp stones and to search blocked out canal orifices.

- Canal orifices are located by precisely removing reactionary dentin covering the orifices.

- Carefully trough and deepen the grooves with ultrasonic tips avoid over cutting of dentin overcutting of dentin result in loss of dentinal map further difficulty in identifying canal orifice.

- Do not hesitate to refer.

Sclerosed pulp chamber

Sclerosed pulp chamber and canals are more common with advance in age orifices and canals are narrow and less patent which makes the negotiating and shaping the canals challenging. Following precautions should be considered.

- Visualization, illumination and magnification are primary requirements
- Dyes can be used to negotiate sclerosed canals.
- long shank burs enhance visualization
- precise careful removal of dentin is recommended to explore orifices
- Over use of chelating agents may cause softening of dentin and results in perforations
- Do not hesitate to refer

2) Armamentarium

a) Tools

Front surface, rhodium coated mouth mirror

Access opening burs

- 3 sizes of round burs no 2,4 and 6 and two lengths regular and surgical are routinely used.

- No 2-round bur - mandibular anterior and most maxillary premolar teeth with small crowns and narrow chambers.

- No 4-round bur –maxillary teeth and mandibular premolars teeth.

- No 6-round bur –used only in molars large pulp chambers

- Extended shank round bur –for calcified canals

- Trans metal bur –used for amalgam, all metal cast restoration and metal coping of PFM

- Diamond burs - access through porcelain without causing it to fracture

- Carbide burs -access through metal

- ZIR cut-access through zirconium

- Endo access burs

- TR 13, TR 24,

- TR stands for round taper

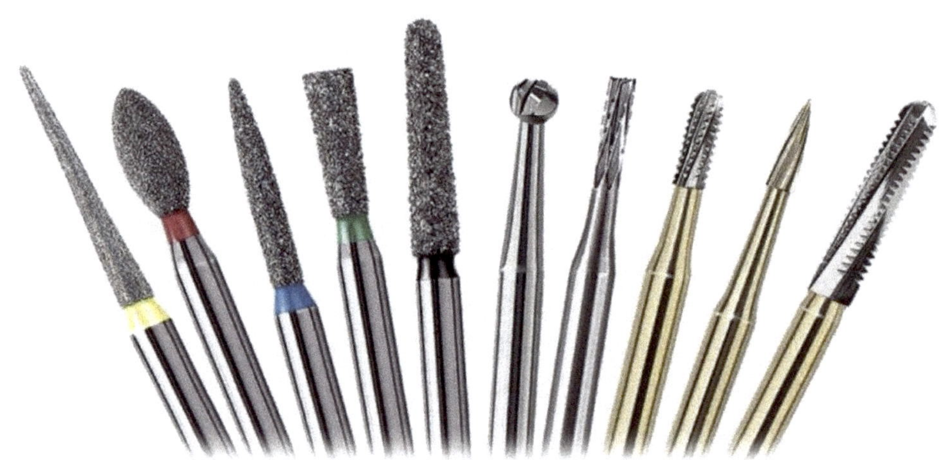

Fig. 9.3:

EX 24

Non cutting tips to avoid damage to pulp floor, safety tips produce wall free gouges and safe for axial walls useful in deroofing the pulp chamber and expansion of access.

SF -11

Straight fissure bur with flat cutting end –less aggressive, line cut or plain cut Use full for penetration in calcified chamber

Access refining burs –these are gut flame shaped, tapered round and diamonds for refining the walls of access cavity preparation.

Explores to search orifices
DG-16

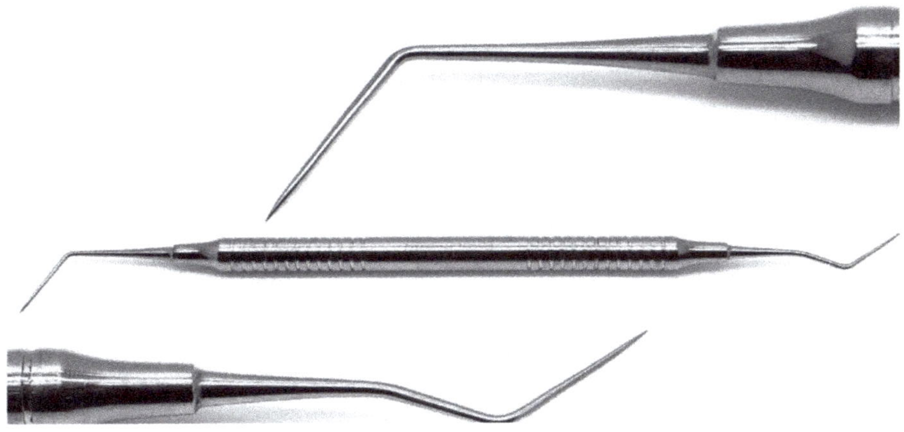

Fig. 9.4:

- Most valuable tool perfect instrument for opening and identify canal orifices and determine canal angulation

- CK-17

- Thinner and stiffer compar to DG-16 used to explore calcified and blocked canals

- Endo spoon

- To remove coronal pulp and carious dentin

Ultra-sonics

- Ultrasonic tips for to trough and deepen developmental grooves to remove tissue and explore canals.

- G3 scaler tip is very aggressive to be used very cautiously under magnification only otherwise it may lead to excessive removal of tooth structure and perforations.

- EN4 tip from credential useful in removing large calcification.

- Tips like RS1 and RS2 from Sybron endo very useful in removing calcification.

Gates Glidden drills

- For enlarging and flaring orifices

- To be used very cautiously in buccal roots of upper molars and mesial roots of lower molars otherwise causes strip perforation useful pre coronal flaring in anterior teeth and larger canals of posterior teeth.

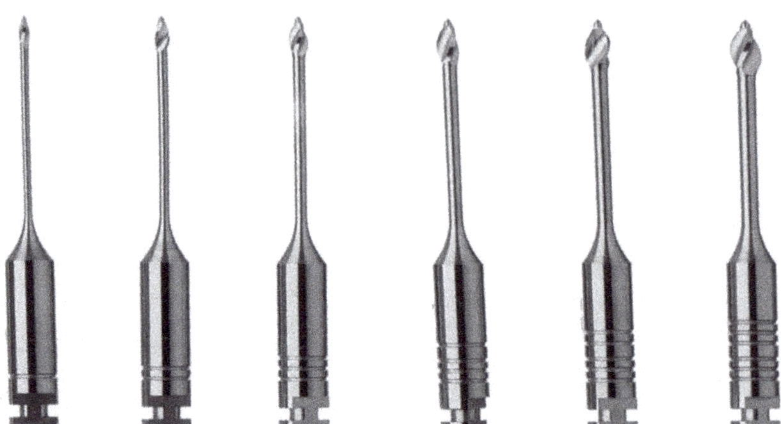

Fig. 9.5:

b) Visualization

- The purpose of visualization is to see the area of interest (anatomical features teeth and oral cavity) clearly while working in a comfortable position.
- Visibility is very important we have to see what we are doing either through direct or indirect vision it is a terrible thing to see and have no vision. Flood the area of interest with light commonly used sources are head light, fiber optic light head mounted light, LED mounted mouth mirrors, bright LED light with push button hand piece.

Following factors influences visualization

- Good quality focusing head light
- Front surface radium coated mouth mirror
- Rubber dam placement
- Use of long shank burs
- Angulation and anatomic position of teeth in the mouth
- Patient mouth opening ability

Poor or Deficient Illumination results in the following

- Treating wrong tooth
- Failure to identify anatomic variation
- Excess removal healthy tooth structure
- Coronal and Cervical perforations
- Muscular pain and back ache
- Eye fatigue and eye sight problems

c)   Magnification

Common way to achieve better vision is to magnify the area of interest. Access opening is no longer a blind procedure, the use of loupes, microscopes and endoscopes in endodontic treatment has enabled the operator to magnify a specified treatment field beyond that of the naked eye. Operating microscope is an invaluable tool in dentistry the resolution of human eye is 0.2mm this can be enhanced up to 6 micrometers with the help of surgical operating microscope.

<u>Surgical microscopes are no longer a luxury but necessary in the field of endodontics.</u>

- Enhances the ability to better identify and treat etiology of endodontic origin
- Identify fracture lines
- Locate canal orifices
- Determine anatomic variations in teeth and supporting structures.

d)   Isolation

Endodontics is all about isolation

Direct methods	Indirect methods
Cotton rolls	Comfortable chair position and patient head posture
Retraction cord	Stress free environment
Lip retractors	Local anesthetics
Saliva ejectors	Drug intervention
Rubber dam	

Rubber dam

"No rubber dam no endo"

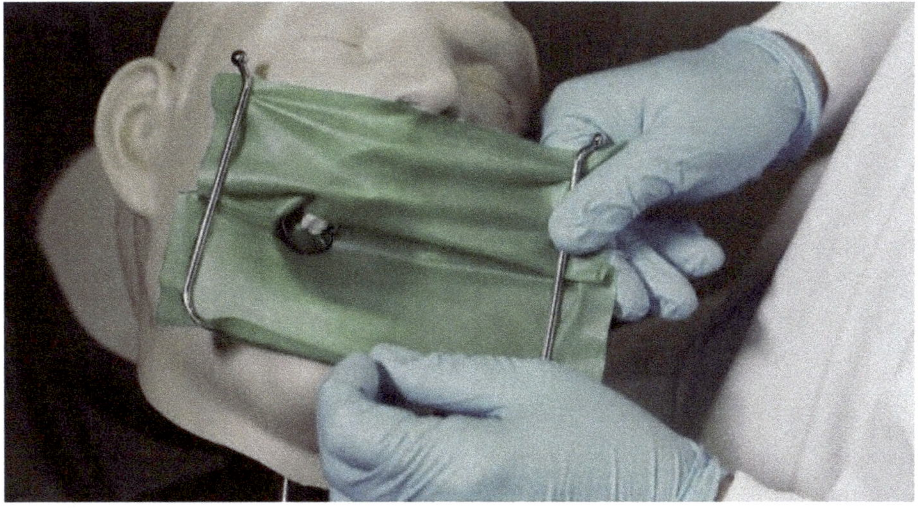

Fig. 9.6:

Advantages

- Patient comfort they don't fear that hands, instruments or fluids are entering their mouth
- Clinician comfort better tactile control no slipping of fingers, good grip with instruments
- Improved safety airway protection
- Improved contrast of adjacent tooth
- Clean surgical field
- Improved moisture control compared to other forms of isolation
- Improved visualization through the retraction of soft tissues
- Time managements no rinsing episodes, no phone calls
- Better patient satisfaction and behavioral management
- Decreases stimulation of the gag reflux in patients that are prone to gagging

Disadvantages

- Learning curve is required
- Time consuming not suitable for busy practices
- Problematic application
- Allergic to some patients
- Patient rejection

Contraindications

- Asthmatic patients
- Claustrophobic patients
- Mouth breathers
- Partially erupted teeth
- Epileptic patients

e) Pre endodontic build up

A tooth that needs a root canal treatment rarely has an intact crown;

It is always advisable to have all the four walls before access opening to:-

- ➤ Achieve stable rubber dam placement and isolation
- ➤ Flood the pulp chamber with irrigating solutions
- ➤ Provide positive seat for interim restorations so that interim restorations do not fracture and get encroached in to interdental papillae between the appointments.
- ➤ Get stable reference points for working length determination

Note :

In cases where emergency drainage of pus through the canals required like acute periapical access first access opening and drainage is accomplished later pre endodontic build up is done.

Procedure

The likelihood of gaining adequate access should be determined. If the access to the tooth is difficult entire treatment may be compromised.

Determination of long axis of root

The long axis of the root should be determined by periodontal probing, A Periodontal probe walked around the gingival sulcus to assess the following

- Angulation of tooth.
- Assess the angulation of crown in relation to the root.
- Assess the coronal restoration in relation to the roots.

Note :- Palpation of roots in upper anterior also aids in assessing the angulation of crown in relation to the root.

Determination of position and shape of cemental enamel junction

The location of CEJ should be determined in order to determine the probable location of pulp chamber floor and orifices of the canals.

Determination of position and orientation of pulp chamber

Position and orientation of pulp chamber should be determined in order to determine the probable location of pulp chamber floor and orifices of canals.

Determination of dimensions of pulp chamber

Depth and width of pulp chamber is determined by pulling out the radiograph on the screen, RVG has calibration device with the help of that following measurements are made or in case of films bur and hand piece held against the film.

- The distance between the occlusal surface of the tooth and roof of the pulp chamber
- The distance between occlusal surface of tooth and floor of pulp chamber
- The distance between mesial and distal of the pulp chamber

Penetration phase

Occlusal reduction of 1.5 to 2 mm is done. The purpose of doing occlusal reduction are.

1)   It aids in the healing of periapical tissues.

2)   It provides stable seat for stopper.

It is necessary to mentally visualize the location of pulp chamber, the bur should be advanced towards the center of mentally imaged CEJ. Penetrate the enamel into the dentin to the pulp chamber with small bites enamel, caries, old restorations if any and dentin are removed in a controlled manner until a thin layer of dentin remains on the roof of pulp chamber. For breaching of roof in calcified teeth straight fissure bur is preferred in non-calcified tooth round bur is preferred at low speed.

Note:

Penetration should be done at the level of the center of CEJ. The law of centrality states that the pulp chamber is located in the center of the tooth at the level of CEJ.

The long axis of the bur should be parallel to long axis of the tooth.

Because the axial walls of the pulp chamber are concentric to the external outline of the crown.

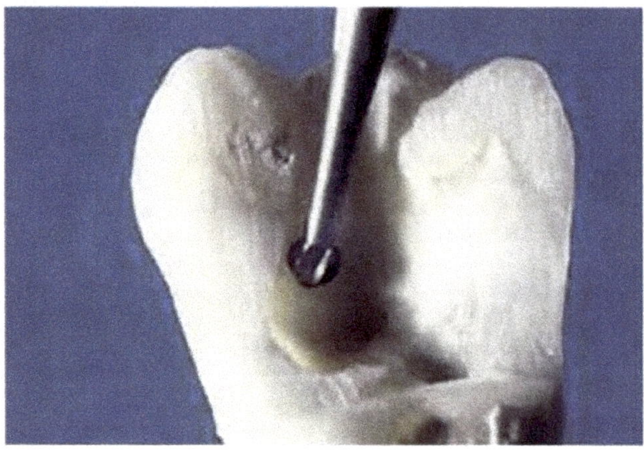

Fig. 9.7: Penetration phase

Complete deroofing phase

Once the roof has been perforated the bur is moved laterally buccal to palatal direction and axially mesial to distal direction to complete internal out line form. the remaining roof is removed by working from inside the chamber to outside the chamber in a scoop out or brushing motion. The purpose of this phase to completely deroof the pulp chamber performed using round bur in high speed contra-angle there are two ways to unroof the chamber are to either place a straight bur and move it laterally while keeping it parallel to the long axis of the tooth, or place a round bur into the access engaging laterally under the remaining overhang and then withdrawing the bur occlusally.

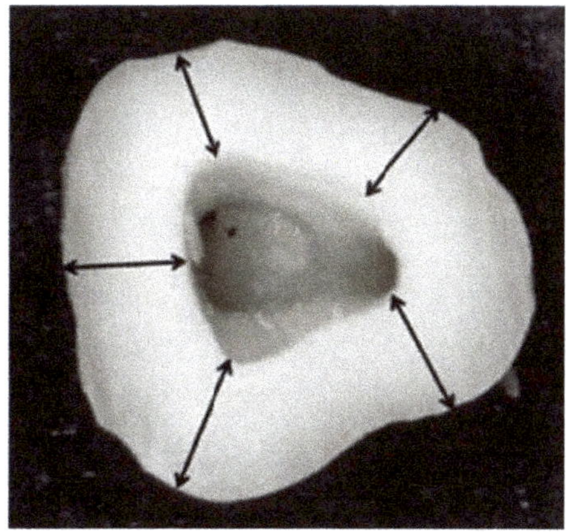

Fig. 9.8: Complete deroofing phase

Enlargement phase / Convenience form

This phase involves the identification and careful removal of dentinal ledges or lips of dentin that are present between the access cavity walls and pulp chamber walls.

Extend the access cavity laterally toward each canal orifice keeping the bur away from the floor until you can see the full circumference of the canals never touch the floor with bur, touching the floor destroys dentinal map and increases difficulty in locating the canals and probability of missing the canals will be more.

Unobstructed access to the canal orifices

We have to identify and remove all restrictions such as dentinal wedges, dentinal triangles cervical hums, overhanging's in and around the orifices interfering in the smooth, clear unobstructed access to the canal orifice. when file is inserted it should get in the orifice freely without touching any other wall of the chamber that is the first contact of file should be the orifice. If any part of the wall is interfering take out only that bit of wall it is not necessary to remove all the wall. The orifice is approached from opposite direction.

Example in lower molars mesial buccal and mesiolingual orifices are approached from distobuccal and distolingual direction respectively and distal orifice approached from mesial direction.

Direct access to the apical foraman

Direct access to apical foramina probably leads to more removal of radicular dentin and weakening of tooth especially if canals are existing from orifice with sharp angles so if we get direct access to at least initial curvature of the canal it's enough.

Cavity expansion to accommodate filling technique

We should have a particular size of cavity preparation so that it can allow free moments of basic filling instruments around the entire circumference of the pulp chamber thereby facilitating the proper flow and adaption of thixotropic filling materials.

Complete authority over the enlarging instruments

Some times our preparation so conservative that part of canal orifice present on the axial wall giving appearance like mouse hole due to this part of the canal present on the vertical wall making the instrumentation stressful and time consuming. We need to push the axial wall to bring the orifice in the corner.

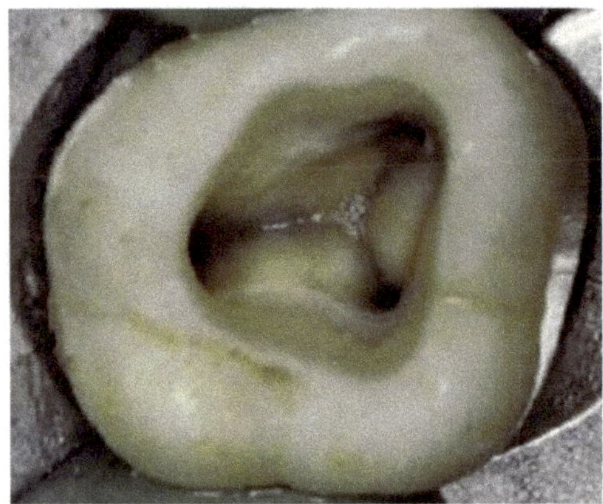

Fig. 9.9: Convenience form

Inspection of access cavity

By using illumination and magnification aids such as loupes, magnifying glasses, operating microscopes.

Should be looked for the following :

- Remnants of vital or necrotic soft tissue.
- Remnants of caries.
- Remnants of fillings like amalgam, gold and ceramic particles
- Remnants of old cements and sealers particles
- Secondary dentin and tertiary dentin
- Pulp stones and calcifications
- Root canal orifices and isthmuses
- Perforations
- Fractures, cracks and craze lines

Refinement of restorative margins

It is a final step in endodontic access cavity preparation which involves removal of undermined weakened enamel overhanging's from cavity walls and smoothing of Cavo surface margins which aids in prevention of coronal leakage of temporary and permanent restorations.

Final axial walls should be parallel or slightly diverging which improves accessibility to pulpal floor and enhances visibility of pulp chamber.

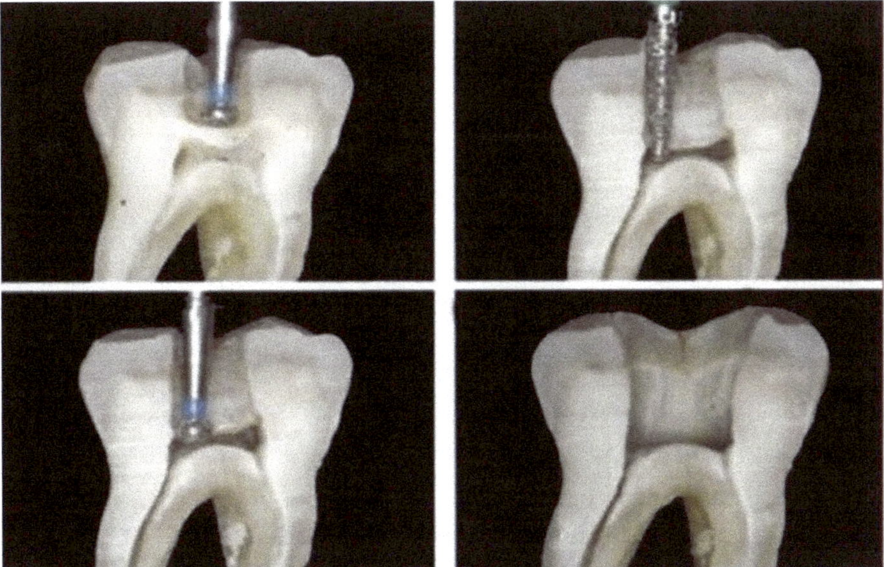

Fig. 9.10: Procedure;- penetration , Enlargement and Refinement

Advantages

Attempted for all the teeth during endodontic treatment

Complete deroofing and direct straight-line access to apical foramina permits adequate access to the root canal system has the following advantages

- Permits direct vision to the pulpal floor

- Facilitates location of all canal orifices and isthmuses if any

- Facilitates complete biomechanical removal all the infected tissue contents of pulp chamber vital or necrotic, particularly tissue of pulp horns thereby decreases the incidence of discoloration especially in anterior tooth.

- Permits the removal of large pulp stones and diffuse calcification safely without damaging the pulp floor.

- Facilities identification remnants of old filling materials and their effective removal.

- Augment thorough disinfection of remaining tooth structure particularly the chronically infected pulp chamber.

Complete deroofing improves straight line access to the canals which in turn facilitates the following.

1. Improved instrumentation control

   - Due to the wide variations of canal morphology many canals curve in two or more directions straight line access usually eliminates at least one of these curvatures hence guarantees an unobstructed direct initial path for the instrumentation leads towards apex and minimizes restorative stress on the file edge and tip of instruments.

- Decreases the effects of canal curvature on instruments minimizes instrument curvature and deflection thereby increases the operator's ability to manipulate files in as many areas of the canal as possible without grossly altering the internal canal anatomy.

2. Improved obturation

   Enable better spreader and plugger penetration makes the obturation and sealing of canal orifices easier and more effective.

3. Decreases procedural errors

   Straight line access decreases procedural errors like

   - Instrumentation separation.
   - Ledge formation.
   - Perforations.
   - Deformation of apical foramina
   - Zipping

4. Avoids errors in determination of correct working length

Disadvantages

1. To discover pulp chamber relays on tactile sense of burs if the chamber is large enough then bur can truly drop into the pulp chamber when chamber is scant like in pulp sclerosis or non-existent like in calcification lead to undesired outcomes.

2. Blindly cutting the tooth structure with large round burs and inverted cone burs without magnification leads inverse funnel shaped preparation which is narrower coronally and wider apically leading to undermine of dentin it is called inverse funneling.

3. Complete deroofing tend create parallel sided wide cylindrical shape preparation with similar coronal and apical width which leads to more loss of peri cervical dentin and weakening of tooth it is called tunneling.

4. Complete deroofing tend to touch the lateral walls of the pulp chamber removes healthy dentin and weakens the tooth is called gouging.

5. Complete deroofing creates surface irregularities on the lateral walls of access cavity which ultimately leads to loss of healthy tooth structure and weakening of tooth.

6. There is no or less chance of preservation of peri cervical dentin.

7. The main cause of failure of root canal treated is the loss of tooth structure traditional access cavity preparation found to be second largest cause of root canal treatment.

Partial deroofing approach or Conservative approach or Contracted access cavity approach

The design of the access cavity is crucial to maintain healthy tooth structure. The smaller access shapes and sizes can meet the biological threshold for resolution of periapical pathology. Conservative approach gives equal importance to both coronal and radicular aspect of access cavity preparation thereby intend to maintain fine balance between operator needs, restoration needs and tooth needs.

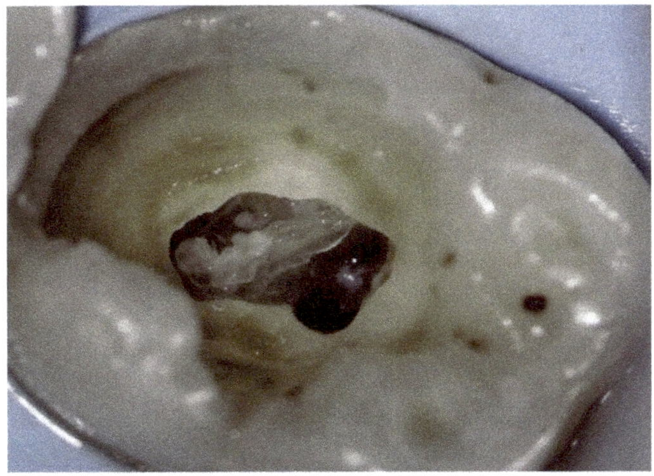

Fig. 9.11:

Principle

Lesser we open the pulp chamber smaller the preparation more will be the preservation of healthy toot structure more we open the chamber wider the preparation more will be the loss of healthy toot structure.

This approach involves partial deroofing and soffit creation. It is tooth centric more importance is given to the preservation of coronal and peri cervical dentin, in this approach the teeth are accessed at central fossa and extended only as necessary to detect canal orifices.

Objectives

To completely eliminate all caries irrespective of its location in the tooth.

To conserve as much as coronal tooth structure as possible

- Cingulum in anterior teeth
- Marginal ridges in lower molars
- Oblique ridge in upper molars
- Functional stress bearing cusps in all teeth

- To conserve as much as coronal dentin as possible (The healthy unaffected dentin overlying the roof)

- To preserve undermined coronal dentin
- To find pulp the chamber
- To partially unroof the dentin covers the pulp chamber
- To Create roof strut to avoid gauging of pulp chamber walls
- To achieve unobstructed strategic straight-line access to the orifice of the canals
- To achieve unobstructed strategic straight line access to the initial curvature of the canals
- To preserve undermined peri-cervical dentin

Shape and Initial out line form

Conservative approach is a tooth centric primarily focuses on the tooth needs and does not have a predetermined shape according to the type of tooth.

The following factors dictate the design (shape and Initial out line farm) :

- Location and extent of caries and Proximity of pulp chamber after complete elimination of caries
- Proximity of pulp chamber after removal of faulty fillings
- Remaining tooth structure after removal faulty prosthesis
- Anatomy of pulpal floor.
- Position of orifice.
- Internal canal anatomy
- Presence of additional roots
- Presence of additional canals
- Angle of emergence of canals from orifice
- Crown to root angulation
- Severity of root curvatures

Initial penetration

Site

- At center of crown
- At central fossa
- Just above the orifice

The roof of the pulp chamber is penetrated through the central portion of the crown at a point where the roof and floor of the pulp chamber are at widest this usually occur at larger diameter canal distal canals of lower molars and palatal canals of upper molar. once the roof of the pulp chamber is breached the bur suddenly drop in to the pulp chamber space.

Partial deroofing and soffit creation

While deroofing some amount of dentin is left ,the three dimensional band of dentin which is formed   after partial deroofing is called soffit which reinforces the tooth or bangs the rest of the tooth structure against the occlusal stresses thereby increases fracture resistance of tooth   can be compared with the metal ring that stabilizes a wooden barrel.

Benefits of soffit or roof strut creation

- It avoids the collateral damage by guiding the rotating bur to the pulp chamber and floor more conservatively.

- It absorbs and transfer the occlusal forces to the radicular dentin thereby increases the fracture resistance of tooth.

Strategic straight-line access

Unobstructed strategic straight-line access to the orifice of the canals

Can be achieved by identifying and selectively removing

- Restrictions such as dentinal wedges and overhanging's created after partial deroofing between cavity walls and pulp chamber walls.

- Interferences such as dentinal triangles and cervical hums in and around the orifices interfering in the smooth, clear unobstructed access to the canal orifice.

When file is inserted it should get in the orifice freely without touching any other wall of the chamber that is the first contact of file should be the orifice. If any part of the wall is interfering take out only that bit of wall it is not necessary to remove all the wall. Then the orifices are approached from opposite direction as follows

<table>
<tr><td colspan="2">Upper premolars</td></tr>
<tr><td>Buccal canal orifice</td><td>Palatal direction</td></tr>
<tr><td>Palatal canal orifice</td><td>Buccal direction</td></tr>
<tr><td colspan="2">Upper molars</td></tr>
<tr><td>Mesiobuccal canal orifice</td><td>Distopalatal direction</td></tr>
<tr><td>Distobuccal canal orifice</td><td>Mesio palatal direction</td></tr>
<tr><td>Palatal canal orifice</td><td>Buccal direction</td></tr>
<tr><td colspan="2">Lower molars</td></tr>
<tr><td>Mesio-buccal orifice</td><td>Distolingual direction</td></tr>
<tr><td>Mesio-lingual</td><td>Distobuccal direction</td></tr>
<tr><td>Distobuccal</td><td>Mesiolingual direction</td></tr>
<tr><td>Disto lingual</td><td>Mesiobuccal direction</td></tr>
</table>

Lower lateral incisors

Lingual canal orifice	Labial direction
Buccal canal orifice	Lingual direction

Can be achieved by identifying and selectively removing restrictions such as dentinal wedges and overhanging's created after partial deroofing between cavity walls and pulp chamber walls.

Removing interferences such as dentinal triangles and cervical hums in and around the orifices interfering in the smooth, clear unobstructed access to the canal orifice.

Unobstructed strategic straight-line access to the initial curvature of the canals

Direct access to apical foramina probably leads to more removal of radicular dentin and weakening of tooth hence if we get unobstructed access to at least initial curvature of the canal it's enough the latest heat-treated files automatically glide in to the sharper curvatures of the canals.

When canals are leaving from orifice with sharp obtuse angles especially in double curved roots coronal widening is performed with Sx, One flare and endomate.

Technique

Occlusal reduction of 1.5 to 2 mm is done. The purpose of doing occlusal reduction are :

1) It aids in the healing of periapical tissues.
2) It provides stable seat for stopper.

Penetrate the enamel into the dentin to the pulp chamber. In calcified teeth straight fissure bur is preferred in non-calcified tooth round bur is preferred in slow speed.

A) Remove all the caries.
B) Remove all the old restorations if any.

Penetration should be done at the level of the center of CEJ. The law of centrality states that the pulp chamber is located in the center of the tooth at the level of CEJ.

The long axis of the bur should be parallel to long axis of the tooth.

Because the axial walls of the pulp chamber are concentric to the external outline of the crown, penetrate with small bites. The roof of the pulp chamber should be penetrated through the central portion of the crown at a point where the roof and floor of the pulp chamber are at widest. This usually larger diameter canal distal canals of lower molars and palatal canals of upper molar once the roof of the pulp chamber is breached the bur suddenly drop in to the pulp chamber space.

Once the roof has been perforated and drop in is felt the bur is moved laterally buccal to palatal direction and axially mesial to distal direction to complete internal out line farm. the remaining roof is removed by working from inside the chamber to outside the chamber in a scoop out or brushing motion. Extend the access cavity laterally toward each canal orifice keeping the bur away from the floor until you can see the full circumference of the canals, never touch the floor with bur, touching the floor destroys dentinal map and increases difficulty in locating the canals and probability of missing the canals will be more, remove undermined tooth structure on walls to remove any steps (no dentinal ledges or lips are present between the access cavity walls and pulp chamber walls.

Partial deroofing is done by leaving some amount of dentin.

The three-dimensional band of dentin which is left after partial deroofing is called soffit or roof strut.

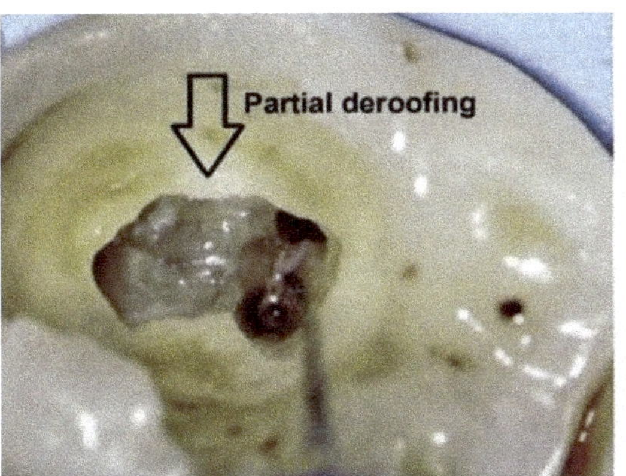

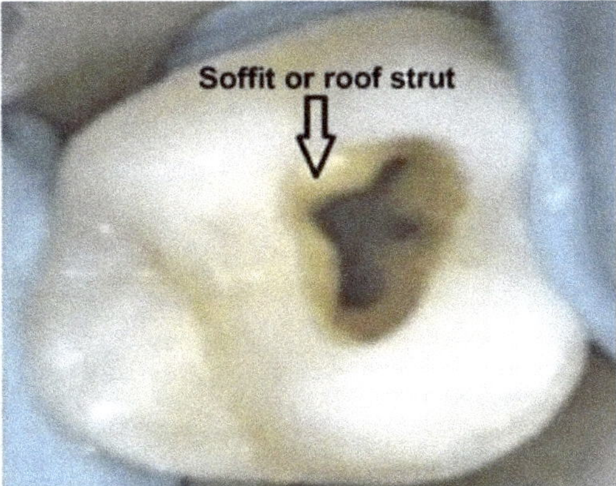

Fig. 9.12: Partial Derooting

Benefits of soffit preparation

1) It guides the rotating bur to the chamber and floor more conservatively.
2) It encloses and embraces all the restoration within thereby reinforces the tooth against occlusal loading.

After partial deroofing, feel the drop. The intensity of drop decreases with age as the height of pulp chamber decreases with advancing age.

- The drop can be better felt by round bur

Enlargement

Is done according to the demands of tooth in question at the time of treatment:

1) To remove soft caries.
2) To remove dentinal wedges to get adequate straight-line axis to the root | apex especially in double curved roots.

Refinement

Done with safe ended straight fissure bur. Safe ended bur has two parts non active cutting tip and active lateral cutting part.

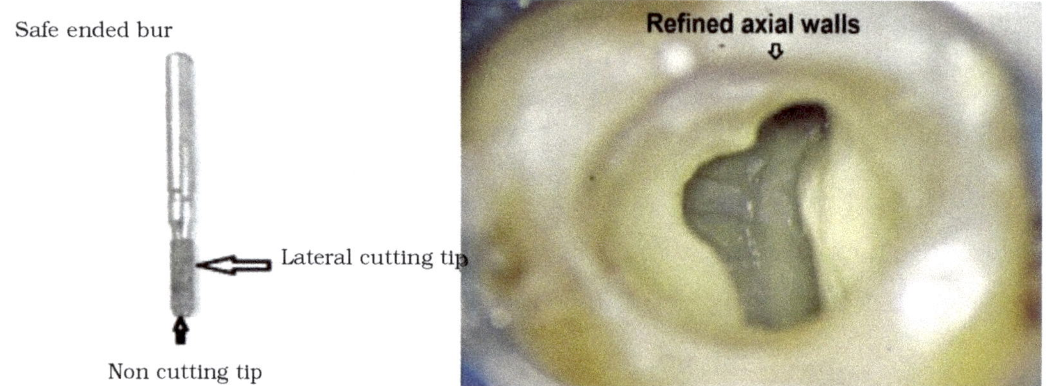

Fig. 9.13:

Non active tip   – Avoids accidental damaging pulp chamber floor.

Active lateral part – Eliminates interferences for a direct access in to the canal

a) Diverging the axial walls occlusally

1)   To increase the visibility of pulp chamber.

2)   To remove unsupported enamel rods and to increase resistance form of the tooth.

b) 45-degree bevel is placed to remove unsupported enamel in order to include enamel and dentinal wall into the restoration. This serves two purpose:

1)   Improves coronal seal

2)   Improves resistance form of the cavity against occlusal forces which in turn prevents fracture of tooth or restoration

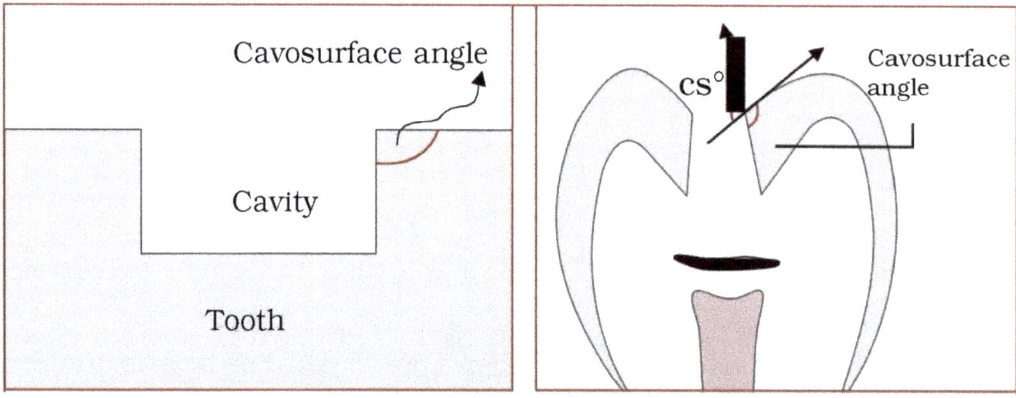

Fig. 9.14: Refinement

Debridement: Removal of all the infected soft tissue

- *Irrigation:* irrigation is done with 2.5% sodium hypochlorite.
- No instrumentation should start until the pulp chamber is completely debrided.

Advantages

Maintain three-dimensional ferrule

- Ferrule means a metal ring which strengthens the end of a handle and prevent it from splitting.
- Facilitates the ferrule effect by avoiding excessive removal of natural tooth structure.
- Ferrule is an axial wall dentin covered by axial of the crown, greater the height and width of the axial wall dentin better the ferrule effect.
- Three components of ferrule
- Vertical component
- The height of the dentin should be minimum 1.5 to 2.5mm
- Horizontal component
- Width or girth of the dentin should be minimum 1 to 2mm
- Total occlusal convergence
- Should be minimum 10 to 20 degree depending upon the height of dentinal wall, if height is more the taper will be more

Soffit or roof strut creation

While deroofing some amount of dentin is left, the three dimensional band of dentin which is formed   after partial deroofing is called soffit which reinforces the tooth or bangs the rest of the tooth structure against the occlusal stresses thereby increases fracture resistance of tooth can be compared with the metal ring that stabilizes a wooden barrel it absorbs and transfer the occlusal forces to the radicular dentin thereby increases the fracture resistance of tooth. Avoid the collateral damage.

Preservation of pericaval dentin

It is the dentin near the alveolar crest the dentin present 4mm above and 4mm below the alveolar crest is called peri cervical dentin it is irreplaceable and sacred for three reasons.

- Ferrule
- Fracturing resistance
- Dentinal tubule orifice proximity from inside out

Preservation of undermining dentin

More the healthy dentin is removed less is the tooth saved dentin is a bimodal composite has a shock absorbing capacity because of its elasticity, orientation of dentinal tubules and fibers its always advice to preserve undermine dentin.

Limitations

- Illumination and magnification in the form at least loupes and/or operating microscope is an absolute must.
- During cavity preparation lack of judgment may lead iatrogenic errors
- Cannot be attempted for all teeth during endodontic treatment
- Possibility of endodontic failure if shaping and cleaning protocol is not followed.

Disadvantages

- Incomplete removal of pulp especially of pulp horn tissue
- Incomplete removal of pulp horn tissue in anterior teeth leads to discoloration of teeth
- Poor visualization of pulp chamber and pulpal floor especially in angulated and tilted teeth
- Difficulty in locating and negotiating canals
- Missing of canals
- Poor debridement and disinfection
- Poor access for placement pluggers and condensers
- Procedural errors like
- Ledge formation
- Perforations
- Instrument separation

Point partial deroofing approach or ultra conservative approach

These designs overlook requirements of traditional and contracted designs and have changed the whole concept of deroofing the pulp chamber and straight-line access. More importance is given to saving crucial dentin and has a stepwise approach that aims at conserving the natural tooth structure prioritize the removal of :

- Restorative material ahead of dentin
- Enamel ahead of dentin
- Occlusal tooth structure ahead of cervical dentin

These designs can be accomplished by employing /using the following

- Pre-operative low FOVs CBCT
- Microscopes with higher level of magnification
- Single dose of narrow tapered highly flexible heat-treated rotary instruments.

- Highly potent irrigation systems.
- Bio ceramic sealers and bio ceramic cements.
- Increased popularity bonded obturation using synchronized hydraulic condensation have made ultraconservative designs possible.

Principle

When the diameter of access preparation decreased by a half the operators remove four time less volume of dentin.

Types

A. Truss cavity design

B. Ninja access cavity design

C. Guided access design

Truss access cavity design or orifice directed dentin conservation design

- Proposed by Ashwin and Ramesh in 2017

- The purpose this design is to preserve the dentin that is leaving a truss of dentin between the two cavities that has been prepared. This cavity design aims at the removal of dentin just above the orifices thereby maintaining the maximum amount of tooth structure.

- In mandibular molars two separate cavities to approach distal canal and mesial canals. Where as in maxillary molars mesiobuccal canal and distobuccal canal approached in one cavity and a separate cavity for the palatal canal is made.

- Pentration started exactly above the pulp horns in case of lower molars access is extended in a buccolingual oval shape.

- Incase of maxillary molars access extended in mesidistal direction.

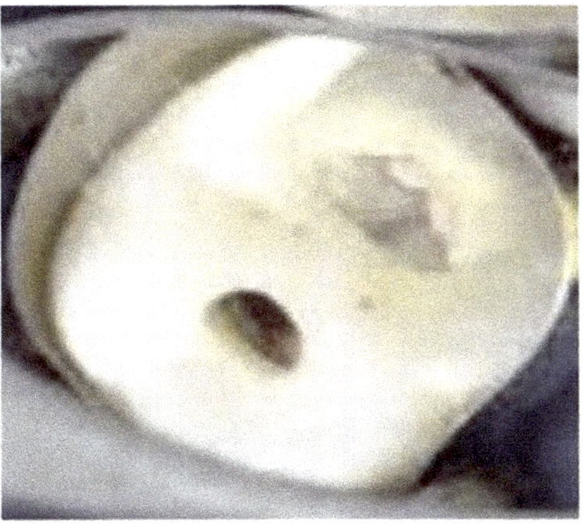

Fig. 9.15: Truss Access

Ninja access cavity design or point endodontic access design

It was proposed by Belogard

It is considered to be most conservative, minimally invasive approach. Penetration started at central fossa following an oblique ridge projection towards the canal orifices, it requires more experience and perfect judgement.

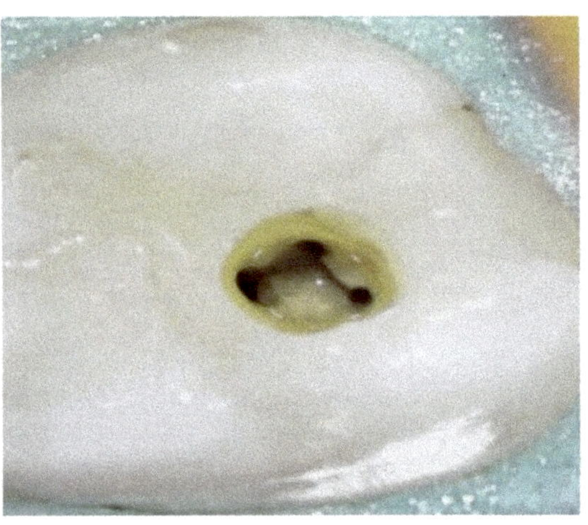

Fig. 9.16: Ninja Access

Guided access design

Guided is in between conservative and ultraconservative design the first case was done in calcified canal in the year 2015.

Take CBCT data, transfer the CBCT images to 3D printer through SD File to create a jig, jig has a hole which directly lead your specifically designed bur to the calcified chamber, a metal barrel inside the jig stabilizes and protect the jig from getting abraded from rotating bur. Place the jig on the tooth and check.

Guided access design aims at combining CBCT and 3-D printer technology a bur is specially designed according to the design as seen by the CBCT image a virtual bur is made and then superimposed on the tooth then 3D printer is used make the specific bur which then helps in making endodontic access cavity.

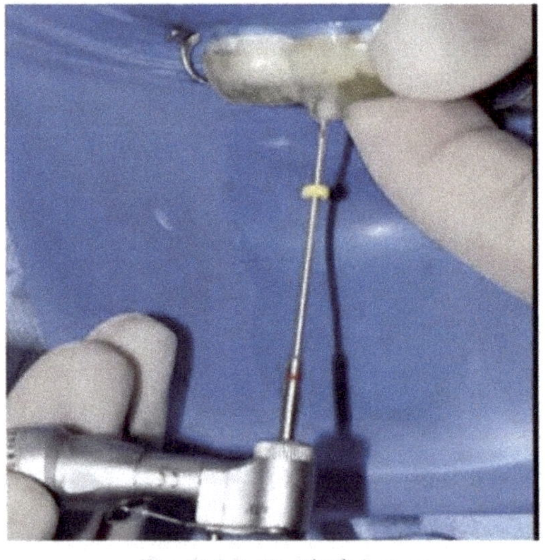

Fig. 9.17: Guided Access

Advantages

- Magnification and illumination in the form of microscopes must
- More preservation of natural tooth structure
- Fracture resistance of tooth is excellent
- No need of placement prosthetic crowns

Disadvantages

- CBCT imaging of tooth is must
- More expensive
- Magnification and illumination in the farm of microscopes must
- Procedural errors
- More stress on instruments
- Unit dose Discord files after single use

Guidelines

- Visualization of the pupal space
- Restorative materials impinging on straight line access should be removed to prevent lodging of debris
- Remove all remaining caries to prevent contamination
- Approach the largest canal first
- Once the roof of the pulp chamber is penetrated always proceeds laterally to avoid perforations
- Locate the canals with the help of a sharp endodontic explorer
- Perform effective toilet of the cavity to remove all debris, necrotic material

B) SELECTION OF FILES

2% STAINLESS STEEL HAND FILES K-FILES

- Files are rigid and more resistant to fracture.
- Made from square blank.
- Number of flutes per mm is more.
- More corrosion resistant

Uses

- To identify and locate root canal orifice.
- To maintain patency throughout the biomechanical preparation of canals.
- To obtain glide path for rotary instruments

Features of files

Available in three different sizes 21 mm, 25 mm, 31 mm. Though the instrument length varies, length of the working blade remains constant that is 16 mm.

- Diameter at the tip of the file is denotated as - D0.
- D0 is in 1/100 of millimetre.

Example:

- Diameter of tip of 2% of 10 size file is 10/100 = 0.1 mm
- Diameter of tip of 2% of 15 size file is 15/100 = 0.15 mm
- Diameter of tip of 2% of 20 size file is 20/100 = 0.2 mm
- Diameter of tip of 2% of 25 size file is 25/100 = 0.25 mm and so on

Do from 10 to 60 increases by 0.05 mm, from 60 to 150 increases by

- 0.1 mm from 6 to 10 increases by 0.02 mm
- 21 mm files used in molars and incisors
- 25 mm files used in canine
- 31 mm files used in very long rooted teeth.

For every increase in 1 mm length of 2% 10 k size file, there is increas in diameter by 0.02 mm.

All files have two features: Taper and diameter. With increase in diameter taper increases. With decrease in diameter taper decreases. Taper is constant and it is available as 2%, 4%, 6%, 8%. Taper helps to prepare larger canals and wider diameter portion of canals without enlarging the apex.

But diameter varies for different sizes files.

From # 6 to # 10 diameter increases by 2 units, from # 15 to # 60 diameter

Increases by 5 units from # 60 to # 150 diameter increase by 10 units.

The angle between the long axis of the instrument and cutting edge is called blade angle which is 75 ± 15.

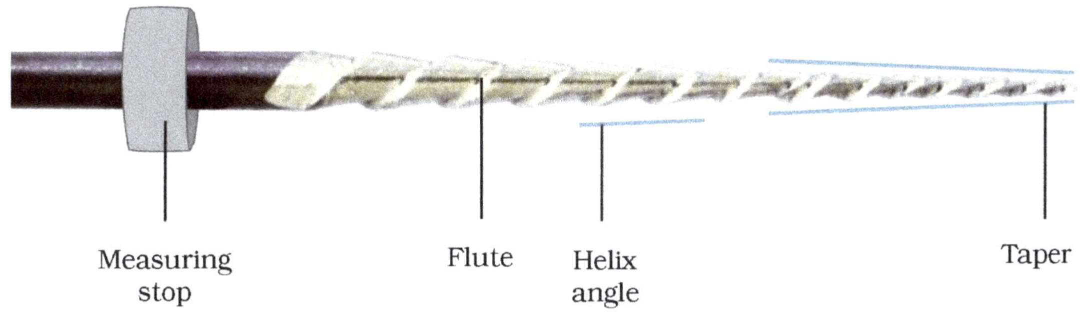

Fig. 9.18:

Colour coding

By 2 units	By 5 units	By 5 units	By 10 units
6 - pink	15 - white	45 - white	60 - blue
8 - grey	20 - yellow	5o - yellow	70 - green
10 - purple	25 - red	55 - red	80 - black
	30 - blue	60 - blue	90 - white
	35 - green		100 - yellow
	40 - black		110 - Red
			120 - Blue
			130 - Green
			140 - Black
			150 - White

TYPES OF FILES

K flex files

Made from rhomboidal or diamond blank increases cutting efficiency and increases flexibility.

Chances of extrusion of debris into periapical area is less.

Usage: Preferred in calcified canals, blocked canals and obstructed canals.

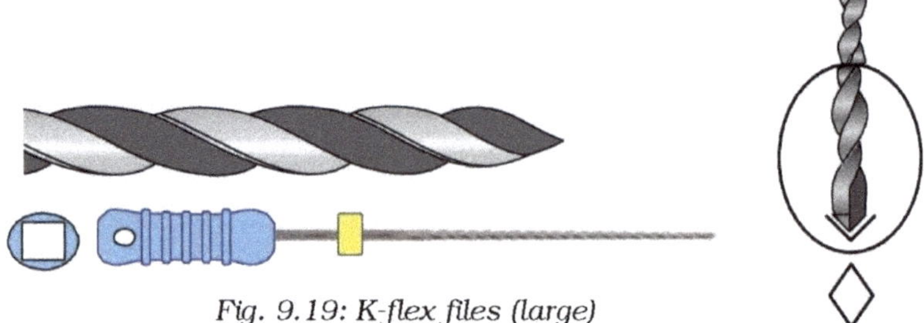

Fig. 9.19: K-flex files (large)

Flexo files

Flexo files made by triangular blank. More flexibility and more cutting efficiency than k flex files.

Used in narrow canals.

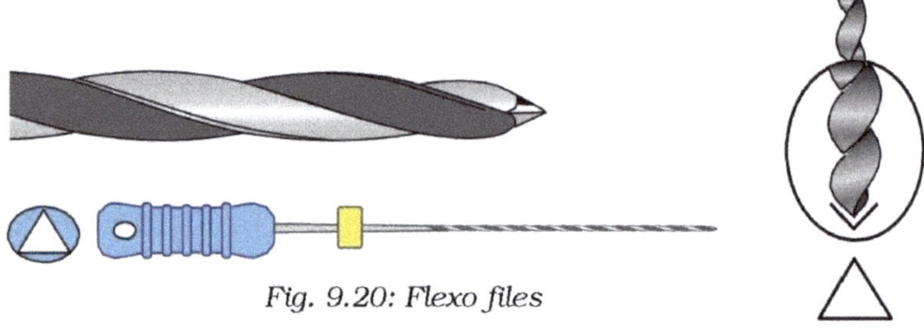

Fig. 9.20: Flexo files

Flex-R files

Stainless steel files have metallic memory, they tend to regain their original shape once the stress is removed and cause ledges. To avoid this Flex-R files are modified at their tips.

Flex-R files have modified cutting edge. These files tend to remain in the centre of the canal thereby preventing any ledge formation and transportation. That is the reason it is used in severely curved canals and in the balanced force technique.

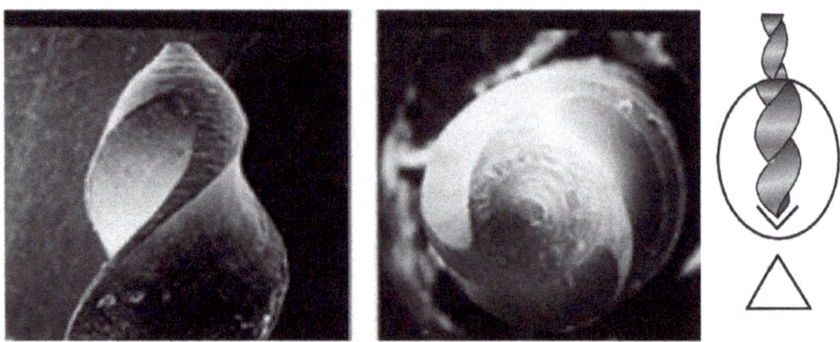

Fig. 9.21: Flex-R file with modified rounded tip

Broaches

Made from round stainless-steel wire. Used in wider canals.

Used to extirpate the pulp tissue and cotton plugs.

Used only when canal is enlarged upto # 20 to # 25 size file.

If decently used in initial stages of cleaning, it helps to remove pulp tissue from complex anatomy of the root. It reduces the chances of apical blockage by removing collagen fibres from apical 1/3 of canal.

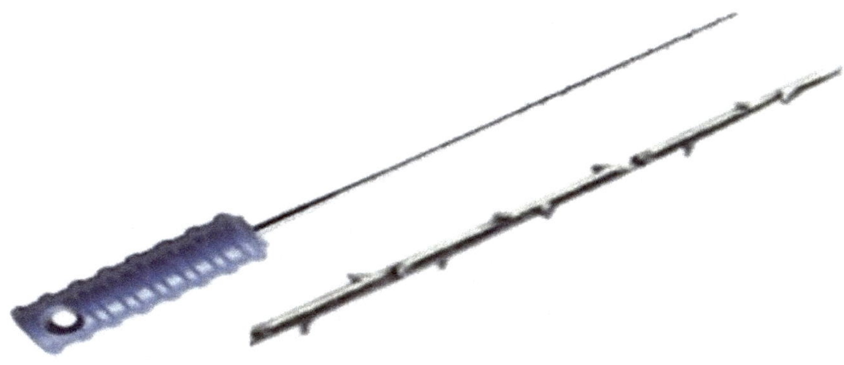

Fig. 9.22: Broaches

H files

H files are made from round stainless steel wire. Looks like a Christmas tree. Flutes are directed coronally. It only cuts by pull and push motion. Never use in circumferential filing motion. Reduces the chances of apical blockage by removing collagen which is the main culprit for apical blockage. If decently used in initial stages of cleaning it helps to remove pulp tissue from complex anatomy of root. (webs, fins laterally and accessory canals).

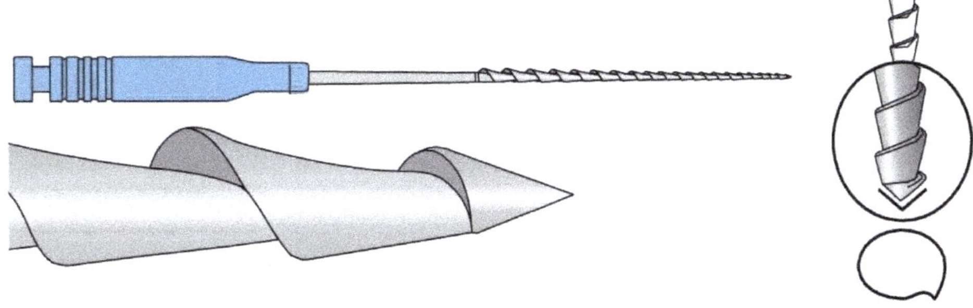

Fig. 9.23: H-files

C) ORIFICE LOCATION

> *WE CANNOT SEE AND ANTICIPATE BEYOND OUR BELIEFS. WE CAN REINFORCE AND AUGMENT OUR BELIEFS ONLY WITH AWARENESS.*
>
> *AWARENESS COMES WITH KNOWLEDGE.*
>
> *KNOWLEDGE IS THE KEY TO BELIEFS.*

Orifice Location is started only after thorough cleaning and debridement of the pulp chamber. Should never be started before complete irrigation of pulp chamber.

For effective location of orifices, we have to rely on some timeless proven success principles which have not changed over centuries.

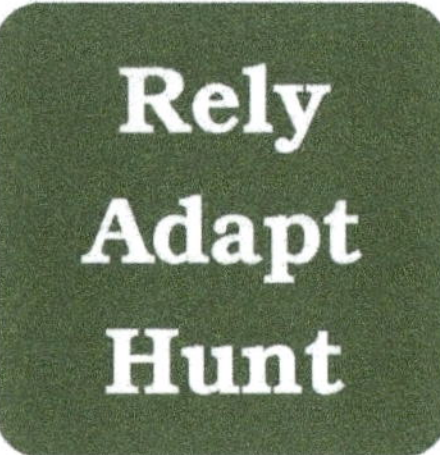

The law of colour change

- The colour of the pulpal floor is darker than the walls of the pulp chamber.

Studying and analysing dentinal map

- Dentinal map can be visualised in all cases except in few cases of total calcification
- The law of centrality states that the pulp chambers is located in the centre of the tooth at the level of CEJ.

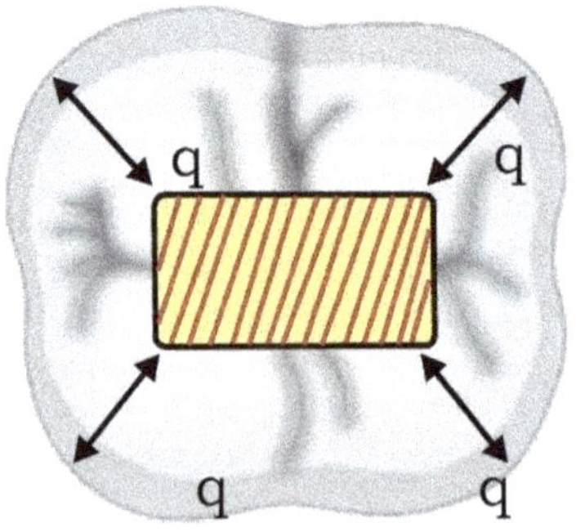

Fig. 9.24: Law of centrality

- The law of concentricity states that the axial walls of the pulp chamber are concentric to the external outline of the crown.

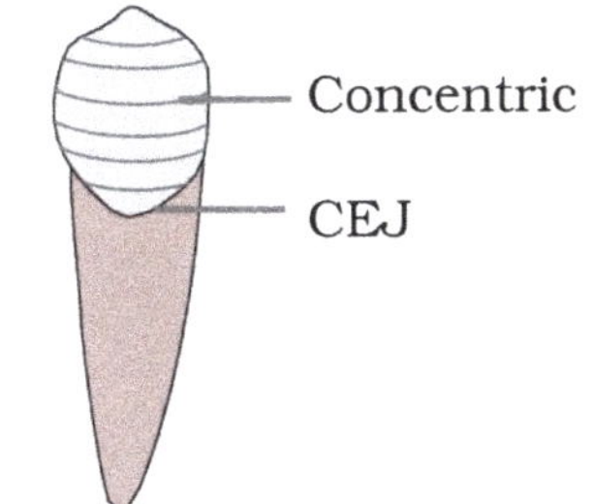

Fig. 9.25: Law of concentricity

- The pulp chamber is almost always directed mesially.

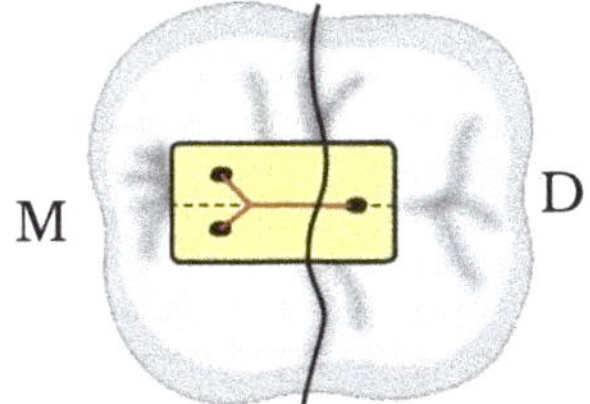

Fig. 9.26: Law of pulp chamber

- **The law of orifice location 1**
- The orifice is located at the terminus of the developmental fusion lines.

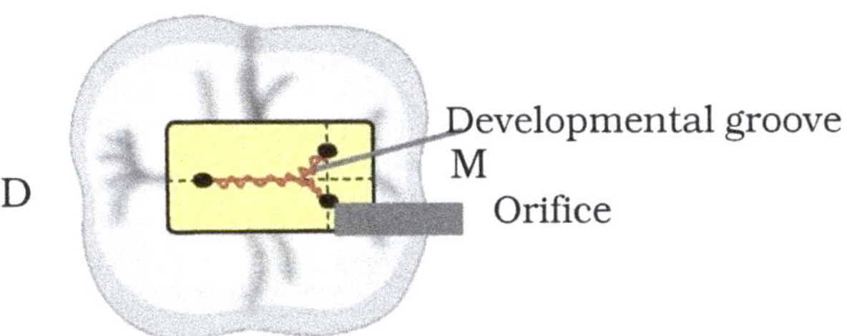

Fig. 9.27: Law I

- **The law of orifice location 2**
- Orifices are located at the junction of walls and the floor (line angles).

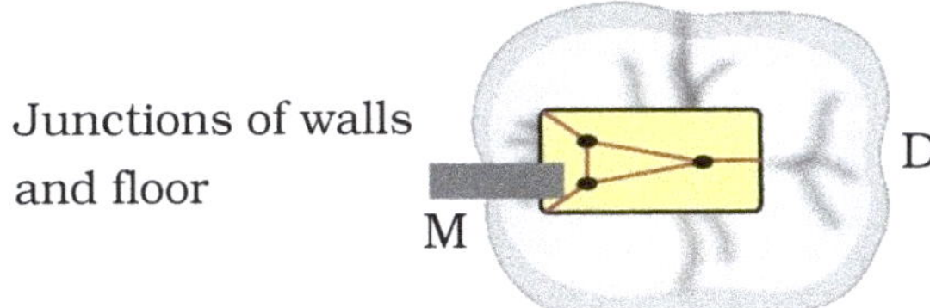

Fig. 9.28: Law II

- **The law of orifice location 3**
- Orifice are located at the angles at the junction of the floor and the walls (corners of the point angles)

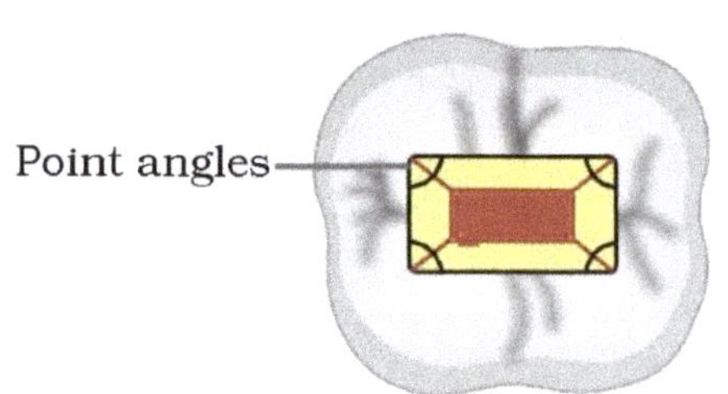

Fig. 9.29: Law III

- **Law of symmetry one**
- In all teeth, the orifice is located equidistant from a mesiodistal line drawn through the centre of pulp chamber except maxillary molars.

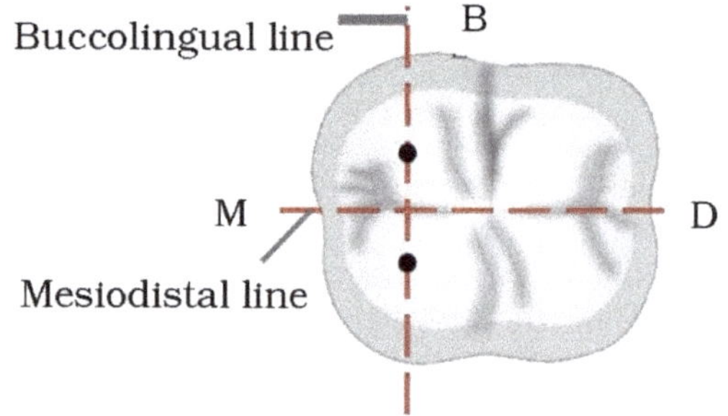

Fig. 9.30: Law of Symetry I

- **Law of symmetry two**
- The canals are located on the buccolingual line drawn perpendicular to the mesiodistal line.

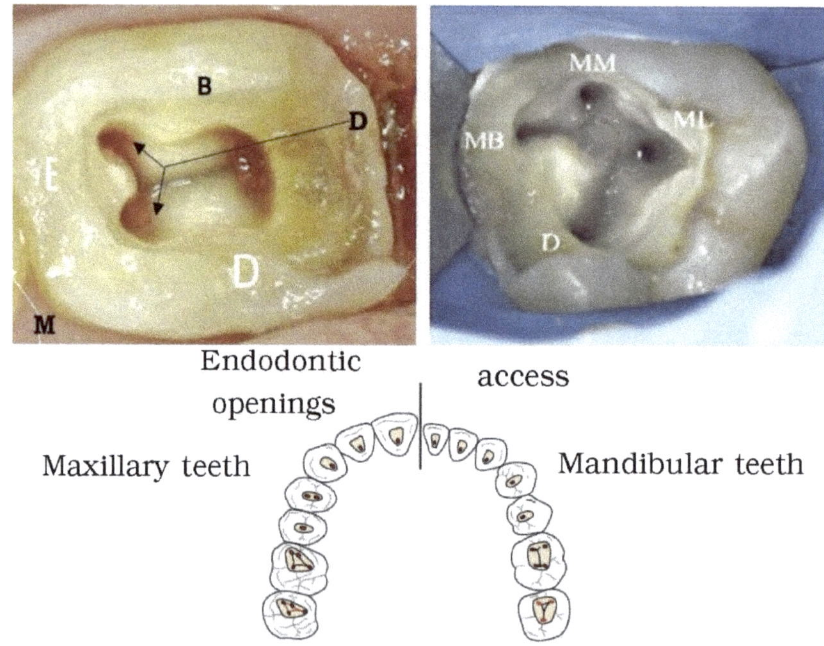

Fig. 9.31: Law of Symetry II

Aids for orifice location

One of the initial steps of endodontic treatment is preparing the access cavity The Holy Grail of the access preparation is to create a minimally invasive preparation that enables the identification of any given orifice and underlying root canal system. There are concepts, strategies, and armamentaria that drive clinical techniques. In turn, these techniques may be utilized for finding root canal orifices. Locating orifices facilitates negotiating and shaping canals, 3D cleaning, and filling root canal systems. The following represents, in no particular order, the more important strategies for identifying any orifice.

Anatomical familiarity: Knowledge, understanding, and appreciation for root canal system anatomy influence predictably successful endodontic treatment outcomes.

Radiographs: Even the best angulated film is a two-dimensional representation of a three-dimensional object. As such, well angulated periapical images should be taken in three horizontal planes: straight-on, mesioblique, and distoblique. For example, another canal is suspected when a file or obturation material is radiographically positioned asymmetrically within the long axis of any given root. Certainly, CBCT technology represents a major advancement in radiographic diagnostics and facilitates identifying aberrant, mineralized, or previously missed canals.

Vision: Magnification plus lighting equals vision. Traditionally, Magnification glasses, headlamps, and transilluminating devices have been used to enhance vision. Today, the dental operating microscope provides unsurpassed vision for identifying orifices.

Surgical length burs: Surgical long-length round burs move the visually-obstructive head of the handpiece further away from the occlusal table. Long-length round burs improve the line of sight along the shaft of the bur, promoting safety when searching for canals.

Access cavities: The access preparation should be prepared so that the operator can look in the mouth-mirror of a furcated tooth and visualize all of the orifices without moving the mirror. Importantly, axial walls should be flared, flattened, and finished to provide straightline access to the orifices.

Piezoelectric ultrasonics: The ultrasonic handpiece eliminates the bulky head of the conventional handpiece, which notoriously obstructs vision. Certain ultrasonic insert tips have abrasive surfaces for sanding away dentin and uncovering hidden orifices.

Micro-openers: Micro-Openers are flexible, stainless-steel hand files attached to an ergonomically designed off-set handle. Micro Openers provide unobstructed vision for initially penetrating and enlarging an offshoot that divides deep within a canal.

Test for orifice location

Dyes: Methylene blue is a water-soluble dye that can be irrigated into a dry pulp chamber. The dye is absorbed into orifices, fins and isthmus areas. This technique serves to visually "map" hard to-find orifices or certain coronal fractures.

Bubble test: When NaCl is flooded into the access cavity, it dissociates into Na+ and Cl- ions and liberates free oxygen. A positive "bubble," or "champagne" test signifies that NaOCl is reacting with pulpal tissue or residual viscous chelator, if used.

Transillumination: A fiber optic wand may be positioned cervically so that light is directed perpendicular to the long axis of a tooth. Identifying an orifice is, at times, improved by turning off any overhead light source.

Explorer pressure: The endodontic hand-held explorer should be strong, thin, and have a durable pointed tip. Firm explorer pressure provides a safe way to punch through a thin layer of secondary dentin and expose a hidden, receded, and more mineralized canal.

White line test: In necrotic teeth, dentinal dust frequently moves into any anatomical space, such as an orifice, fin, or isthmus, when performing ultrasonic procedures without water. This dust can form a white dot or line that provides a visible roadmap to, for example, an MB2 orifice/canal.

Red line test: In vital teeth, blood frequently emanates from an orifice, fin, or an isthmus area. Like a dye, blood serves to map and visually aid in the identification of the underlying anatomy below the pulpal floor.

Restorative disassembly: Removing a full-coverage dental restoration provides direct visualization of the underlying tooth preparation. Coronal disassembly improves the predictability of safely watering the pulp chamber and identifying any given orifice.

Perio-probing: Circumferentially probing the sulcus around a tooth is another important strategy for locating canals. Intersulcular probing can provide important information as to the emergence profile of the clinical crown and the orientational alignment of the underlying root.

Symmetry: In a furcated tooth, the orifices on the pulpal floor should be symmetrically positioned in relationship to each other and the external root surfaces. Appreciating the rules of symmetry will help to confirm that all the orifices and underlying canals have been identified. • Color: A dark, narrow line on the pulpal floor of a multirooted tooth provides a visual trail of color that leads to a canal orifice. Visually, an orifice or fin will generally appear darker in color compared to the surrounding dentin.

Use of dyes in locating root canal orifice location

Dyes: Methylene blue is a water-soluble dye that can be irrigated into a dry pulp chamber. The dye is absorbed into orifices, fins and isthmus areas. This technique serves to visually "map" hard to-find orifices or certain coronal fractures.

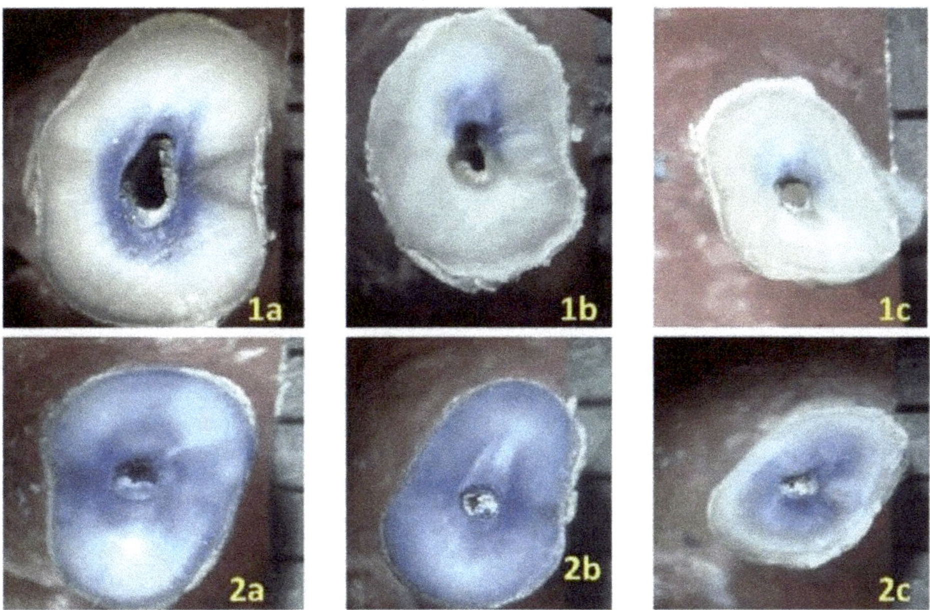

Fig. 9.32 :

The relationship between uninstrumented root canals and endodontic treatment has been studied extensively.

Locating all the canals, then subsequently shaping and cleaning them in their entirety has shown to be essential for predictable clinical and biological success.

High visual magnification and fibre optic illumination incorporated in the surgical operating microscope has revolutionized endodontic therapy.

The use of the SoM has facilitated the ease with which root canals are found in their typical as well as aberrant positions during orthograde endodontic treatment.

Although SOM is an indispensable aid in visualizing the detailed anatomy of the pulp chamber. It is essential to develop the visual acuity to appreciate the subtle differencesthat aid in the location of root canals.

The inherent colour differences between axial dentin and pulpal floor dentin, the coronal dentin and radicular dentin, as well as the differences in color and consistency between soft tissue and hard tissue will assist in locating the root canal orifice.

Although SOM is an indispensable aid in visualizing the detailed anatomy of the pulp chamber. It is essential to develop the visual acuity to appreciate the subtle differencesthat aid in the location of root canals.

The inherent colour differences between axial dentin and pulpal floor dentin, the coronal dentin and radicular dentin,as well as the differences in color and consistency between soft tissue and hard tissue will assist in locating the root canal orifice.

This is of even great importance in teeth with full coverage where the orientation markers of natural tooth cannot be seen, such as cusp tips, grooves and the external contours of the root outliners.

Other situations where the pulpal road map have been altered are teeth that have been previously endodontically treated where canals have been missed, where prior occlusal access has been made, altering the chamber floor anatomy and teeth with pulp chamber obliterations and canal calcifications.

Any help in terms of 'marking' the pulp tissue in canal orifices will facilitate the location of canals as both conventional and retreatment cases.

Fluorescein sodium is available as clear, orange red solution as sterile single dose disposable drops in cartons of 10 units.

There are no serious contraindications reported for its use topically except possible hypersensitivity.

How they work?

When dyes come in contact with vital or nonvital pulp tissue they are readily absorbed by the connective tissue elements of the pulp in the chamber and rootcanal system.

When exposed to blue light, these dyes dramatically fluoresce showing scattered tissue segments that contrast with surrounding monochromatic dentin.

It is the quality that makes them useful in location of pulp tissue I root canals especially in those that are calcified and have tissue remnants.

Technique

One straight line access is achieved and the coronal pulp tissue is removed, the pulp chamber is flooded with fluorescein sodium and allowed to contact all the walls for a couple of minute.

The excess is then suctioned away, with the incident light from the SOM turned off, blue light is used to illuminate the chamber.

With the aid of SOM the operator can now visualize the bright green fluorescence emitted by the pulp tissue that has absorbed the dye.

D) DETERMINATION OF WORKING LENGTH

*THERE IS NO LIMIT TO HUMAN POTENTIAL. EVERY
HUMAN DNA CARRIES MICROSCOPE IN IT
THERE IS NOTHING AS ACCURATE AS HUMAN SENSES ON FIRE.*

Introduction

Root canal treatment is a step by step procedure each step plays vital role in the outcome of treatment. Once the access cavity preparation is done, as soon as orifices are located we should know the exact length of the canal to confine our biomechanical preparation and obturation within the dentin, in order to accomplish this we need to determine the apical limit of the canal first, the proposed apical limit of the canal is cemental dentinal junction. If we terminate our biomechanical preparation and obturation short of cemental dentinal junction it will lead to incomplete disinfection, underfilling, poor apical seal, apical leakage and finally failure of root canal treatment. If we terminate our biomechanical preparation and obturation long, behind cemental dentinal junction that will lead to over instrumentation, over filling, poor wound healing ultimately poor prognosis. Hence precise determination of cemental dentinal junction and exact termination our procedure at it is most crucial for the success of treatment.

Definition

It is distance from a reference point on the coronal surface of teeth and cemental dentinal junction at which we must terminate biomechanical preparation and obturation.

Importance

1. Determines how far into the canal instruments are placed and worked.

2. Determines how far into the canal debridement, irrigation, disinfection and obturation are to be done.

3. It affects the degree of pain and discomfort the patient will feel during and after the treatment.

4. Limits the depth of obturation.

    Finally, it aids in determining success or failure of treatment.

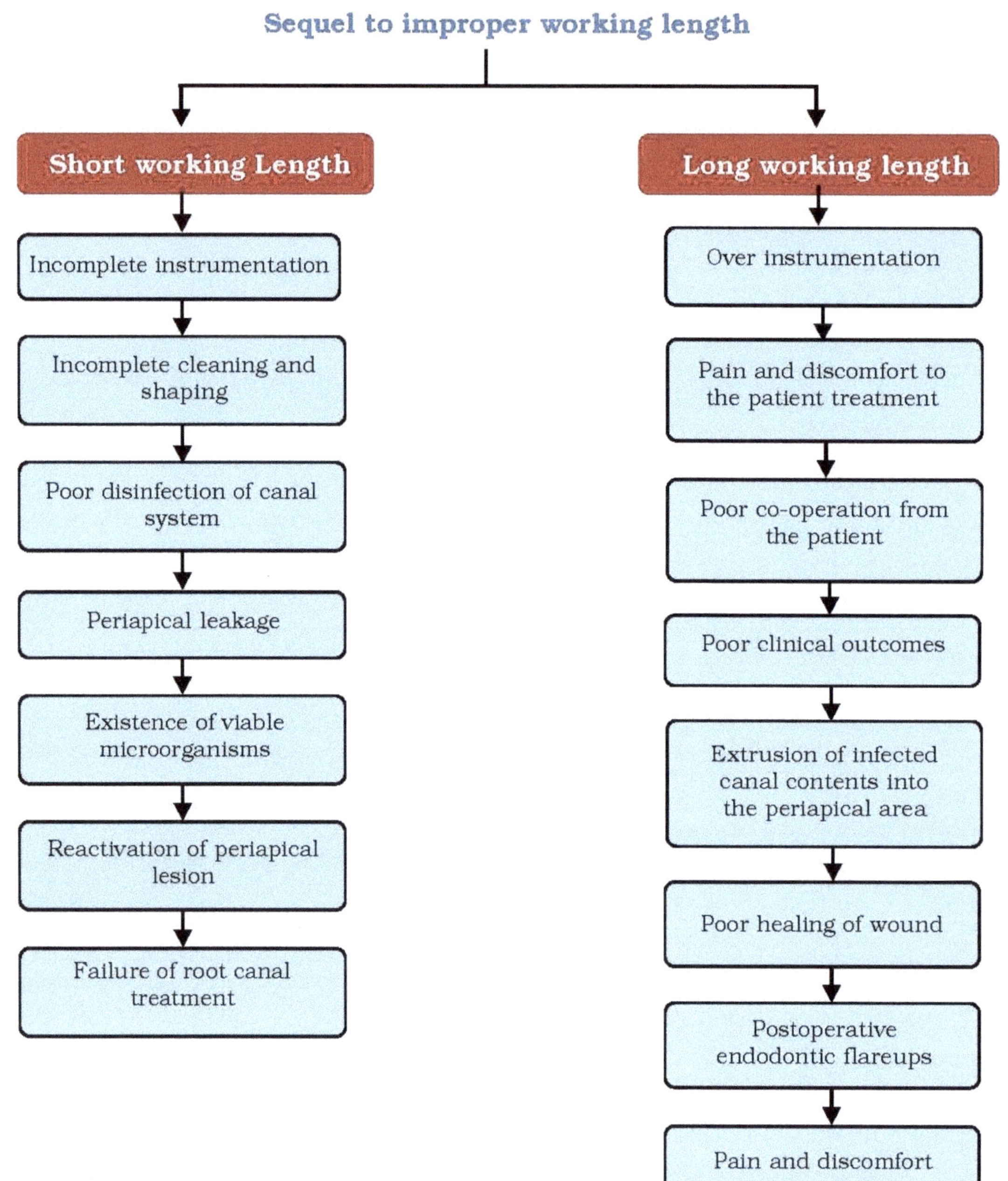

Methods of determining working length

Working length is a distance between a coronal reference point and cemental dentinal junction. Unless the working length determined precisely, disinfection and obduration of the root canal system cannot be accomplish accurately.

Prerequisite
Meticulous understanding of anatomy of root apex and able to determine cement dentinal junction.

The foundation to determine working length is to able to determine the end point of root canal. The recommended point is cemental dentinal junction for the following reasons it is challenging to determine the cemental dentinal junction.

It is a histologic land mark can be seen only in histologic sections

It is not a definite or defined point

It cannot be seen clinically or radiographically

It can be felt with digital tactile sense only when apical constriction coincides with it this occurs in 50 to 60% of cases

Knowledge of average anatomic length of all the teeth
Maxillary Central Incisor:

Length of tooth   :   Average: -23.3mm

Max Lateral Incisor :

Length of tooth   :   Average: -22.8mm

Mandibular Anterior Teeth :

Central Incisors: Length of tooth   :   Average-21.5mm

Lateral Incisors: Length of tooth   :   Average-22.4mm

Mandibular Canine: Length of tooth   :   Average-25.2mm

Average length of maxillary canine-27mm

Average length of mandibular canine-26mm

Pre-operative radiographs
Good, undistorted angled radiographs showing the total length and all roots of the involved tooth.

When two superimposed are present; either

A.   Take two individual radiographs with instruments placed in each canal.

B.   Take radiographs at different angulations usually 20-40 at degree horizontal angulations.

C.   Take radiographs applying slob rule that is exposed tooth from mesial or distal horizontal angle, canal which moves to same direction is lingual, whereas canal which moves to opposite direction is buccal.

D.   Insert two different instruments, K file in one canal, H file in another canal take radiographs at different angulations.

Straight line access to the root apex

It can be achieved by removing the dentinal triangles in the coronal segment and preflaring the cervical 1/3 of the canal. Straight line access reduces the effects of canal curvature on instruments like buckling and avoids the errors in working length determination.When small file is inserted in to the canal the handle position of the initial file should be upright paralleling on the long axis of the tooth.

Small stainless-steel K-file with stopper

The file must be small enough to facilitate the exploration of canal and negotiate the total length of canal and large enough not to be loose in the canal.

Definite reproducible reference points and stops

Coronal reference points

It is the site on the occlusal or incisal surface from which measurements are made :

For anterior teeth - incisal edges

For posterior teeth – buccal cusp tips.

As reference point is used throughout the canal preparation and obturation a definite reproducible plane of reference to an anatomic landmark on the tooth is necessary.

Must be stable -Don't use weakened enamel walls, diagonal lines of fracture and transitional restorations eg cements.

Diagonal surfaces should be flattened to give an accurate site for reference. weakened cusps or incisal edges must be reduced to well supported tooth structure.

Should not change between appointments and easy to identify and monitor between appointments.

Stops

Stopper should seat on the file perpendicular to long axis of handle of the file not oblique, tear drop shaped silicon stopper is preferred for the following reasons

It is radio-opaque

Does not need to be removed during sterilization

Enhances the visibility especially in curved canals

Apical reference point

Cemental dentinal junction

Note :

In long standing chronic periapical infections 0.3 to 0.6 mm beyond cemental dentinal junction better.

Practice and experience

Non electronic method

This method utilizes both radiographs and digital tactical sense to determine final working length

1. Radiographas

In this method radiographic apex root end is used as reference point hence quality of image is important for accurate interpretations.

The foundation of this method is <u>assumption</u> that cemental dentinal junction is located 1mm short of radiographic apex hence using this method solely to determine final working length is not recommended as it often gives inaccurate readings. It should be used in conjunction with other methods.

Advantages

1. It is the most popular and commonly used method
2. On radiographs we can see the anatomy of tooth, curvature of the canal, relationship between adjacent anatomic tooth structure and thus we can determine radiographic end of the tooth in a mesiodistal dimension easily.
3. Used in conjunction with other methods.
4. Gives estimated working length
5. Confirms final working length

   Comparatively inexpensive requires knowledge of anatomy of tooth and good quality radiographs and endodontic file with stopper.

Limitations

➢ Limited accuracy, a working length 1mm short of the radiographic apex may result in over or under instrumentation.

➢ Two-dimensional representation of a three-dimensional object.

➢ Technically sensitive in both its exposure and interpretation.

➢ Magnification (shortening or elongation) even with paralleling technique elongation of image has found to be 5%

➢ Distortion of image

➢ Apical foramina may exist buccally or lingually

➢ Superimposition of anatomical structures

➢ Time consuming

➢ Radiation exposure

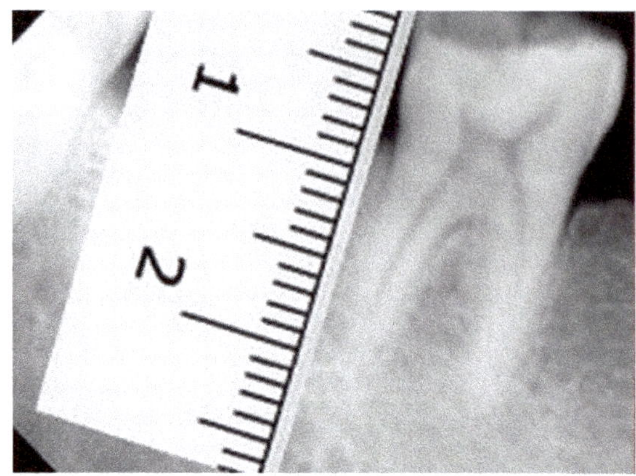

Fig. 9.33: Radiographic Tooth Length (RTL)

2. Digital Tactile sensation methods

In this method apical constriction is used as apical reference point which usually coincides with cemental dentinal junction and also the site of cemental dentinal junction is widely accepted as being 0.50mm to 0.75mm coronal to the apical constriction. This suggests most of the time cemental dentinal junction either located coronal to apical constriction or at apical constriction.

The foundation of this method is based on feeling of digital tactile sense against resistance. Although it may appear simple its accuracy depends on sufficient experience.

Technique

After access cavity preparation and establishing patency, an appropriate size file introduced in to the canal slowly in watch winding motion at around 1 to 2mm near the apex a tug or resistance will be felt, the area where resistance is felt is considered as apical constriction.

Advantages

a. Simple method

b. Not expensive gadgets only require attention and utilizes patience.

c. It develops with practice more the practice more the accuracy.

d. If done properly in conjunction with radiographic method it can be a most reliable method which gives final working length when used in conjunction with radiographs.

Limitation

It is ineffective in the following conditions

    ❖ In cases of open root apices

    ❖ In incompletely formed root apices

    ❖ In blunder buss canals

It is inaccurate in the following conditions

- ❖ If canal is constricted throughout its length
- ❖ In case of calcification.
- ❖ In sclerosed canals,
- ❖ In blocked canals especially at apical 1/3

Note :

If coronal segment of canal is constricted especially in curved canals pre coronal flaring coronal 1/3 canal is recommended.

Procedure of obtaining working length

Step 1

Determination of estimated working length by radiographs

The tooth is measured on the good quality radiograph to get radiographic tooth length RTL.

Subtract at least 1 mm "safety allowance" from radiographic tooth length to compensate for possible image distortion or magnification to get estimated working length EWL.

Example:

Suppose the RTL is 23 mm

EWL = 23mm – 1mm = 22 mm

This 22mm estimated working length is transferred to endodontic file with the help of devices like Endbloc, file mate and stopper is adjusted at this level.

Step 2

Determination of actual working length by digital tactile sense

Gently insert the file with preadjusted estimated working length into the canal. Go all the way until the stopper at the plane of reference and employ digital tactile sense near the apex usually within the range of 1 to 2mm you can feel the tug or resistance. The point where you feel the tug is minor constriction which is usually coincides with CDJ or located coronal to cemental dentinal junction, Expose, develop and clear the radiograph. On the radiograph the distance between tip of the file and radiographic apex is analyzed.

If the distance between tip of the file and radiographic end of apex is 0.5 mm then it is your final working length.

If the file has ended short and the distance between tip of the file and radiographic end of apex is more the difference is correct by adding that much differed length to the file and 0.5 to 1mm is subtracted from adjusted length to get final length a confirmatory radiograph is taken.

Example

Suppose the file is 2mm short the 2mm is added to estimated working length to get adjusted working length 24mm

$$2mm + 22mm = 24mm$$

from this 24mm adjusted working length 0.5 mm subtracted (CDJ is located 0.5 to 1mm from radiographic apex) to get final working of 23.5mm

$$24mm - 0.5mm = 23.5mm$$

This new final working length is transferred to endodontic file and a confirmatory radiograph is taken.

If the file has gone long beyond the apex and the distance between tip of the file and radiographic end of apex is negative the difference is correct by subtracting that much differed length from the file and a confirmatory radiograph is taken.

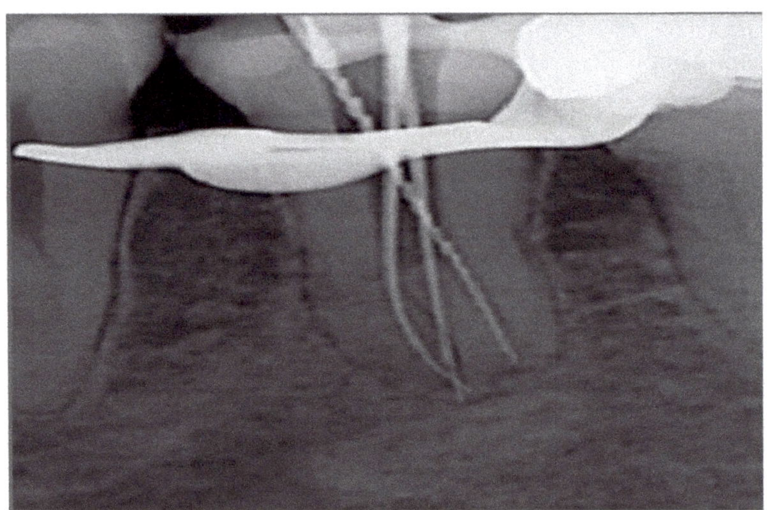

Fig. 9.34 : Actual working length and final wr---- length

Paper point method

This technique useful in open apex cases or towards the end preparation particularly in blown out apex cases. Recently millimeter markings have been added to paper points these paper points have markings at 18,19,20,22, and 24mm from the tip and can be used to estimate the point at which the paper point passes out of the prepared apical stop.

Indications

-    Root canal with immature apex
-    Cases in which apical constriction lost due to perforation or resorption
-    Blown out apices due to over preparation

Technique

Gently pass the blunt end of the paper point into the canal knowing that the canal has been cleared of all its contents, minute amount of blood or tissue fluid at the end of point is an indication that it has been inserted beyond cemental-dentinal junction or apical stop.

Note: Repeated points are used to determine the wet /dry points.

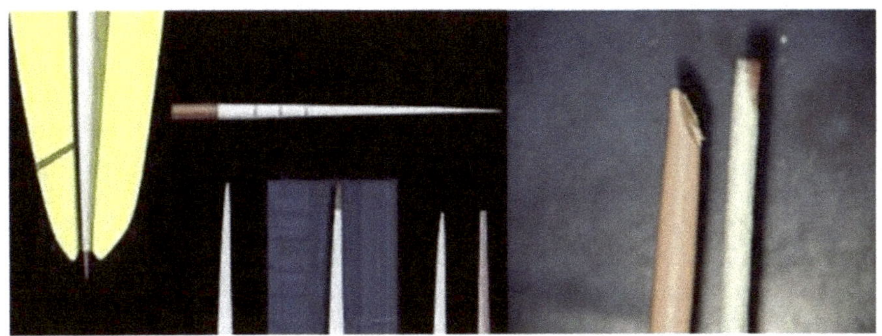

Fig. 9.35: Paper point method

False readings or unreliable data

- If the pulp not completely removed
- Periapical lesion rich in blood supply
- If the paper point left for a long time

Weine's modification

Based on the radiographic evidence of root and/or bone resorption

If no root or bone resorption is evident preparation should terminate standard 1mm from apical foramina.

If bone resorption is apparent but there is no root resorption shorten the length by 1.5mm as apical constriction would have been destroyed by resorption and would have moved coronally.

If both root and bone resorption is apparent shorten the length by 2mm as apical constriction would have been destroyed by resorption and would have moved more coronally.

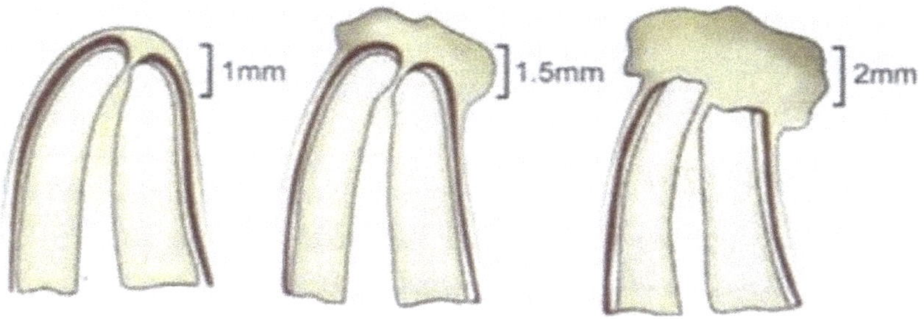

Fig. 9.36: Wein's modification

Electronic method

Apex locators or electronic apical foramen locator or electronic root canal length measurement device.

Introduction

It is challenging to determine the cemental dentinal junction first, it is a histologic land mark can be seen only in histologic sections, cannot be seen clinically or radiographically. Second, it is not a definite or defined point for the following reasons.

➢ Cemental dentinal junction is very rarely located at the apical constriction.

➢ The thickness of cementum varies greatly from one tooth another and between patents.

➢ The thickness of cement changes with physiology due to continued deposition of cementum with advancing age the cemental dentinal junction moves more coronally from the radiographic apex. The thickness of cement changes with pathologies such as preapical resorption due to periapical granulomas, periapical cysts, impacted tooth...etc.

Why apex locators?

90% of the time radiographical apex and anatomical apex do not match.

The major apical foramen deviates in the buccal and/or lingual plane difficult to locate its position even with multiplane angles.

Definition

An electronic device used to determine the position and location major apical foramen in order to determine the working length of the root canal.

Mechanism

The electrical resistance between the periodontal membrane and the oral mucosa is a constant of 6.5 kilo -ohms. The working length is determined by comparing the electrical resistance of the periodontal membrane with that of mucous membrane of the lip both of which should be similar.

Principle

Resistance: - complete opposition of electric current in direct current circuit is called resistance. Resistance does not depend upon frequency of direct current.

Impedance: - complete opposition of flow of current in alternate current circuit because of resistance and capacitance is called impedance. Impedance comprises of resistance and capacitance. Impedance depends upon frequency of alternate current, change in frequency leads to change in impedance, frequency can be single or multiple and it can be low or high, frequency can be used as simultaneously or separately.

Electronic apex locators use an electric circuit traversing through the endodontic canal and the patient's oral mucosa, to determine the location of apical foramen.

When circuit is complete, periodontal tissue contacted by the tip of the file resistance decreases markedly and current suddenly begins to flow and the event will be singled by a beep, buzz, flashing lights and digital readouts.

History

The idea of using apex locators was born when Custer in 1918 used electric current to measure length of root canals. Suzuki, in 1942 an experiment was conducted in dogs using direct current and discovered that electrical resistance between periodontal ligament and oral mucosa had a constant value of 6.5k ohm according to this postulation it was possible to design a device to measure the length of root canals electronically. An ohmmeter was used with one electrode connected to oral mucosa and as another electrode connected to endodontic file as the file moved into canal the tip of the file was just touching the PDL at apical foramen level the device registered 40 MA regardless of patient age or shape and length of tooth from these findings it is explanatory that it was necessary to pass the file through apical foramen to obtain accurate measurements. This would produce erroneous measurements as the variable could get eliminated. Based on these principles, first apex locators were introduced in reality these devices operate using human body one of the components to complete electric circuit. One of the electrodes of apex locators is connected to an endodontic file while the other is connected to labial mucosa of patient through the clip. Once the file is inserted into root canal the circuit partially completed and as file reaches upper electric circuit is completed. In 1962 Sunanda adopted the Suzuki principle, Inoue's significant contributions lead to the evaluation of sono-explorer.

The first generation of apex locators used direct current. Unfortunately, they were very inaccurate and unpredictable. Therefore in 1969 a Japanese company designed a device that used alternating current. This apex locator was called root canal meter and worked at frequency of 150 Hz; electrode therefore electrolytic substance sodium hypochlorite causes erroneous measurements when using these devices. The presence of electrolytes within in root canals prevents proper operations of all these devices. A significant breakthrough was achieved with introduction of new generations of apex locators. This third generation of electronic apex locators such as "index" calculates difference between 2 electrical impedances in canal using an alternating current composed of two different frequencies this apex locator can accurately measure the length of root canals even in presence of electrolytes. In this method EALs work in such way that if there is an electrolyte in canal two impedances are measured simultaneously by two electric current with different frequencies . Thus, if one of the impedances changes in canal the second one also changes in same proportion as ratio between frequencies is not affected even in presence of electrolytes. This device has the advantage of not having to be calibrated for each patient and makes it one of the efficient and versatile to use.

First generation apex locators

These apex locators use the resistance method for determining the working length basically these instruments measured the opposition to the flow of current hence the name resistance-based apex, based on the principles of Suzuki and Sunanda

Resistance value 6.5 kilo ohms eg. Root canal meter, Dento- meter, endodontic meter and endo Radar.

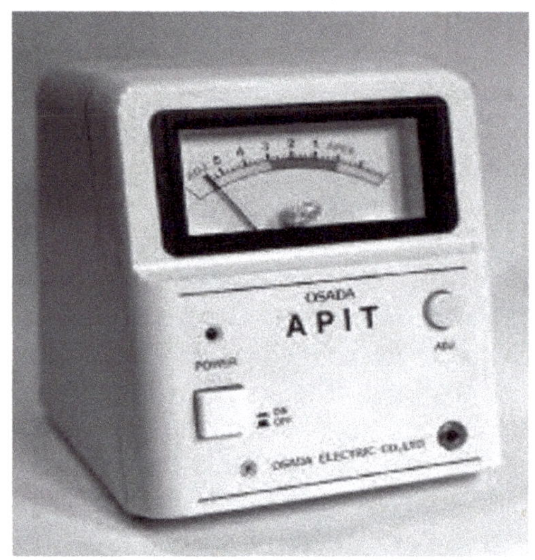

Fig. 9.37:

Advantages

1) Easy to operate
2) Uses K-type files
3) Digital readout -audible indications
4) Detect perforations
5) Built in pulp tester

Disadvantages

1) Requires a dry environment
2) There should be no caries or defective restorations
3) Requires calibration
4) Requires a lip clip with good contact
5) Patient sensitity and pain was felt during earlier models
6) Perforation can give false reading
7) Contraindicated in patient with pacemaker
8) Unreliable, electrolytes, exudates, hemorrhages, vital pulp tissue and excessive moisture caused inaccurate results.

Second generation of apex locators

These apex locators use the impedance method for determining working length basically these instruments measure the opposition to the flow of electric current (impedance) hence name impedance apex locators. Increasing electrical impedance across the walls of root canal greater apically than coronally CDJ level of impedance drops eg. Sonoexplorer, Endocater and Apex finder.

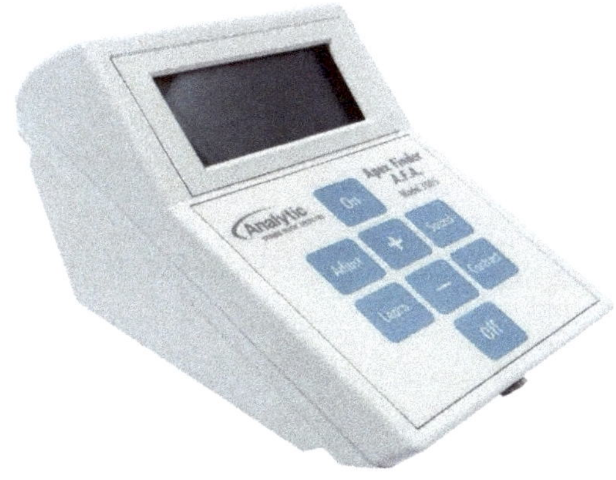

Fig. 9.38 :

Advantages

1)   Operate in fluid environment.
2)   No patient sensitivity
3)   Operated with RC Prep
4)   No lip clip
5)   Defect bifurcated canals
6)   Detect peroration
7)   Analogue meter

Disadvantages

1)   Requires calibration.
2)   Requires coated probes
3)   No digital readout
4)   Difficult to operate

Third generation

These apex locators use two frequencies instead of a single one to measure the impedance in order to determine the working length hence, name comparative impedance type. Measures impedance of tooth at two different frequencies. Coronal portion is constant. As the file advances the difference in the impedance value begins to differ greatly with maximum differences at apical area. eg Endex /Apit Root zx Apex finder AFA.

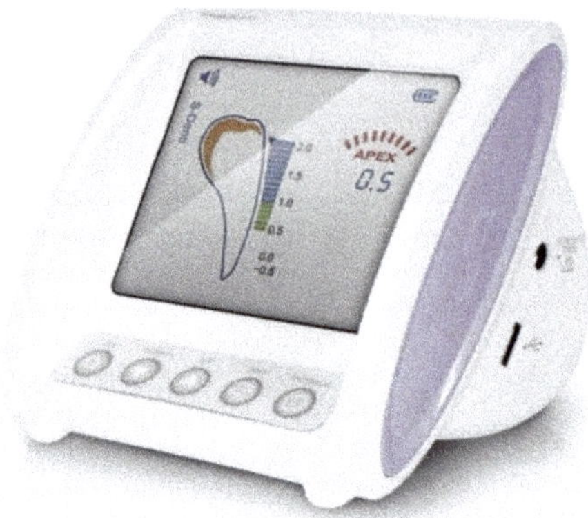

Fig. 9.39 :

Advantages

1) Easy to operate
2) Operates in fluid environment
3) Operates with RC prep
4) Low voltage electrical output
5) Analog readout
6) Audible indication
7) Uses K file

Disadvantage

1) Must calibrate each canal
2) Sensitive to canal fluid level
3) Needs fully charged battery

Fourth generation

These apex locators use multiple frequencies (2-5) to measure the impedance in order to determine the working length. Measures resistance and capacitance separately the **eg** Bingo 1020 / Raypex 4, elements diagnostic units.

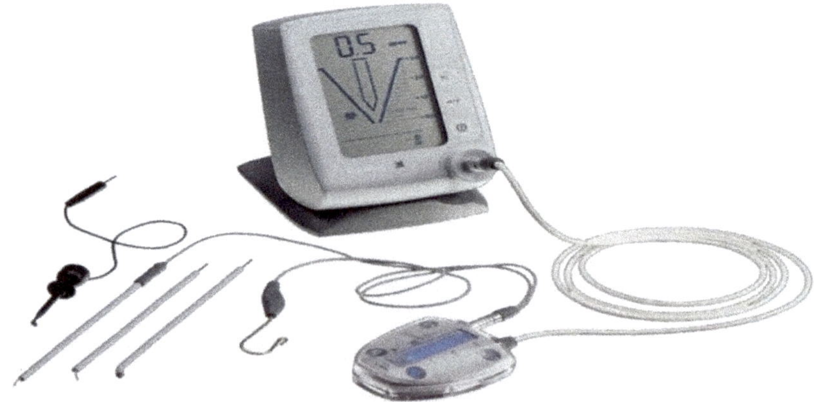

Fig. 9.40 :

Fifth generation

These apex locators use multiple frequencies rather than the dual frequencies of the third and fourth generation of apex locators to measure the impedance in order to determine the working length. Works in dry and wet canals and requires no calibrations.

Eg Ray apex 5 and propex II

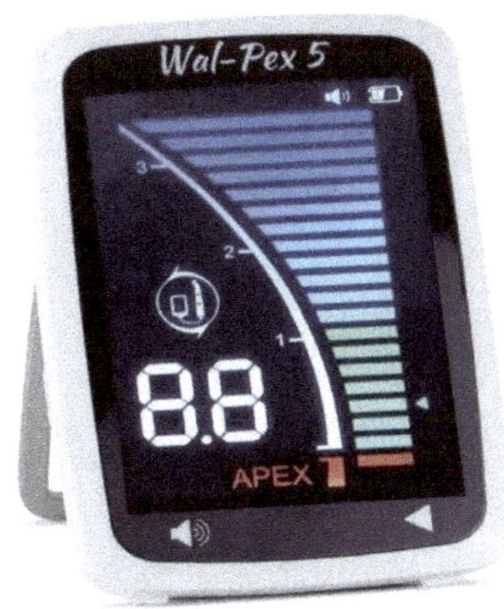

Fig. 9.41:

Sixth generation

Adaptive type

Classification based on type of current

1) **Direct current**

   OHM meter used by Suzuki and Sunanda

2) **Alternating current**

a) **Resistance type**

   Root canal meter, Dento- meter, endodontic meter and endo radar

b) **Impedance type**

   Sonoexplorer, Endocater and Apex finder

C) **Frequency type**

   1) **Ratio type**   a) Two frequencies

   Root ZX

   b) Five frequencies

   AFA and apex finder

   2) **Subtraction type**

   Endex and neosono ultma EZ

Uses

1) Particularly useful to determine the working length when the apical portion of the canal system is obscured by certain anatomical structures.
   - Impacted teeth
   - Tori
   - Zygomatic arch
   - Excessive bone density
   - Overlapping roots
   - Shallow palatal vault

2) Invaluable tool for
   - Detecting site of root perforations
   - Determination of perforations caused during post preparation,
   - Detecting all types of fractures
   - Detecting all types of resorption

3) Used in patients with gag reflexes and cannot tolerate X-ray films in patient with acute gag reflex taking radiographs is challenging EALS can provide invaluable assistance in such cases.

4) Useful in children, disabled patients, heavily sedated patients.

5) Can be used in teeth with incomplete root formation requiring apexification and to determine working length in primary teeth.

6) In pregnant ladies to reduce radiation exposure.

Basic conditions for accuracy of apex locators

- Canals should be relatively dry
- Canals should be free from debris
- There must be no cervical leakage
- No blockage or calcification of canals
- Proper contact of files with canal walls and peri apex

Parts of apex locators

- It is an electrically operated device which is usually battery-operated, has four parts
- The lip clip - needs to attach to the lip of patient
- The file clip –holds a file
- Electronic device with display screen - monitor display some markings in millimeter that shows apical anatomy of tooth
- A cord which connects the above three parts

Clinical technique/ Clinical steps

Routinely regular endodontic therapy starts with anaesthetizing the region and rubber dam isolation. Then an endodontic access is prepared, pulp tissue is removed from chamber and canal orifices are located then the chamber and canal are irrigated with sodium hypochlorite solution.

Step 1

Choose a no 6/8/15 size K file depending upon the size of canal, the file should be snuggly fitting (contact the both walls of canal) and longer size file is chosen as we need some space for the file holder and file.

Step 2

Attach the file to the file clip, there is a push button on file holder of file clip, place hook between stopper and handle.

Step 3

Attach lip hook on the opposite of root canal treating tooth, make sure that the lip clip is in stable contact with the lip.

Step 4

Put the apparatus on and checking the battery of apex locators and calibrating, it if required (most recent models of EALS do not require to be calibrated).

Step 5

The file is gently introduced in canal until, it reaches estimated working length. The Files can also be introduced to EWL following coronal pre-flaring of canals. It is always helpful to remove calcification and dentinal savings which may have negative impact on accuracy of EALS. Pre-flaring of canals prior to working length measurement may increase the accuracy of these devices.

Step 6

- As the file progresses deep in the canal the apex locator beginning to indicate that file is short, beyond or at working length. It needs to be adjusted accordingly until indicates the file is at working length.

- A faster beeping means it is at the apical constriction - first half the green zone

- A solid tone means it is long beyond the apical constriction - Red zone

- A slow beeping means it is short of apical constriction - Blue zone

- For an accurate reading it is recommended to introduce file slightly beyond the foramen in order to make sure that file has reached the PDL and then pull the file back to adjust the working length at apical constriction. That is go long in to the red zone, and back out to the first half the green zone, keep pulling and pushing in watch winding motion until the screen displays 0.0 reading.

- Usually 0.0 reading happens at the junction end of green zone and beginning of red zone or may vary between bars of green zone.

- Procedure is repeated several times until we confirmed 0.0 reading on the screen. Once the reading has been confirmed, remove the file holder adjust the silicon rubber stopper to the referral cusp or plane. Take the file out of the canal carefully without moving the rubber stopper. Measure the length of the file on endobloc and subtract 0.5mm from it. That will be our final working length.

- It is noteworthy that if their sudden changes in reading it is possible that there is flooding or a lot of liquid in the chamber or the file is touching a metal restoration. Drying the chamber may overcome this problem. Special attention is made to remove any metal restoration that comes into contact with the files that are used to make measurements, the contact of these files with metallic elements transmits electricity directly to adjacent periodontal area. There the apex locator will provide wrong measure.

Precautions

- Pulp chamber must be dry: -Should not be wet
- Canals should be dry or relatively moist: -should not be completely dry
- Always use the largest endodontic file possible; -the file should be in contact with both walls of canal
- Make sure the decay in the tooth is completely removed: - electric resistance of decay is different when file touches decay the apex locator may read it as apex
- Pull your file away from metallic fillings or crowns before taking your readings: -cover the shaft of file with Teflon or rubber sleeve
- Check the batteries regularly before use
- Go to zero readings then subtract
- Use your apex locator throughout the procedure

Problems associated with electronic apex locators

1) Unstable electronic signal with rapid wandering signs

Unstable electronic signal with rapid wandering signs can happen due to presence of metallic restorations in crowns or leakage of fluids through the cervical portion of crown.

Remedy: - If it is due to metallic restorations –Remove the metallic restoration or cover the shaft of the file with plastic shelves.

If it is due to cervical leak do pre-endodontic build up and blow the air into chamber.

2) Sharp drop of signal at apical foramen

Sharp drop of signal at apical foramen can occur due to very dry canals resultant from no electric contact is happening drop abruptly occur when it reaches apical foramen this phenomenon called as "Apex -circuit breaks out".

Remedy: - Make the canals slightly moist then measure the working length.

3) Apex sign from beginning

If you see that apex sign right from the beginning it may be due to severely bleeding or exudation from the canals.

It can also be due to excessive electrolyte in the canals.

Remedy: - If it is due to severely bleeding or exudation from the canals. Irrigate the canals gently with sodium hypochlorite and saline until drainage stops.

If it is due to too much electrolytes: - Reduce quantity of electrolytes.

4) Premature reading, open apex

Sharp drop in impedance due to thin dentinal walls.

Remedy: - Relay on non-electronic methods of working length determination.

Effects of some conditions on accuracy of apex locators

Regardless of the mechanism of the device, the best results were found when electronic root canal length measurement was performed at the apical foramen.

Pulp conditions

Electronic apex locators were more accurate in vital teeth than in necrotic ones, pupal conditions did not affect the accuracy of EALS.

Periodontitis

Ability of the root ZXII to detect the apical foramen in teeth with apical periodontitis

Presence of defects in the periapical area did not affect the accuracy of the root ZXII.

Canal patency

Canal patency appears to be more important as dentin debris may disrupt the electrical resistance between the inside of the canal and the periodontal ligament. Constant recapitulation and irrigation ensure accurate electronic length reading during instrumentation.

Size of apical foramen

Size of apical foramen has an influence on electronic length determination, the root ZX apex locator is accurate under a diameter apical size of 0.6mm. In case of 0.7 to 0.8 mm, we must adjust the files to the foramen to maintain accuracy whereas above size 0.9mm the device is not accurate.

Immature apex

In immature apex or blunderbuss apices tend to give short measurements electronically due to the instruments not touching the apical dentine walls.

Resorptions

Possible destruction of apical constriction and loss of surrounding PDL, dependent on operators experience   root ZX locate root end consistently even with resorption lacunae.

Root fractures

Any connection between the root canal and the periodontal membrane will be recognized by the EALS are excellent tool in these circumstances.

The root ZX was more accurate in the detection of horizontal root fractures and vertical root fractures than the other EALS tested.

Presence of calcium hydroxide in the canals

Presence of calcium hydroxide residues did influence the accuracy adversely.

Pacemakers

The recent apex locators (those developed after 2002) did not interfere with the functioning of any of the cardiac devices tested.

Advantages: -

1.   Provide objective information with high degree of accuracy
2.   Used when apical portion of canal is constricted
3.   Beneficial in reducing number of radiographs required to determine WL
4.   Patient exposed to radiation is reduced
5.   Provides greater precision in locality apical foramen.
6.   54% reduction of times is reported compared to conventional radiographs.
7.   Apex locators can be used at any stage if required for several times during instrumentation to verify whether WL remains stable.
8.   In multirooted teeth EALS can be helpful in lessening uncertainties
9.   Devices are mobile, light weight and easy to use.
10. 93 to 97 % accuracy.

Limitations: -

Apex locators do not work properly in the following conditions

a.   Presence of metallic restoration

b.   Presence of fluids

c.   Saliva in contact with file

d.   Presence of calcium hydroxide in the canals

e.   Profuse bleeding

f.   Open apices

g.   Lack of patency, due to the accumulation of dentinal debris, calcifications, blockage of canals with remnants calcium hydroxide, sealers, gutta-percha.

Other limitations

1.   Some patients have sensed electrical impulses when apex locators are used although common

2.   They are expensive than their predecessors

3.   Technique requires operator to be familiar with the equipment and learn how to interpret it.

4.   Learning curve is required:-

   like any new instrument the apex locators require a period of learning to use them effectively.

Disadvantages

a.   Accuracy limited to mature root apices.

b.   Extensive periapical lesion can give faulty readings.

c.   Weak batteries can affect accuracy.

d.   Though latest designs apex locator cannot interfere with the functioning of artificial cardiac pacemakers should be used cautiously.

Clinical consideration

It is most important critical step in endodontic therapy because improper working length leads to either under shaping which results in inadequate cleaning, poor disinfection and under obturation or over shaping which results in over instrumentation and over obturation thereby leading to failure of root canal hence following factors should be considered.

➤   Before determining a definitive working length, the coronal access to the pulp chamber must provide an unobstructed straight-line pathway into the canal orifice.

➤   Modifications in access preparation may be required to permit the instruments to penetrate unimpeded up to the apical constriction.

➢ Monitor the working length periodically and maintain the same working length throughout the entire length of root canal procedure. Because working length may change as curved canal is straightened

Causes of loss of working length

- The accumulation of dentinal and pulpal debris in the apical 2 to 3mm of canal.
- Failure to maintain the apical patency of canal.
- Failure to do recapitulation, skipping the instrument sizes, or failing to irrigate apical one third of canal.
- Occasionally, working length is lost owing to ledge formation or to instrument separation and blockage of the canal.

Working width

Endodontic Working Width: Current Concepts & Techniques

- In a relatively round canal, Minimum initial working width and Maximum initial working width are approximately same.
- In an oval, long oval, or flat canal, Maximum initial working width is several times larger than Minimum initial working width at different levels of the canal.
- In a maxillary cuspid (before instrumentation), Minimum initial working width may be the same as Maximum initial working width at zero, whereas Maximum initial working width at 2, may be four times larger than Minimum initial working width. On the other hand, after instrumentation, Minimum initial working width at zero may be the same as Maximum initial working at zero (considering no significant transportation). However, the ratio between Maximum initial working at 2 and Maximum initial working width at 2 may be altered by mechanical preparation of the canal.

Descriptions of the Horizontal Dimensions (Cross Sections) of the Root Canal

1) **Round (circular) canal :** Maximum initial working width equals Minimum initial working width.

2) **Oval canal :** Maximum initial working is greater than Minimum initial working width.

3) **Long oval canal:** Maximum initial working is two or more times greater than Minimum initial working width.

4) **Flattened (flat, ribbon) canal:** Maximum initial working is four more times greater than Minimum initial working width.

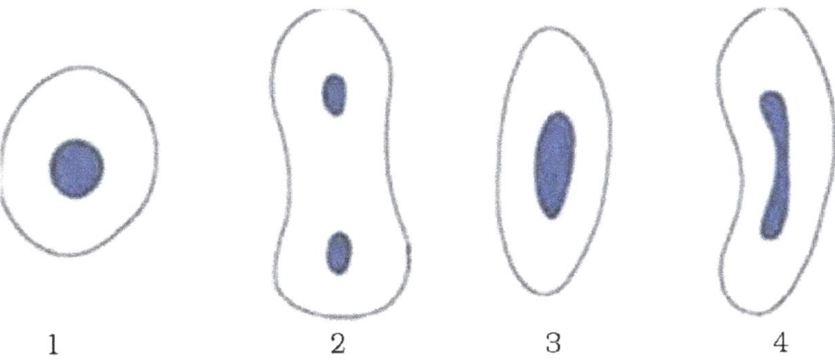

Fig. 9.42:

- ## Determination of Initial Working Width at Working Length

First determine the preoperative canal diameter by passing consecutively larger instruments to the WL until one bind. This initial apical file estimation is referred to as the determination of Maximum initial working width at zero. Then, the master apical file size is suggested to be three ISO file sizes larger than that initial binding file. But this concept is being questioned as recent studies suggest that the first K file that binds at the WL did not accurately reflect the diameter of the apical canal. The inaccuracy and discrepancy is the result of various morphologic and procedural factors as each of the factor discussed further can affect the clinician's tactile sense.

Canal morphology

Canal morphology is a critically important part of root canal therapy. Various in vitro studies have recorded the scales and average sizes of root canals, but only few clinical attempts have been made to determine the working width (WW). Sectioning of all levels of the teeth and making section plane exactly perpendicular to the canal curvature is a difficult task. Therefore, most morphometric studies cannot exactly depict the horizontal dimensions of root canal system. Until recently, most investigations have involved counting the number of canals and foramina and categorizing the canals on the manner in which they join or split. Current studies focus more on the shape of the canal systems and its clinical implications than on the actual preoperative size of the canal (8). The horizontal dimension of the root canal system is not only more complicated than the vertical dimension but also more difficult to investigate because it varies greatly at each vertical level canal.

The Round canal can be measured more easily because the minimum initial working width and maximum initial working width are the same however, other factors make initial working width (WW) determination difficult, even in straight canals. To determine the minimum initial working width of the oval, long oval, and flat canals, we may need instrumentation and tactile sensation. The presence of undetected lingual canal or an untreated isthmus may be responsible for endodontic failure of lower incisors. The prevalence of two canals in mandibular incisors has been found to be 11.5% -44.1%, although many merge into single canal in the apical 1-3 mm of the root, factors affecting the determination of working width at working length. Sectioning of root is the most common method for evaluating the shape of the canal. Cross sections at different levels in a root allow direct viewing of canal shape and position with regard to the borders of the root surface.When using an instrument to measure working length (WL), the longer the canal, the higher the friction resistance, In a very lang canal (>25 mm), the friction resistance may increase to affect the tactile sense of the clinician to determine the IWW correctly. In addition, if the coronal flare is foo conservative or limited to the coronal third of the canal, then shaft of the instrument may engage the canal wall and lead to a false premature conclusion regarding WW.

Canal taper

Any discrepancy between the gauging instrument and canal due to tapering can cause an early engagement of the canal wall with the instrument, leading to a false sensation of apical binding.

The tapering or the canal may increase due to early coronal flare, however, the tapering discrepancy between the gauging instrument and canal wall may decrease the last 3-5 mm of the canal has parallel walls, making accurate determination of WW. The root canal content may be fibrous or calcified material (calcific metamorphosis) creating different degrees of frictional resistance against the gauging instrument. This eventually affects the tactile sense of the clinician to determine the WW accurately.

Canal curvature

Curved canals can cause deflection of the gauging instrument and increase friction resistance. The curvature of the root canal can be categorized into two dimensional, three dimensional, small radius, large radius, and double curvature (S-shaped, Bayonet shaped) and with different degree of severity. Each of these curvatures has a different effect on a clinician's tactile sense. The combination of these curvatures make correct determination of Initial Working Width extremely difficult, if not possible. In curved mandibular premolars, the study indicated that the first K file and the first speed instrument that bound at the Working Length failed to accurately reflect the diameter of the apical canal. Careful canal preparations is an important part of successful root canal therapy.

The ability to enlarge a canal without deviation from the original canal curvature in a primary objective in endodontic instrumentation. It has been stated that the final preparation should be an exact replica of the original canal configuration in shape, taper and larger. After studying the effects of several instrumentation techniques, it is noted that every file, whether precurved or straight, tended to straighten within the canal they reported at the largest amount of apical canal preparation occurred at the outer portion of curvature, away from the furcation.

An attempt to solve this problems has led to the development of various instrumentation technique like step back, crown down, balanced force, and curvature filling etc in addition several instruments like K flex, flex arc, flex-o, Protaper, race files, light speed, hero shaper hands and rotary files have been designed. This instruments aim at alleviating procedural difficulties at coronal, middle, apical regions.

The Schneider method is the primary technique used to measure Canal wall irregularities.

Attached pulp stones, denticles and reparative dentin can create convexities on the canal wall surface.

Resorption can produce concavities on the canal wall surface. These phenomena conserve as an impacting factor that induces a false estimation of the true canal dimension at working length and other levels.

Instrument for determining initial working width.

The rigidity and tapering of the instrument used for determining WW can affect accuracy. Any tapering discrepancy between the gauging of instrument and canal may lead to an early instrument engagement of the canal wall altering the tactile sensation.

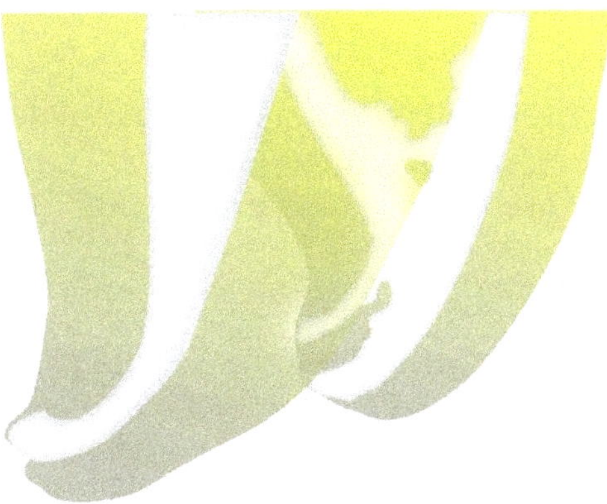

Fig. 9.43:

Eliminating the influence of affecting actors

Prior to determining the initial working width (WW), the orifices should be widened for early coronal flaring (crown down, double flaring), which ensures effective irrigation and minimizes any interferences with tactile sensation.To avoid interference and to achieve better results, an adequate instrument with maximal flexibility and minimal taper should be used. The exact outline of the horizontal dimensions of the root canal should be followed by root canal preparation at every level of the canal. To minimize incomplete cleaning of the root canal system, circumferential preparation or instrumentation need to be taken into consideration. A continuous reaming action of most of the nickel titanium (NITI) rotary instruments makes the canal relatively circular. Incomplete cleaning of the root canal system may be a result of imprudent use of the NiTi rotary instruments alone, which leads to failure of the endodontic therapy.

Determination of the Minimal and Maximal Final Working Width at Working Length

A final working width is required for bacteria and their substrates removal, and also for dead pulp tissue removal. Further, it is necessary to increase the capacity of the root canal to retain a larger sterilizing agent and also to prepare the tooth to receive the canal filling to increase the success rate of the treatment, it is essential to remove the infected dentin.

For this purpose, the instruments and techniques used in retaining the original shape of the canal to maximize the cleaning effectiveness and minimize unnecessary weakening of tooth structure.

How Do We Know When The Final Apical Instrument Size Is Reached?

By instrumenting and cross sectioning many teeth, it has been concluded that no technique is perfect, and a correct WW is a clinical judgment. However, instrument that meets resistance 45 mm short of working length (WL) and then requires a firm push to reach WL closely approximates the correct WW.

The instrument that approximates the correct WW the final apical size.

Rotary system has been found to be very important for achieving larger apical preparations safely. In its original form (stainless steel and hand driven). NITI rotary system evolved through the 1990s and 2000s from improvements made to the earlier versions.

Majority of rotary systems comprise a very short cutting blade, a non-cutting pilot tip, and a smooth flexible taperless shaft. This provides maximum flexibility to negotiate curves and cut dentin from canal walls, maintaining canal anatomy without the need for excessive mid-root or coronal over enlargement. Because only the very tip of the instrument comes in contact with canal walls, the tactile sensation is incomparable. Rotary system is extremely safe because of its safety release feature aids the instrument to separate at the handle instead of at the tip when excessive twisting forces are encounterd.

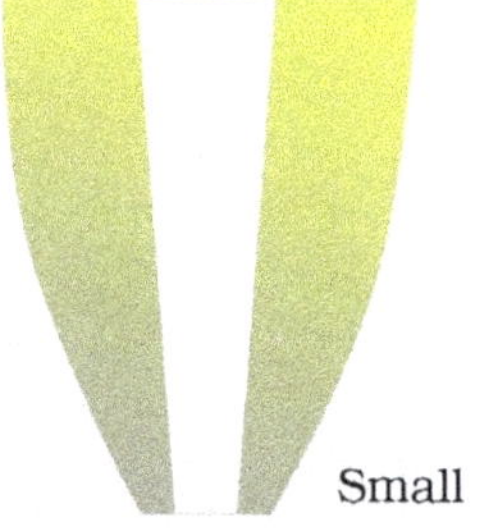

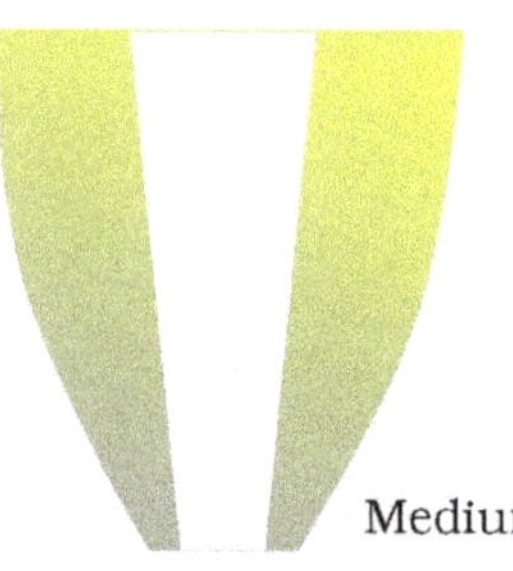

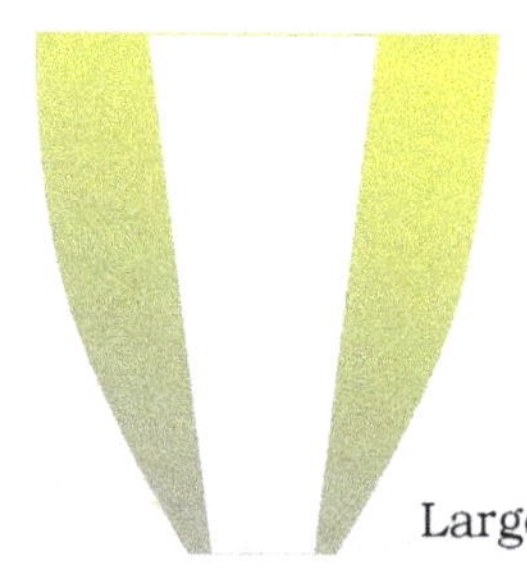

Fig. 9.44:

E) SHAPING

> MORE THE HEALTHY DENTIN REMOVED LESS IS THE TOOTH SAVED.
>
> WITH THIS AWARENESS, COMES CHOICES.
>
> CHOICES CREATE STRATEGY.
>
> STRATEGY IS THE KEY TO SUCCESS.

Shaping serves the objective of endodontics that is eliminating and preventing apical periodontitis by facilitating three-dimensional disinfection and air tight obturation of the root canal system. Too large shapes more than required compromises the integrity of tooth by removing excessive dentin there by influences the long-term surveillance of tooth. Too small shapes less than required compromises effective three-dimensional disinfection and air tight seal (obturation) leading to poor prognosis. We propose adequate shaping not too large or not too small, the tip of the irrigating needles should reach till apex or part way till apex to effectively eliminate biofilm from canal walls especially at apical 1/3. We should consider following factors before shaping.

The adequate shaping technique is determined by the following factors:

1) Purpose of shaping
2) Status of tooth in question
3) Age of patient
4) Severity of infection
5) Anatomy of canals
6) Type of material used during obturation
7) General health of patient

1) Purpose of shaping

Intentional root canal treatment	–	Before placing prosthetic bridges in patient with highly placed pulp horns, large pulp chambers, patients with hypersensitivity and patient with deep bites
In smaller canals (narrower)	–	Maximum preparation with 2% taper
In larger canals (broader)	–	Maximum preparation with 4% taper

2) Status of tooth

Vital non necrotic tooth requires less taper preparation smaller canals with 2% taper and larger canals with 4% taper. Whereas non-vital necrotic tooth requires more taper preparation minimum 4% and maximum 6% to 8% depending upon severity of infection.

3) Age of patient

The taper decreases with advance in age because:

A) Size and width of canals decreases with age.

B) Number of accessory canals, lateral canals, multiple foramina decrease with age.

C) Number and diameter of dentinal tubules and their permeability decreases with age.

   All these factors create less favorable environment for bacterial surveillance and multiplication

4) Severity of infection

More the severity of infection greater the taper preparation to eliminate

biofilm on the canal walls – minimum 6% and maximum 8%

Examples

In cases of Acute alveolar abscess, chronic alveolar abscess, periapical granuloma, infected radicular cyst, phoenix abscess and Re-root canal cases.

Lesser the severity of infection, smaller the taper preparation – minimum 4% and maximum 6%

Examples

In cases of initial and late stages of irreversible pulpitis, chronic hyperplastic pulpitis, internal resorption.

5) Anatomy of canals

Narrow and smaller the canal lesser taper preparation is required – Minimum 2% and maximum 4%.

Examples

In cases of Mesial roots of lower molars, Buccal roots of upper molars, Multi rooted premolars or any other multi rooted teeth, Mandibular incisors.

Broader and larger canals require more taper preparation. Minimum 4% and maximum 6%

Examples

In cases of Palatal roots of upper molars, Distal roots of mandibular molars, Upper anteriors, Lower cuspids.

6) Type of obturating materials

- Gutta percha requires continuous tapering funnel with round apical seat at apex. Due to its semi solid soft flexible nature more the taper easier and better would be the condensation.
- Bio ceramic exhibits flow and dentin bonding properties, even in narrow taper it easily slides and adheres to the canal walls nicely.
- Metal cones like silver points, stainless steel points and platinum points easily get into the narrowest taper due to their rigidity.
- So gutta percha requires more taper preparation compared to bio ceramic materials.
- Bio ceramic require more taper preparation compared to metal cones.

7) General health of patient

Patients with compromised immunity requires more instrumentation to disrupt and remove the biofilm.

Examples:

In cases of: uncontrolled diabetes, Patient on long term corticosteroids therapy, HIV and other immune deficit patients.

In pediatric patients and children unnecessary over shaping should be avoided because thickness of dentin is less, pre-existing natural taper is more and finally immunity and healing ability is high.

OBJECTIVES OF SHAPING

Biological

- Complete elimination of infected tissues.
- Should facilitate smooth and effective irrigation.
- Should provide adequate space for obturating materials.
- Should facilitate three-dimensional air tight seal.
- Should provide adequate space for intracanal medicaments.

Mechanical

- Should flow with the natural curvature of the canal.
- Apical constriction should be as small as possible. (avoid apical perforation). Original position of apical foramina should be maintained. (avoid zipping and apical transportation).
- Overall preparation should be as conservative as possible.

F) MANUAL SHAPING TECHNIQUES

> *CARE IS THE CORNERSTONE TO SUCCESS.*
> *CARE DEMANDS RIGHT CHOICES.*
> *RIGHT CHOICES REQUIRE RIGHT KNOWLEDGE, PATIENCE,*
> *COMMITMENT AND CONCERN.*

1. Step back technique/telescopic technique/bottom to top technique/apexo coronal technique/manual technique.

   It is the basic most important and commonly used method of shaping.

Indications

- If there is no access to rotary files like in cases of trismus and patient with limited mouth opening.

- Mesio angularly angulated 2nd & 3rd molar teeth where there is more risk of separation of rotary files.

   Inability to own glide path. (minimal canal preparation which is must before using rotary due to various reasons like very narrow canals, ledge formations, broken instruments so on).

- To shape and disinfect the canal surfaces untouched by rotary files

   like Bucco lingual canal surfaces of upper and lower anterior.

- Teeth with elliptical or oval root apices in conjunction with rotary files.

- Preparation of apical 1/3 of doubly curved canals as much as possible before introducing rotary files to prevent instrument separation.

- Negotiation and preparation of extremely curved canals like S shaped canals, ribbon shaped canals and C shaped canals.

- In sudden sharp curves which starts at the cervical or middle third of the canal.

Advantages

- Better tactile awareness.
- Keeps the apical preparation small.
- Avoids stripping and zipping.
- Conservation of more dentin.

It is done in two phases

1) Apical one third preparation

The apical one third is enlarged to develop the apical stop of size of three times larger than the first binding file. If the first binding file is 2% 6k ile then the master apical file would be 10. (sequence 6, 8, 10).

Suppose first binding file is 2% 10 K size file then the master apical file would be 20. (sequence 10, 15, 20).

Suppose first binding file is 15 then master apical file would be 25 (sequence 15, 20, 25).

2) Preparation of coronal two third (cervical one third and middle one third)

It involves the preparation of the rest of thecanal by sequentially increasing the size of the files by decreasing the working length. It involves preparation of continuous widening taper. Suppose master apical file is 20 then the sequence would be 25, 30, 35.

Suppose master file is 15 then the sequence would be 20, 25, 30.

Suppose the master apical file is 10 then

The sequence would be 15, 20, 25.

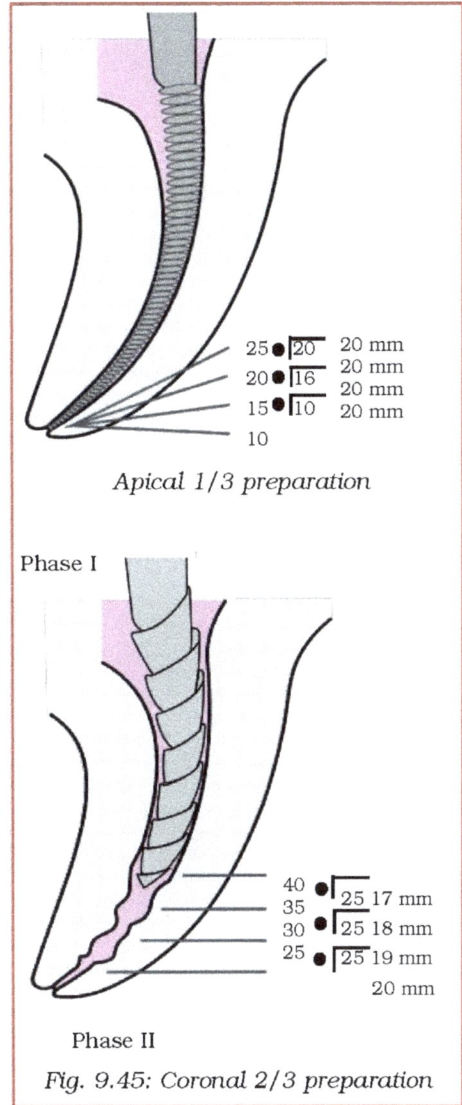

Fig. 9.45: Coronal 2/3 preparation

Procedure:

Insert the selected file into the canal and go all the way till the exact working length. Engage the file to the dentin. Apply lateral pressure. (circumferential filing). Withdraw when one cutting cycle is completed. Do minimum 2 to 3 cutting cycles with same file. By now the canal have started getting the shape. Insert the next larger file, engage in the dentin with apical pressure do circumferential filing. Do 2 to 3 cutting cycles. Repeat the procedure with the sequentially larger files. In between do the recapitulation to maintain the patency and working length. This helps in preventing the blockage of apex with the dentinal debris. Recapitulation means stepping back to previously used files.

G) MECHANICS OF SHAPING

1) Reaming

- Means enlarging or widening
- Act of doing repeated clockwise rotations with reamers is called reaming. The resultant shape after reaming will be roughly round or circular. So with reaming motion round canals or circular portion of the canals are effectively shaped.

Examples

- Apical 1/3 of almost all root canals are roughly circular.
- Lower Half of middle 1/3 of almost all root canals are roughly round.

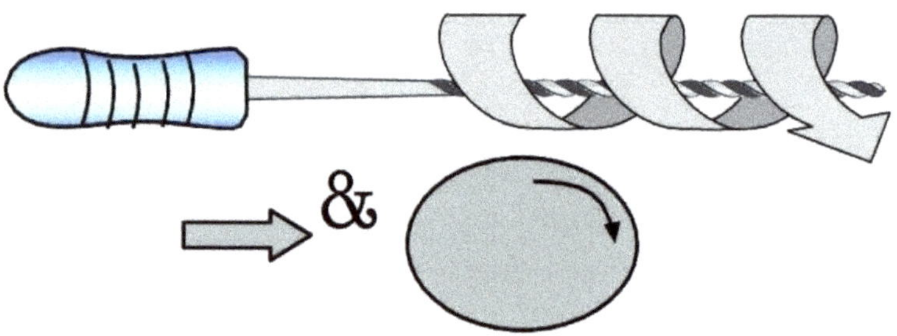

Fig. 9.46: Reaming

2) Filing

- Means rubbing.
- Act of doing repeated push pull actions without rotations with files is called filing.
- The resultant shape after filing will be irregular or roughly oval so with filing action oval or elliptical portion of the canals are effectively shaped.

Example

- Cervical 1/3rd of almost all root canals are roughly oval or elliptical.
- Upper half of the middle 1/3rd. of almost all root canals are roughly oval or elliptical.

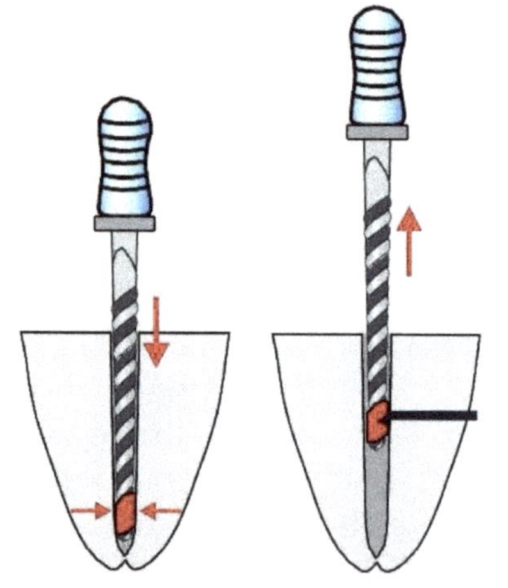

Fig. 9.47: Filing

Note

For effective shaping, step back technique utilizes both reaming and filing actions.

3) Recapitulation

Recapitulation includes the following:
a) Using the files in a sequential order
b) Re-entry and reuse of each previous file
c) Skipping back to smaller size files in between larger size files

Example

- Suppose the sequence is 10k, 15k, 20k.
- After using the 15k file, again go back to the 10k file instead of proceeding to 20k file.

Advantages

- Maintains patency by preventing accumulation of dentinal mud and soft tissue remnants of pulp.
- Maintains correct working length
- Prevents ledge formation.
- Prevents apical perforation and zipping.
- Prevents file breakage.

4) PRECURVING OF FILES

- All root canals have bends to some extent. Canals are curved mesio- distally or Bucco-lingually.
- Apical 1/3rd. almost all teeth show curvatures. Buccal roots of upper molars sometimes show sharp bends in the body of canal.

Definition

Bends are placed on the files to negotiate the curvature of canals is called pre curving.

Types

J bend or quarter bend - Apical 2-3 mm of file is curved called j bend. C bend or full Bend - Bend is placed along the full length of file is called full bend.

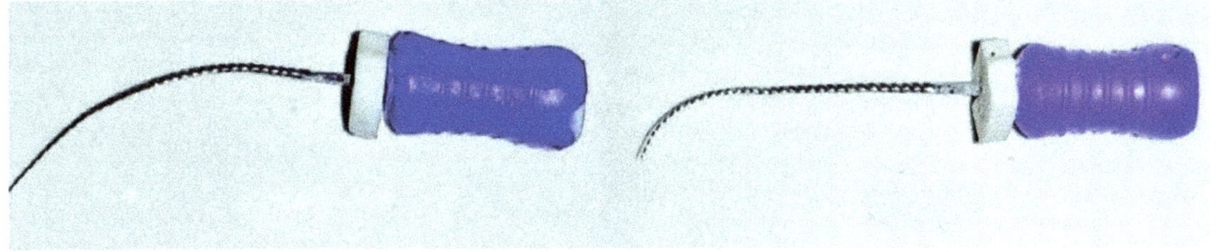

Fig. 9.48: Precurving

Advantages of pre curving

- Effectively negotiate and prepare curved canals or curved portion of canals.
- Maintains correct working length in curved canals.
- Prevents apical blockage and maintains patency in curved canals. Prevents lateral perforations in curved canals.
- Prevents ledge formation
- Prevents file separation

5) APICAL PATENCY

Shaping and cleaning of apical 1/3 of the canals, plays pivotal role in determining the success of root canal treatment. It is the apical patency which facilitates the effective cleaning and shaping of apical 1/3 of canals by maintaining correct working length and enhancing drainage of periapical infection.

Definition

Ability to keep the apical constriction open throughout the shaping and cleaning process is called apical patency.

Establishment of apical patency

- Established by passively passing the smallest file through the apical foramina without widening it.
- After the initial binding file, carry and set the smallest file 0.3 to 0.6 mm beyond the apex.

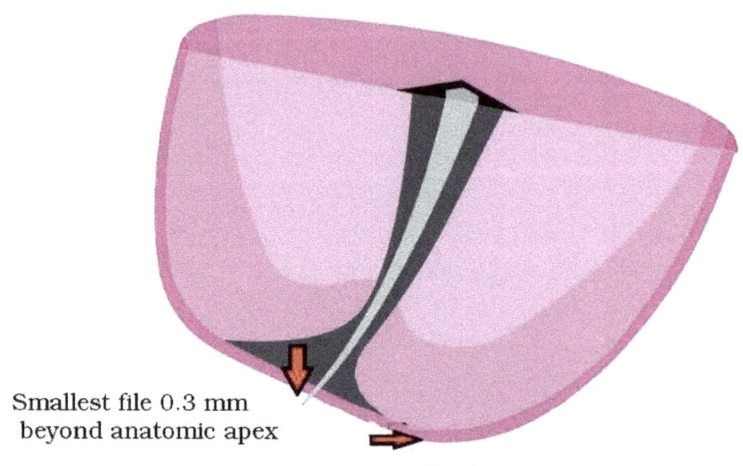

Fig. 9.49 : Apical patency

Maintenance of apical patency

Apical patency can be effectively maintained throughout the cleaning and shaping procedure by the following:

1)   By doing regular recapitulation
2)   Carrying out copious irrigation
3)   Using chelating agents
4)   Pre-curving the files

Advantages

Improves tactile sensation Avoids loss of working length Facilitates peri apical drainage Enhances periapical healing Enhances irrigation.

Prevents apical blockage.

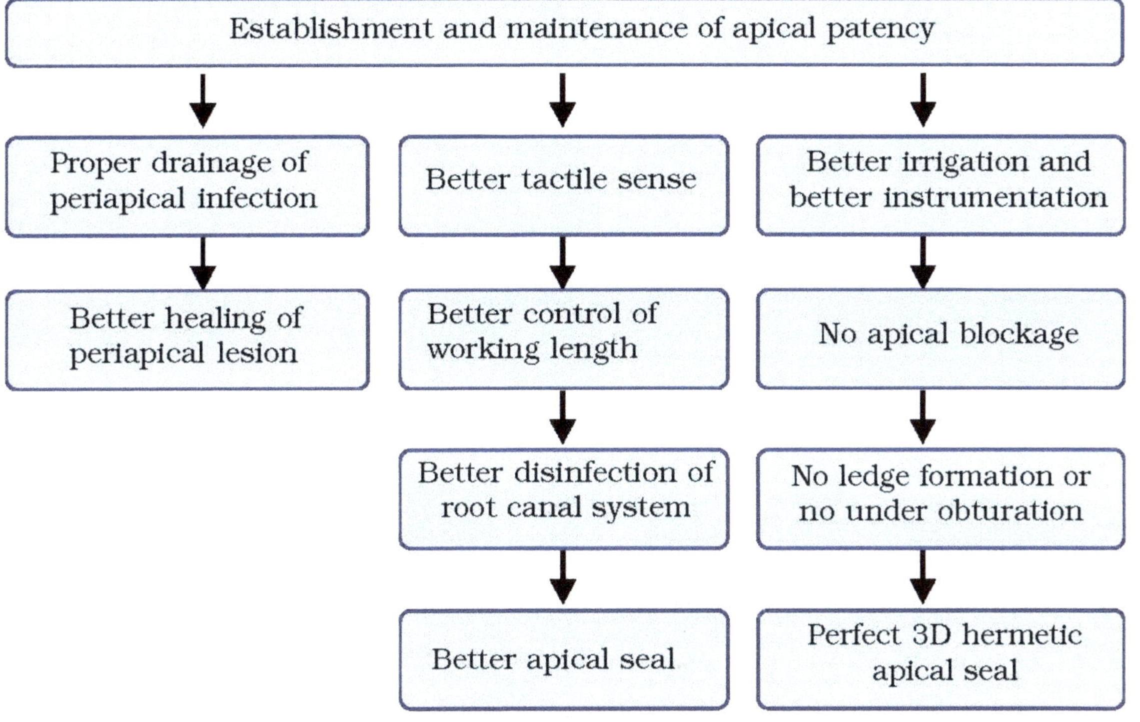

6)   BALANCE FORCE CONCEPT

This concept was proposed by Roane and Sabala in 1985. It involves the following:

1)   Use of flex-R files
2)   Balancing of apical positioning force and lateral cutting force.

1) *Flex-R files*

Stainless steel files have metallic memory and tend to regain their original shape once the stress is removed and cause ledges. To avoid this, files are modified at their tips. Flex-R files have modified cutting edge. These files tend to remain in the center of the canal thereby preventing any ledge formation and transportation. That is the reason it is used in severely curved canals.

2) *Balancing of apical positioning force and lateral cutting force.*

Apical positioning

-   The file is passively positioned between the dentinal canal walls without applying apical pressure.

-   In severely curved canals the file is positioned with less than quarter turn with no apical pressure.

-   In medium curved canals the file is positioned with quarter turn 45 degree with no apical pressure.

-   In straight canals the file is positioned with full turn 90 degree with no apical pressure.

Lateral cutting

With adequate or sufficient apical force, the file is completely rotated in counter - clockwise direction at 180 to 360 degree to cut.

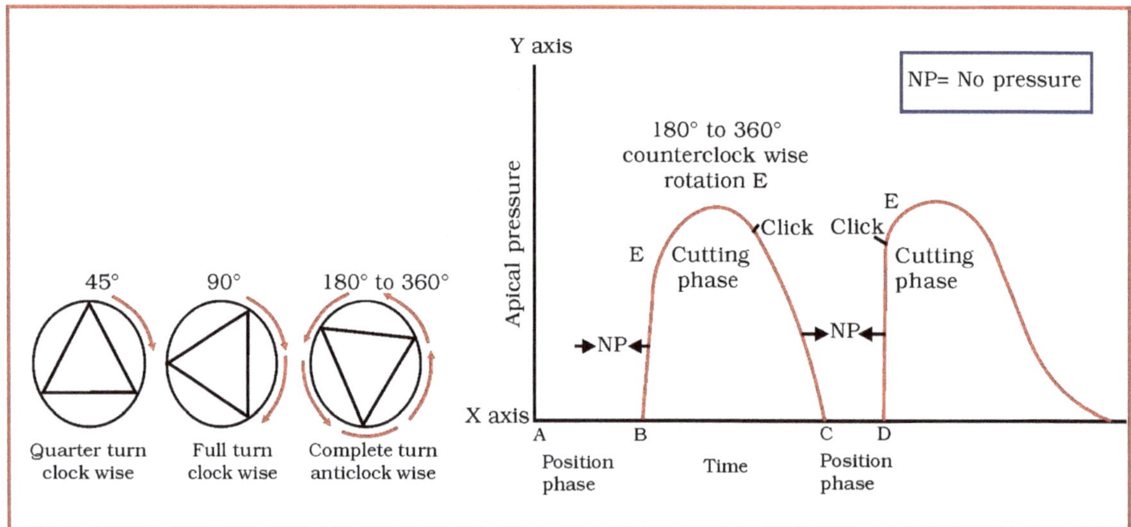

Fig. 9.50 : Balance force concept

- Y axis - Denotes apical pressure

- X axis - Denotes time or phase of canal preparation

- AB and CD on X axis denotes apical positioning of file without apical pressure (zero pressure phase)

- BE on Y axis denotes adequate apical pressure.

- EC on Y axis denotes lateral cutting in counter clockwise direction at 180 to 360 degree.

- CD on Y axis denotes relief phase

Advantages

- More efficient cutting saves lot of time

- Minimizes canal straightening

- Prevents ledge formation especially in curved canals

- Eliminates apical zipping

- Avoids apical transportation

Disadvantages

- Technique sensitive
- File breakage in inexperienced hands

H) IRRIGATION

DEFINITION

It is the process of cleaning and disinfecting the three-dimensional root canal system with the help of diluting and antiseptic agents.

Mechanisms and mode of action of irrigants

The only effective solution to pollution is dilution.

Physical

Hydrodynamic forces of fluids with their erosive action.

Mechanical

1) **Effervescence:** Bubbling effect of nascent oxygen released from mechanical agitation of sodium hypochlorite pushes the debris out coronally.

2) **Effect of nascent oxygen on dentinal tubules:** Dilates and increases the permeability of dentinal tubule there by removing the bacteria clogged inside the dentinal tubules.

3) **Disruption the biofilm:** The kinetic energy of molecules of irrigants disintegrates and dissociates the biofilm present on the canal walls.

Chemical

Dissolving of soft tissues by sodium hypochlorite. Chelation of hard tissues by EDTA.

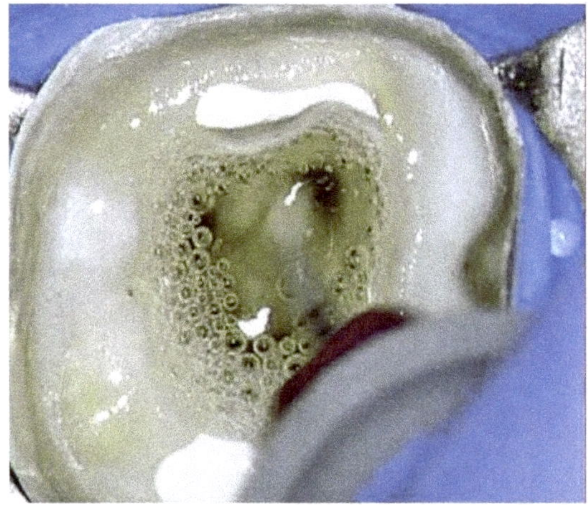

Fig. 9.51: Bubbling effect of NaOCl (Sodium Hypochlorite)

Biological

Bactericidal action.

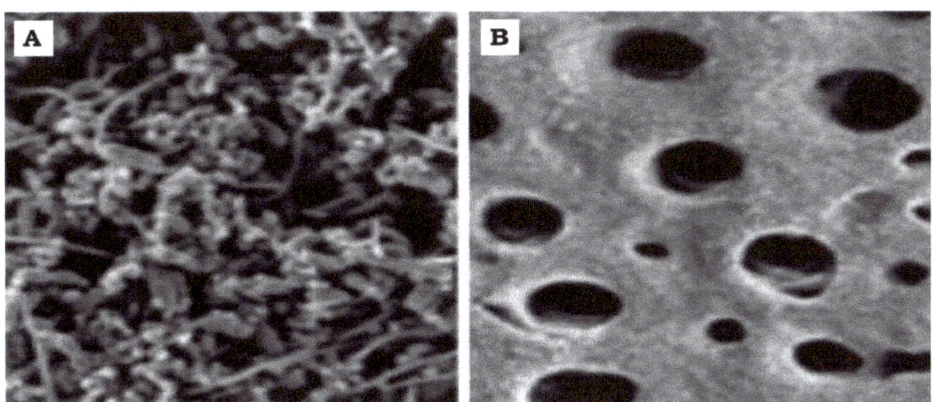

Fig. 9.52: (A) Canal surface before irrigation; (B) Canal surface after irrigation

Diagram A shows biofilm and diagram B shows clean disinfected surface.

OBJECTIVES

To achieve clean and dry canals. (bacteria free canal system). Clean and dry canals enhance bonding of the sealers to the canal walls which improves cervical and apical seal.

Clean and disinfect inaccessible areas like fins, webs, isthmuses, lateral canals, accessory canals, furcal canals and multiple foramens which are untouched by instrumentation.

Facilitates smooth instrumentation by lubricating action there by prevents ledges, blockages and instrument separation.

Ideal requirements of root canal irrigants

1) Have a broad antimicrobial spectrum high efficacy against anaerobic and facultative microorganisms organized in biofilms
2) Dissolve necrotic pulp tissue remnants.
3) Inactivate endotoxins
4) Prevent the formation of smear layer during instrumentation or
5) Dissolve the smear layer once it has formed
6) Be systemically non toxic
7) Be non-caustic to periodontal tissue
8) Be little potential to cause an anaphylactic reaction

2 ml syringes.

30- and 31-gauge needle with side vent.

Master apical file or master apical GP. Ultrasonic files from 15 to 30 size

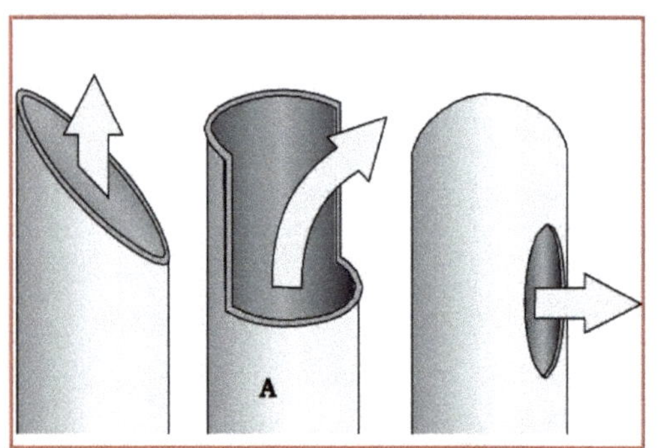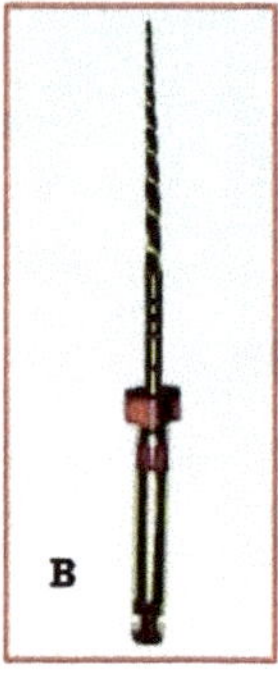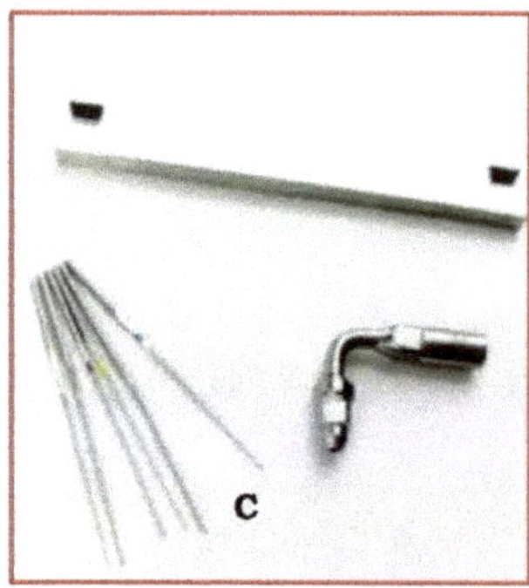

Fig. 9.53 : (A) Side vent needles; (B) Master apical file; (C) Ultrasonic files

Prerequisite

Shaping of canals to get irrigating needles part way or to full working length should be determined by sizes of irrigating needles.

1) In case of narrow canals like Mandibular incisors, Buccal roots of upper molars, Mesial roots of lower molars, Multirooted premolars or any multirooted tooth:

   - If you are choosing 31 (thinner) gauge needles the minimum canal preparation should be with 2% taper till 30 size K file.

   - If you are choosing 30 (thicker) gauge needle till 35 size K file - With 4% taper till F1 finishing file for 31-gauge needle and till F2 for 30-gauge needle.

2) In broader canals like, Upper anterior, palatal roots of upper molars, Distal roots of lower molars, Lower cuspids:

   - If you are choosing 31 gauge needle the minimum preparation should be with 4% taper till F1 finishing file. If you are choosing 30 gauge needle the minimum preparation should be till F2 finishing file with 6% Taper If you are choosing 31 gauge needle the minimum preparation should be till F1 finishing file.

   - If you are choosing 30 gauze needle minimum preparation should be till F2 finishing file.

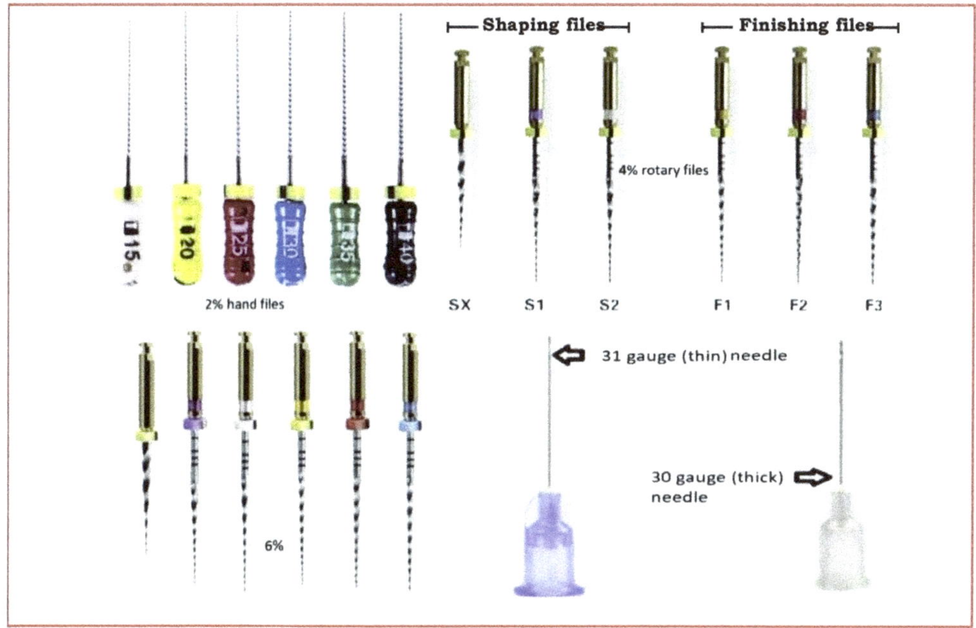

Fig. 9.54 :

Measures to avoid extrusion of irrigating solutions in to the periradicular area

-   Pre-bend the needles.

-   Adjust stoppers of ultrasonic files to the Desirable length.

-   Selecting correct gauze needles to the correct volume syringes.

-   Avoid forcing solutions with high pressure especially in open apices.

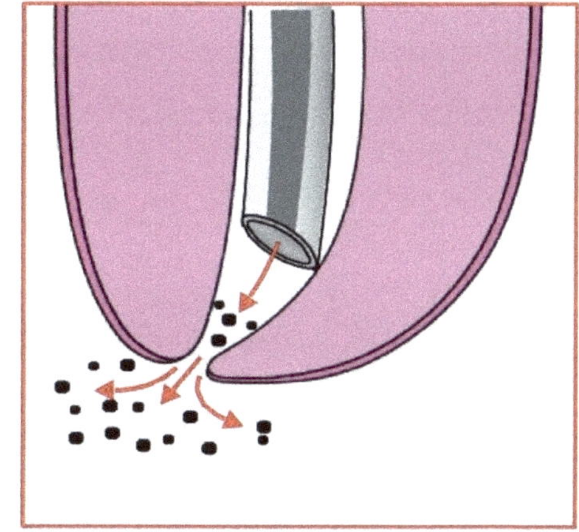

Fig. 9.55:

Irrigating solutions

1)   Sodium hypochlorite 3%

-   Available as 0.5%, 1%, 2.6%, 3%, 5.25%

-   Sodium hypochlorite acts by dissociating into hypochlorous acid and hypochlorite ion.

-   It dissolves the pulp tissue within few minutes. It is a bactericidal agent.

-   It is a lubricant.

- It flushes out the debris.
- It disinfects the pulp with its anti-bactericidal activity.
- It removes debris from irregular spaces at the isthmus area.

2) EDTA: 17% (Ethylene diamine tetra acetic acid)

- It is a chelating agent
- It acts by removing calcium ion of dentin. The dentin becomes more fragile and softer.

Uses:

i) Softens the dentin and clears the patency in case of calcification and blockages.

ii) Removes the smear layer.

iii) Poses broad spectrum anti-microbial activity.

iv) Very effective against E. coli and candida species.

3) Chlorhexidine gluconate: 2%

- Available as 0.1%, 0.2%, 0.6%, 0.12%, 2%
- Chlorhexidine exhibits substantivity (persistence of effect)
- Possess broad spectrum anti-microbial activity.
- Very effective against E. coli and candida species.

Used: in severe infections and re-root canal cases.

4) Doxycycline

- Broad spectrum effective against gram positive and gram-negative Bacteria and atypical microorganisms like chlamydia, micro plasma and rickettsia.
- Bacteriostatic. Act by inhibiting bacterial protein synthesis.

Used as an irrigants in multi visits re-root canal treatment cases and as an intracanal medicament in necrotic non vital tooth and severe serious infections.

INJ Doxol

PROCEDURE

It is done with a disposable syringe with side vent needle. Care must be taken not to force the irrigating solution into peri-radicular area. The needle is inserted part way or 3-4 mm short of apex in case of vital tooth and tooth with open apex.

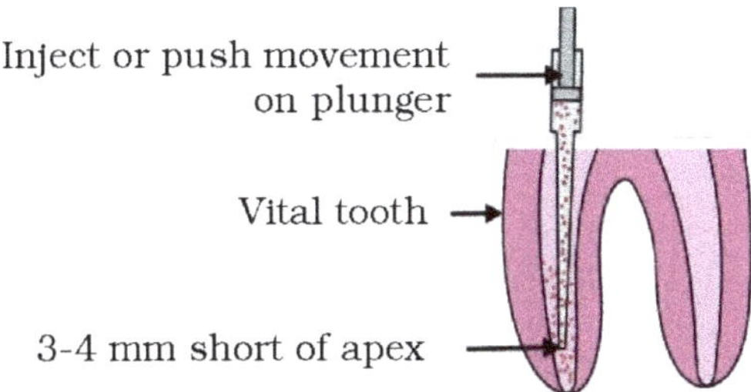

Fig. 9.56 : Vital Tooth

In case of non-vital tooth, the needle is inserted to full working length.

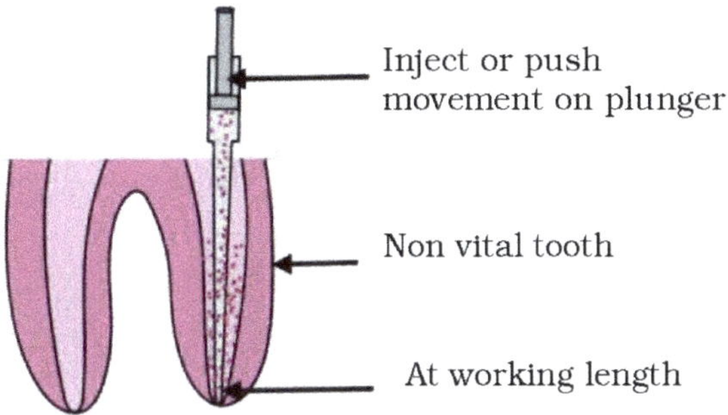

Fig. 9.57: Non-Vital Tooth

Push the solution with mild to moderate pressure into the canal. In case of very narrow and fine canals like extra canals in mandibular lateral, mb2 in upper molars and canals in 3rd molars, the tip of needle is placed near the root canal orifices, the irrigants disposed until it fills the chamber. The solution is then pumped into the canal with the files.

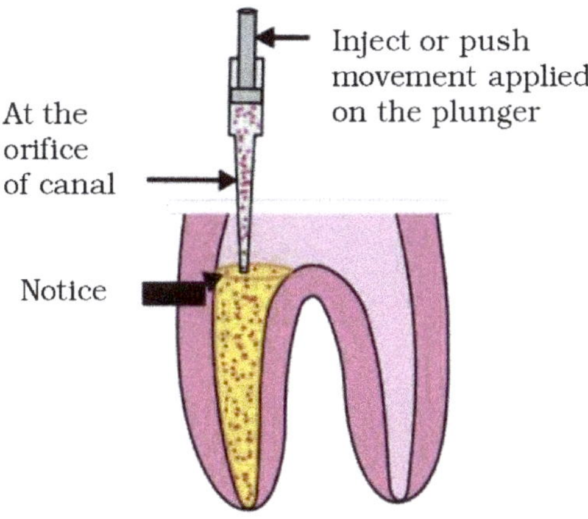

Fig. 9.58: Tooth with open apex

The solution is agitated manually with master apical file or master gutta percha point.

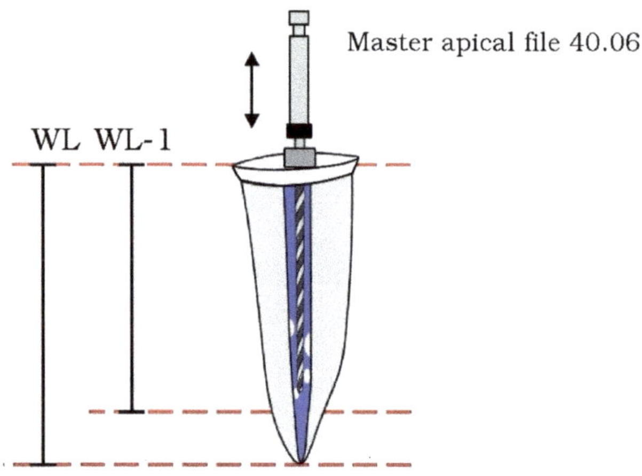

Fig. 9.59: Agitation

Finally, ultrasonic irrigation is done with ultrasonic files in sequential order from #15 to #45, each file for one minute (only in and out motion).

Sonication with ultrasonic files is done cautiously and wisely because it creates ledges and removes dentin which weakens the tooth.

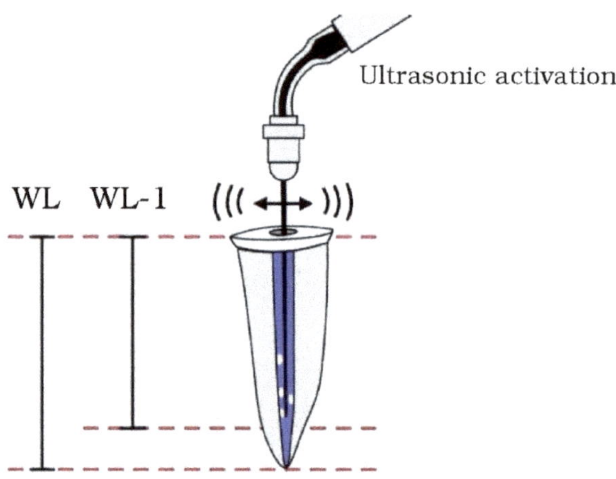

Fig. 9.60: Agitation

In case of open apex for example in immature young permanent tooth negative pressure irrigation is recommended.

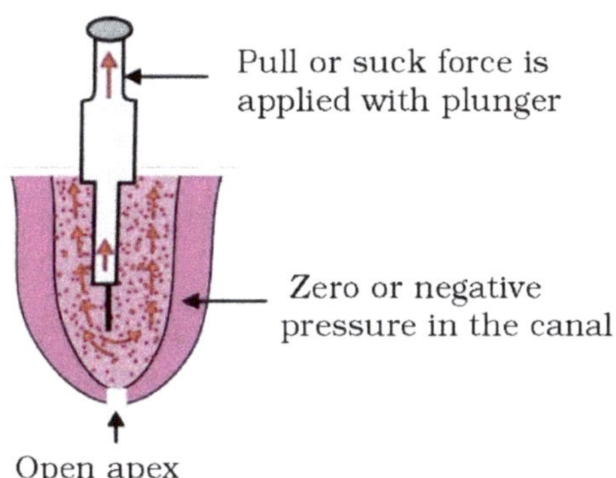

Fig. 9.61: Inmature tooth

Factors affecting irrigating solution

- Concentration of the irrigants.
- Type of irrigants.
- Frequency of irrigation.
- Volume of irrigating solution.
- Temperature of irrigating solution.
- Diameter of prepared canal.
- Size of the irrigating needle.

Pressure alteration techniques in endodontics

Introduction:

- Debridement of root canal system is essential for endodontic success.

- Irrigation is a vital part of root canal debridement; it is impossible to shape and clean the root canal completely because of the intricate nature of root canal anatomy.

- Even with the use of rotary instrumentation, the nickel titanium currently available only act on the central body canal, levin the fins, isthmus and cul-de-sacs untouched after completion of preparation.

- These areas might harbor tissue debris, microbes, and their byproduct, which might prevent close adaptation of obturation material and result in persistent peri-radicular inflammation.

- An ideal irrigant should reduce instrument friction during preparation, facilitate dentin removal, dissolve inorganic and organic tissue, penetrate to canal periphery, kill bacteria and yeasts and least irritating to periapical tissue.

- However, there is no such unique irrigant that can meet all these needs, even with the use of lowering pH, increasing the temperature, as well as addition of surfactants to increase the wetting efficacy of the irrigant.

- More importantly, these irrigants must be brought into direct contact with the entire canal wall surfaces for effective action, particularly for the apical portions of small root canals.

- To accomplish these objectives, there must be an effective delivery system to working length. An improved delivery system for root canal irrigation is highly desirable.

- Such a delivery system must have adequate flow and volume of irrigant to working length to be effective in debriding the canal system without forcing the solution into periradicular tissues.

- In selecting an irrigant and technique, consideration must be given to their efficacy and safety.

- Today's irrigation armamentarium presents a diverse variety of tools and technique that can assist the practitioner in reducing bacteria and debris within the canal system.

- However, currently there is no universally accepted standard irrigation technique. Since most research comparing the efficacy of different irrigation technique are in vitro studieswith low levels of clinical evidence, caution is advised when considering the purchase of these devices.

A) Manual agitation techniques

Syringe irrigation with needles or cannulas

- Conventional irrigation with syringes has been advocated as an efficient method of irrigant delivery before the advent of passive ultrasonic activation.

- This technique is still widely accepted by both general practitioner and endodontists.

- The technique involves dispensing of an irrigant into a canal through needles cannulas of variable gauges, either passively or with agitation.

- The latter is achieved by moving the needle up and down the canal space.

- Irrigation tip gauge and tip design can have a significant impact on the irrigation flow pattern, flow velocity, depth of penetration and pressure on the walls and apex of the canal.

- Irrigation tip gauge will largely determine how deep an irrigant can penetrate into the canal.

- A 21-gauge tip can reach the apex of an ISO size 80 canal, a 23gauge tip can reach a size 50, a 25-gauge tip can reach a size 35 canal and a 30- gauge tip can reach the apex of size 25 canal.

- 27 -gauge needle is the preferred needle tip size for routine endodontic procedures.

- Irrigant has only limited effect beyond the tip of the needle because of the dead water zone or sometimes air bubbles in apical root canal, which prevents apical penetration of the solution.

Needle tip design

- The smaller needles allow delivery of the irrigant close to the apex, this is not without safety concerns.

- Several modifications of the needle tip design have been introduced in recent years to facilitate effectiveness and minimize safety risks.

- Open ended tips express irrigant out the end towards the apex and consequently increase the apical pressure within the canal.

- Close ended irrigant tips are side vented and thus create more pressure on the walls of the root canal and improve the hydrodynamic activation of an irrigant and reduce chance of apical extrusion.

- This allows irrigant to reflux and causes more debris to be displaced coronally, while avoiding the inadvertent expression of the irrigant into periapical tissue.

- One of the advantages of syringe irrigation is it allows comparatively easy control of depth of the needle penetration within the canal and the volume of irrigant that is flushed throughthe canal.

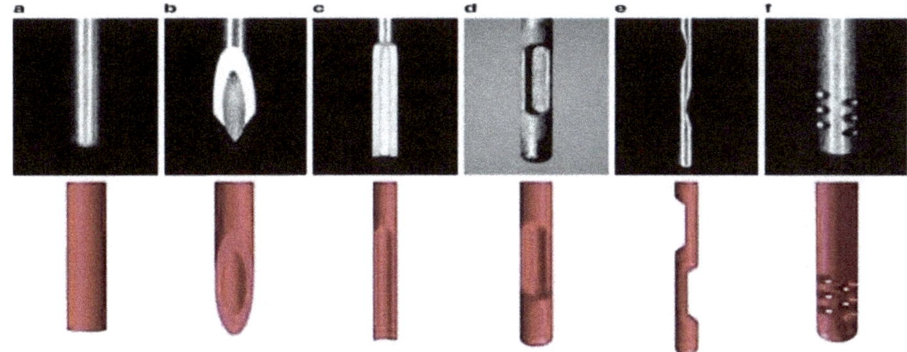

Fig. 9.62 :

Syringes

- Plastic syringes of different sizes are most commonly used for irrigation. Although large volume syringes potentially allow some time-savings, they are more difficult to control for pressure and accidents may happen.

- Therefore, to maximize safety and control use of 1-5ml syringes is recommended instead of the larger ones.

- All syringes for endodontic irrigation must have a luerlok design.

- Because of the chemical reactions between many irrigants, separate syringes should be used for each solution.

Brushes

- Brushes are not directly used for delivering an irrigant into the canal spaces. They are adjuncts that have been designed for the canal walls or agitation of root canal irrigant. They might have also been indirectly involved with transfer of irrigants within the canal spaces.

- Also, friction created between the brush bristles and the canal irregularities might result in dislodgement of the radiolucent bristles in the canals that are not easily recognized by practitioner, even with use of surgical microscope.

- Vapor lock effect

- Air entrapment by an advancing liquid front in close-end microchannels is a well-recognized physical phenomenon and has been reffered to as the vapor lock effect.

- The ability of liquid to penetrate these close-end-channels is dependent upon the contact angle of the liquid and the depth and size of the channel.

- Because endodontic irrigation is performed within a time frame of minutes instead of hours and days, air entrapment in the apical portion of the canal might preclude this region from contact or disinfection by irrigant.

- It is a fact that NaOCL reacts with organic material in the root canal and quickly forms micro gas bubbles at the apical termination that coalesce into an apical vapor lock with subsequent instrumentation.

- Because the apical vapor lock cannot be displaced within a clinically relevant time frame through simple mechanical actions, it prevents further irrigants from flowing into the apical region.

- More importantly, acoustic streaming and cavitation can only occur in a liquid phase.

- Therefore, once a sonic or ultrasonically activated tip leaves the irrigant enters the apical vapor lock, acoustic microstreaming and cavitation becomes physically impossible.

- A simple method to disrupt the vapor lock might be achieved via the use of a hand activated well-fitting root filling material, that is introduced to working length after instrumentation with the corresponding NiTi rotary instruments.

- This method although cumbersome, eliminates vapour lock because the spaces previously occupied by air is replaced by the root filling material, carrying with it a film of irrigant to the working length.

Manual dynamic irrigation

- An irrigant must be in direct contact with the canal walls for effective action. It is often difficult for the irrigant to reach the apical portion because of the so called vapour lock effect.

- Well-fitting gutta percha master cone up and down inshot 2-3mm strokes within an instrumented canal can produce an effective hydrodynamic effect and significantly improve the displacement and exchange of given reagent.

- Studies revealed that manual dynamic irrigation is more effective than automated dynamic irrigation.

Factors affecting manual dynamic irrigation

- The push pull motion of a well-fitting gutta percha point in the canal might generate higher intracanal pressure changes during pushing movements, leading to more effective delivery of irrigant to the untouched canal surfaces

- The frequency of push pull motion of the gutta percha point is higher than the frequency of positive negative hydrodynamic pressure generated by RinsEndo, possibly generating more turbulence in the canal.

- The push pull motion of the gutta percha point probably acts by physically displacing, folding and cutting of fluid under "viscously dominated flow" in the root canal system. The latter probably allows better mixing of the fresh unreacted solution with the reacted irrigant.

- Although manual dynamic irrigation has been advocated as a method of canal irrigation as a result of its simplicity and cost effectiveness, the laborious nature of this hand–activated procedure still hinder its application in routine clinical practice.

- Therefore, there are a number of automated devices designed for agitation of root canal irrigants that are either commercially available or under production by manufacturers.

Mechanical Agitation Techniques

Rotary brush

- A rotary handpiece attached micro brush has been used to facilitate debris and smear layer removal from instrumented root canals. The brush includes shaft and a tapered brush section. The latter has multiple bristles extending radially from a central wire core.

- During the debridement phase, the micro brush rotates at about 300 rpm, causing bristles to deform into the irregularities of the preparation. This helps to displace residual debris out of the canal in a coronal direction.

Sonic irrigation

- Sonic irrigation operates at a lower frequency and produces smaller shear stresses than ultrasonic irrigation.

- The endoactivator is one form of the sonic irrigation that uses non-cutting polymer tips to quickly and vigorously agitate irrigant solutions during treatment.

Vibringe

- Vibringe is a new sonic irrigation system that combines battery-driven vibrations with manually operated irrigation of the root canal.

- Vibringe uses the traditional type of syringes or needle but adds sonic vibration.

Ultrasonic irrigation

- Ultrasonics is another group of instruments that can be used for irrigation in the ultrasonics and subsonic handpieces.

- Ultrasonic handpieces pass sound waves to an endodontic file and cause it to vibrate at 25000 vibrations/s.

- It cuts dentin as well as causes acoustic streaming of the irrigant.

- It was also found that debris dislodgement from canal walls occurs through cavitation occurring within the irrigating solution.

- The dental literature has described two types of ultrasonic irrigation. The first one is a combination of simultaneous ultrasonic instrumentation and irrigation.

- The second one operates without simultaneous instrumentation and is reffered to as passive ultrasonic irrigation.

  Passive ultrasonic irrigation is more effective than syringe needle irrigation at removing pulpal tissue remnants and dentine debris. These may be due to the much higher velocity and volume of irrigant flow that are created in the canal during ultrasonic irrigation.

- Ultrasonics can effectively clean debris and bacteria from the root canal system, but cannot effectively get through the apical vapor lock.

Positive pressure versus apical negative pressure

- These are two apparently dilemmatic phenomena associated with conventional syringe needle delivery of irrigants.

- It is desirable for the irrigants to be in direct contact with canal walls for effective debris debridement and smear layer removal. Yet it is difficult for these irrigants to reach the apical portions of the canals, because of air entrapment, when the needle tips are placed too far away from the apical end of the canals.

- Conversely, if the needle tips are close to the apical foramen, there is increased possibility of irrigants extrusion from the foramen that might result in severe iatrogenic damage to the periapical tissues.

Pressure Alteration Devices

The RinsEndo irrigation system and the EndoVac irrigation system are examples of negative pressure irrigation.

- The RinsEndo irrigation system irrigates the canal by using pressure suction technology. It is composed of a handpiece, a cannula with a 7mm long exit aperture, and a syringecarrying irrigants.

- The EndoVac system is regarded as an apical negative pressure irrigation system composed of three basic components, a Master Delivery tip, the Microcannula, and the Microcannula.

- The MDT delivers irrigants to the pulp chamber and evacuates the irrigant concomitantly.

- Both the microcannula and microcannula are connected via tubing to a syringe of irrigant and the highspeed suction of a dental unit.

- The Macrocannula is made of plastic flexible polypropylene with an open end of 0.5mm in diameter, an internal diameter of 0.35mm and a 0.02 taper, used to suction irrigants up to the middle segment of the canal.

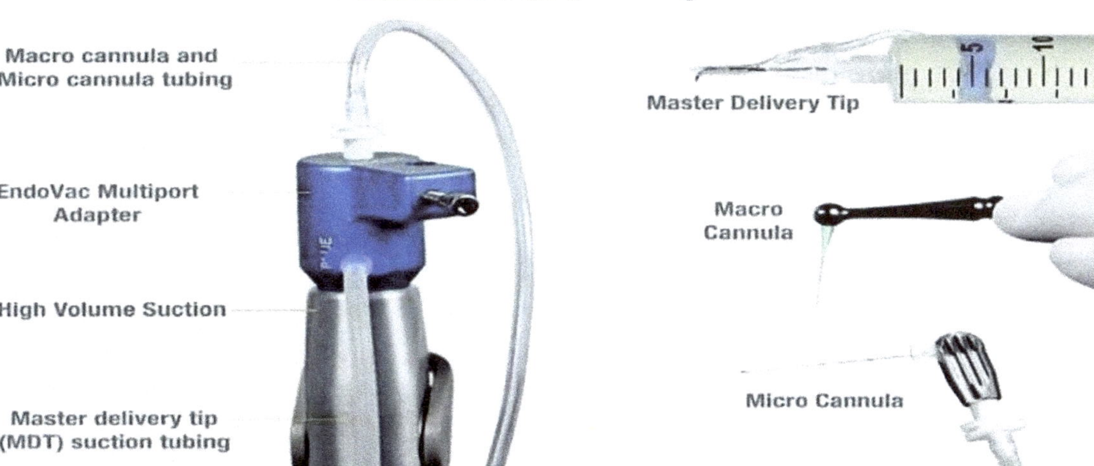

Fig. 9.63:

- Lastly the Microcannula is made of stainless steel and has 12 microscopic holes disposed in four rows of three holes, laterally positioned at the apical 1mm of the cannula. Each hole is 0.1mm in diameter, the first one int the row is located 0.37mm from the tip of microcannula and the distance between holes is 0.2mm.

- The microcannula has a close end with external diameter of 0.32mm can be used in the canal that are enlarged to size 35 or larger and should be taken to the working length to aspirate irrigants and debris.
- During irrigation, the MDT delivers irrigant to the pulp chamber and siphons of the excess irrigant to prevent overflow.
- The cannula in the canal simultaneously exerts negative pressure that pulls the irrigant from its fresh supply in the chamber by the MDT, down the canal to the tip of cannula, into the cannula, and out through the suction hose.

  Thus, a constant flow of fresh irrigants is being delivered by negative pressure to the working length.

Recent trends in irrigation of endodontics

1) MTAD, [Mixture of tetracycline acid and detergent]
2) Tetra-clean
3) Photo activated disinfections
4) Electrochemically activated solutions
5) Ozonated water
6) Herbal irrigants

MTAD: - [Mixture of tetracycline acid and detergent]

MTAD was enhanced when NAOCL issued as an intracanal irrigant before use of MTAD as a final irrigant.

- MTAD does not seem to change structures of dental tubules and MTAD effective against E faecalis less toxic compare to other medicaments.

- MTAD is effective against removing smear layer along whole length of root canal and in removing organic and inorganic debris and does not produce any signs of erosion or physical changes in dentine.

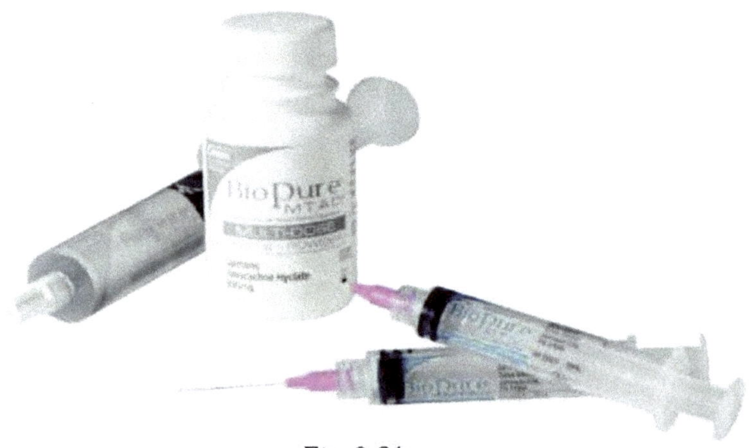

Fig. 9.64:

Electrochemically activated solution

Electrochemically activated solutions are produced from tap water and salt solutions of lower concentration. Principles of EAC is transferring liquids into metastable state via anode or cathode action by use of an element/element reactor

- The element or reactor is called as FEM i.e. flow through electrolyte module.

- The FEM consists of anode and cathode. Anode, a solid titanium cylinder with special coating that fits coaxially inside cathode. These electrodes are separated by ceramic membrane. FEM is capable of producing solution that have bactericidal and sporicidal activity. They are odorless, safe to human tissue and no corrosive for most metal surfaces. Electrochemically treatment in anode and cathode chambers is anolyte and solution produced in cathode chamber is catholyte.

- Anolyte solutions containing solution containing mixtures of oxidizing substance demonstrate pronounced microbiocidal effectiveness against bacteria virus and fungi as well as protozoa.

Tetra clean:-

Like MTAD tetraclean is a mixture of an antibiotic, an acid and a detergent. However, the concentration of antibiotic doxycycline (50 mg / ml), and the type of detergent (polypropylene glycol) differ from those MTAD. Only the NaOCI could disaggregate and remove the biofilm at every time interval tested although treatment with tetra clean caused a high degree of biofilm disaggregation at each time interval when compared with MTAD.

Photo activated disinfections:

Photodynamic therapy is based on concept that nontoxic photosensitizer can be preferentially localized in certain tissue and subsequently activated by light of appropriate wavelength to generate oxygen and free radicals that are cytotoxic to cells of target tissue methylene blue is a well-established photosensitizer that has been used in photodynamic therapy for targeting gram negative and grampositive bacteria. Along methylene blue tolonium chloride had also been used as a photo sensitizing agent. It is applied in infected area and left in situ for a short period of time. This agent binds the cellular membrane of bacteria which will then rupture when activated by a laser source emitting radiation at an appropriate wave length. Tolinomium chloride dye is biocompatible and does not stain dental tissue.

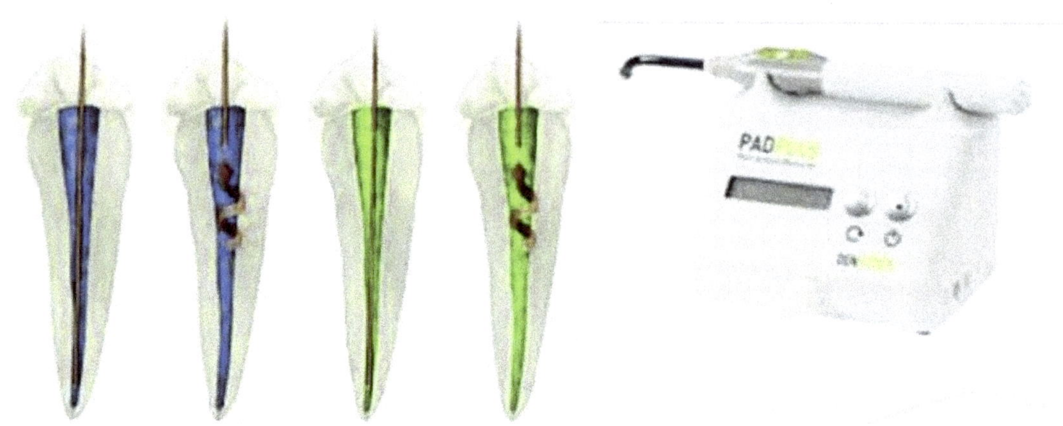

Fig. 9.65:

Ozonated water:

Ozone is very powerful bactericide that can kill microorganism effectively. It is an unstable gas capable of oxidizing any biological entity. It was reported that ozone at low concentration,0.1 ppm, is sufficient to inactivate bacteria cells including their pores. It is present naturally in air and can be easily produced by ozone generator. Although ozonated water is powerful antimicrobial agent against bacteria fungi protozoa and virus less attention had been paid to the antibacterial activity of ozonated water in bacterial biofilm and hence in root canal infections.

Herbal: Ayurvedic herbal formulation is known as triphala is a combination of dried and powdered fruits of three medicinal plants and green tea polyphenols

- 3 medical plants are terminalia bellerica, terminalia chebula and embelica officinalis

- Triphala and green tea polyphenols shows similar antibacterial sensitivity on E Faecalis.

But triphala shows more potency on E Faecalis bio film.

I) GLIDE PATH

Obtaining and managing glide path

Whoever owns the glide path wins the game of endo.

Introduction

A glide path is a preexisting part of root canal, once occupied by healthy pulp. It needs to be followed not artificially made.

Once the glide path is obtained everything falls in to place. Glide means to move smoothly without obstruction.

It is the smooth unobstructed reproducible path from the canal orifice to the exact working length of the tooth. It may be single or multiple. It may be straight or curved. It may be partial or total. It provides the blue print map for rotary instruments. It is the minimum preparation required before introducing rotary instruments into the canal. Glidepath determines the size and sequence of rotary instruments. We should not use rotary unless until we have glide path.

A vital step in the instrumentation process is preparation of the glide path to allow all subsequent instruments to move smoothly from the coronal orifice of the canal in an unimpeded progression to the apical constriction. Glide path management is considered to be the shaping success in endodontic treatment. Hence, it is of prime importance that we slip, slide, and glide through the canal from the orifice to the apical constriction, so that the root canal system is successfully and three-dimensionally cleaned and shaped to a tapering funnel shape to receive the obturating material.

Definition:

The endodontic glide path is a smooth radicular tunnel from canal orifice to physiologic terminus (foraminal constriction).

What should be the size of initial glidepath?

- Its minimal size is super loose" no. 10 k file

- But, the recent international protocol for GPM suggests, that terminus of any given canal should be at least 0.15mm before rotary shaping to safely accommodate the tip of first rotary file.

- So no.15 k file at full working length is the ideal size of glide path

Importance of glide path

A successfully secured glide path means a smooth passage exists that is reproducible by successful larger files. During cleaning and shaping of the root canal system, no rotary instrument should be used where a hand instrument has not been placed before. The other significance is the coronal preflaring, which considerably decreases the separation of instruments. Use of small hand files prior to the use of rotary Ni-Ti instruments will confirm patency as well as maintain sufficient space, thereby, improving the safety of the rotary or reciprocating endodontic files. The presence of intracanal calcifications or denticles poses severe problems during endodontic therapy, especially, in the aging population.These denticles may be present at the coronal, middle, or apical third of the root canals. Instrumentation beyond these calcification is an ardent task, which can effectively be accomplished with successful glide path management. Failure to achieve patency beyond the calcifications leads to ledge formation, which is one of the most important reasons for retreatment."

- Allows more safer and effective rotary shaping by creating sufficient root canal space to accommodate the first rotary file.
- Reduces risk of instrument separation.
- Maintains the original root canal anatomy.
- Minimizes risk of iatrogenic mishaps

Steps in glide path preparation

1) Access opening
2) Removal of coronal restrictive dentin
3) Debridement of pulp chamber
4) Orifice location
5) Initial scouting of canals
6) Removal of restricitive radicular dentin or Precoronal flaring
7) Following the canal to radiographic terminus
8) Working length determination
9) To create a reproducible glide path.

Debridement of pulp chamber

In medical terms, debridement is the removal of damaged tissue and/or foreign objects from a wound. In dentistry pulpal debridement, also referred to as a pulpectomy or partial root canal, is an endodontic treatment for the removal of diseased or damaged pulp tissue, the soft area at the center of a tooth which contains the blood vessels, nerves, and pink connective tissue. Pulpal debridement is the first step of a root canal treatment where all of the pulp tissue is removed, or in the case of a partial root canal, it is done before a complete root canal treatment can be completed in order to relieve serious pain caused by swelling from an infection of the dental pulp and nerve This relieves pressure and pain by providing room for the dental pulp to expand. However, the complete root canal treatment must still be done, can be, and almost always is done in one visit, because a root canal is the only way to save the tooth.

Initial scouting of canals

- Canal scouting is the first phase of canal instrumentation, during which procedural errors might occur frequently.

- The manual preflaring creates a glide path for safer use of hand files and NiTi rotary instrumentation.

- Scouting coronal two-third provides information about root canal system anatomy and gives feedback regarding canal degree of curvature, recurvature or if there is presence of dilacertion.

- There are commonly five encountered anatomical forms which include canals that merge, curve, recurve, dilacerate or divide.

- When straight line access has been completed and all the orifices have been identified, attention is directed towards preparing the root canal.

- If the pulp is vital and bleeding, the chamber is filled brimful with viscous chelator, when the pulp is necrotic the chamber is irrigated and completely filled with 5% NaOCL which should be warm.

- With the scouting the smaller stainless steel files are measured on the pre-op radiograph and prebend to confirm to the anticipated full length and curvature of the root canal.

- Stainless steel 10K file is used to scout the coronal two-third of canal.

- After negotiation the coronal two third, the canal is flushed with NaOCL and may be preenlarged using hand instruments, gates gladden drills, utilized like a brushes, or rotary NiTi shaping files.

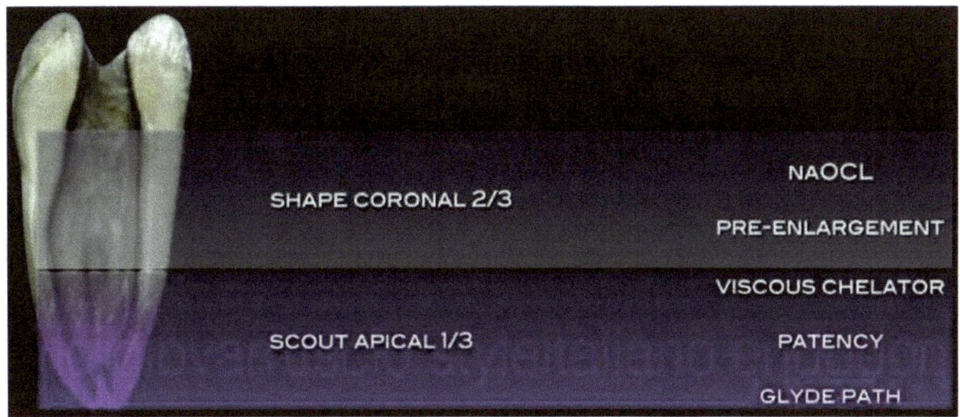

Fig. 9.66:

- With coronal two-third optimally prepared and filled with irrigant, the apical one-third is then scouted and reconnaissance information is gathered.

- Small hand files like 8K-10K files are used to negotiate the rest of the canal.

- Confirm a smooth glide path to the terminus and establish patency.

- In complex anatomy with small, long and potentially multiplanar canals, it is not possible to immediately pass a 10K-file initially to the root end.

- Subsequently the clinician with scouting may try to use smaller files to the apex.

- However 6K-8K files typically are not needed to enlarge the glide path to the apex, unless it is an extraordinary difficult case.

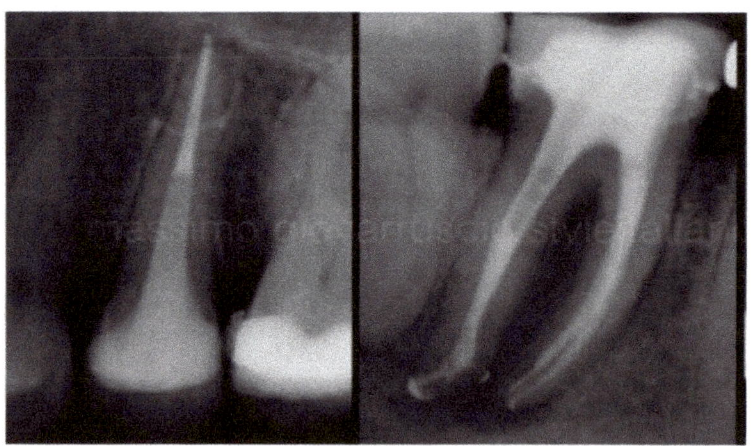

Fig. 9.67:

- The apical foramen will always be larger than a 10K file; therefore any resistacemet prior to the apex is likely due to curvature or irregularity in the canal. As a result, opening up the canal with a 10K file in small increments can be an efficient way to follow a reproducible glide path, while minimizing the likelihood of creating a ledge or blockage in the canal.

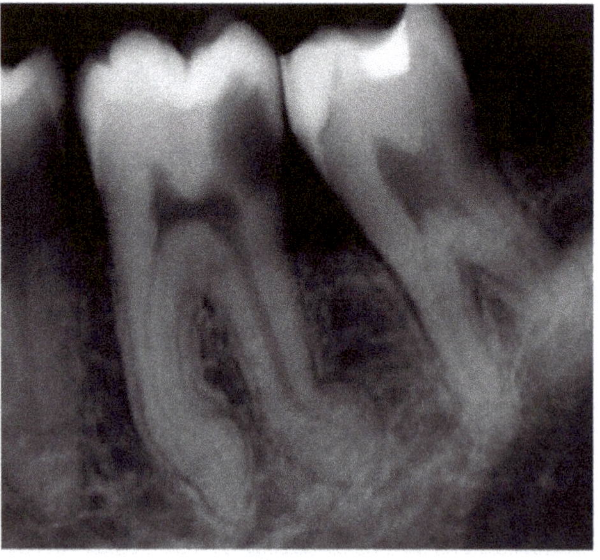

Fig. 9.68:

- The TIP of the SCOUTING is that the file should never be forced apically because the risk of creating a ledge is greatly increased. If the tip of the file never binds into the canal wall, it is impossible to make a ledge.

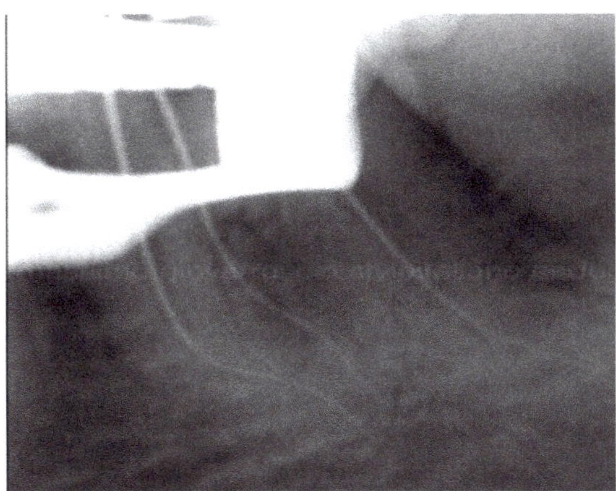

Fig. 9.69 :

- The Post-Op radiograph shows how the original anatomy has been preserved after root canal instrumentation. Preflaring and Scouting guarantee a well respected of the entire root anatomy.

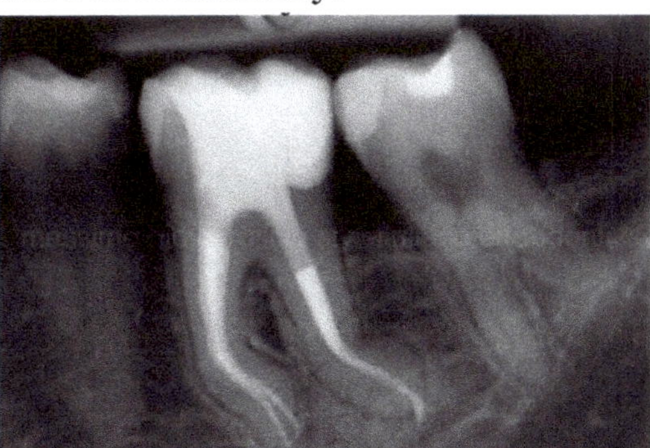

Fig. 9.70 :

- Canals just present with anatomic impediments such as straight canal with apical irregularity, curved canal with irregularity and abruptly bent canal.

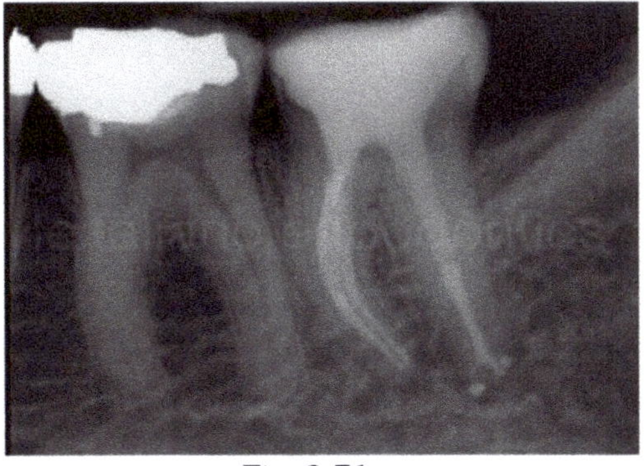

Fig. 9.71 :

- This canals require cleverness and persistence to traverse.

  Impediments are identified by the tactile sense (felt through the file handle) of loose resistance to apical file placement. This occurs because the tip of the file is hanging up in a irregularity, rather than grinding to length and beyond.

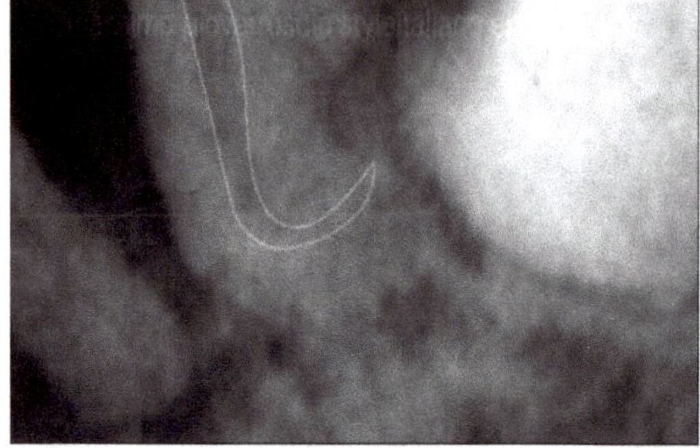

Fig. 9.72:

- When an impediment to apical progress is met, remove the file, smoothly bend the very last 2mms with file bending plier (EndoBender), align the directional mark on the silicon stop toward the file bend, and you are able for a path around the impediment.

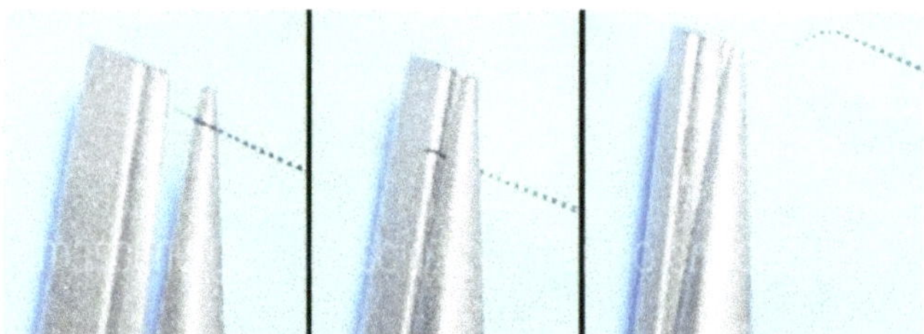

Fig. 9.73:

- When scouting a careful watch-winding motion is used to advance the file trough the impediment. When the impediment is met, pull back a mm, turn the file tip in a new direction, move it apically with a wiggle and see if it advances. If not pull back, redirect the bent file tip and see if it drops. Repeat, if apical progress is seen, until patent. An apex locator and a radiograph control is essential to check whether the terminus has been reached after an impediment is successfully.

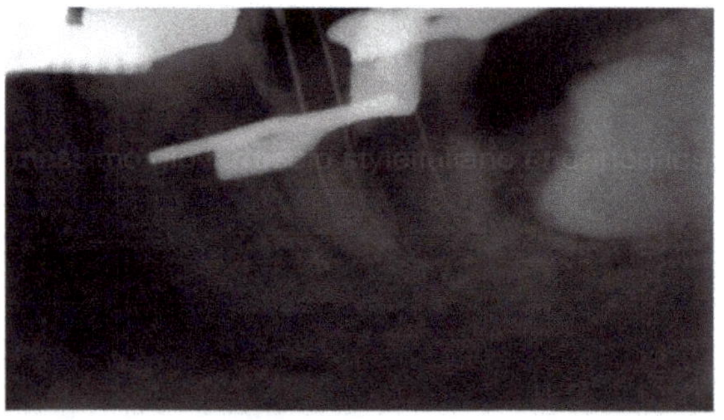

Fig. 9.74:

- Post operative radiographs shows a complete tridimensional root canal filling and the respect of the complex anatomy.

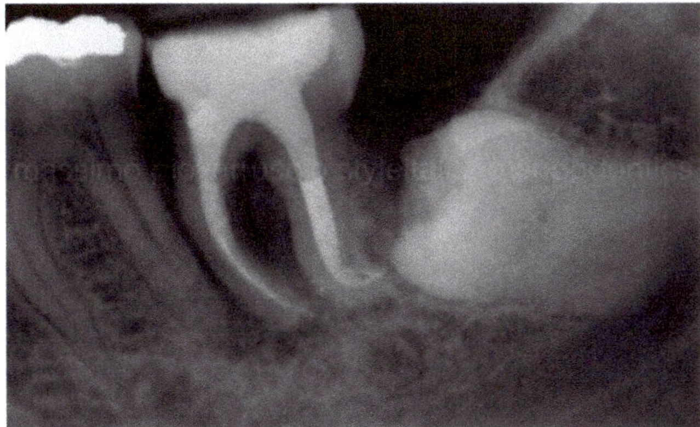

Fig. 9.75:

- In challenging cases, many attempts may be required when scouting the canals. As soon as the file tip moves beyond the impediment, it will drop deeper into the canal.

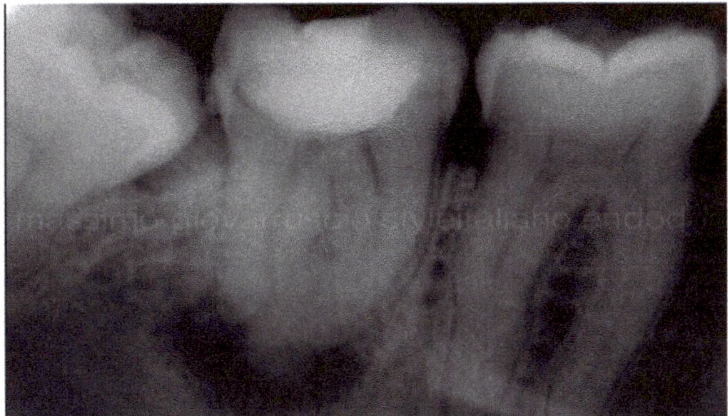

Fig. 9.76:

- During this scouting, the directional on the silicone stop informs the clinician about the direction of the bent file tip as it traverses the impediment, in essence, mapping the path. Wiggle the file and move deeper, and work it, checking it with an apex locator lead until length is reached.

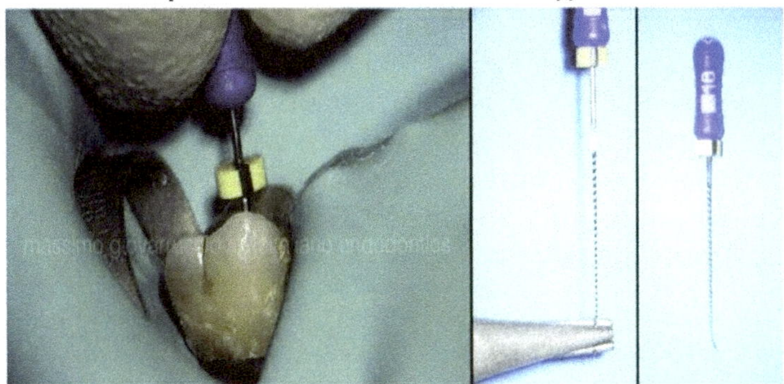

Fig. 9.77:

- Once past the impediment, avoid withdrawing the file to the impediment level as the file has inevitably straightened and will no longer traverse it without being withdrawn, rebent, and re-inserted. In the canal with a double impediment of S-shaped curvature, the present fill will drop when directed around the first bend in the canal but will again meet loose resistance to apical file placement as it encounters the second canal bend. In this case, pull the file back slightly, turn it 180 degrees, give it a wiggle, and see if it catches or just drops to length.

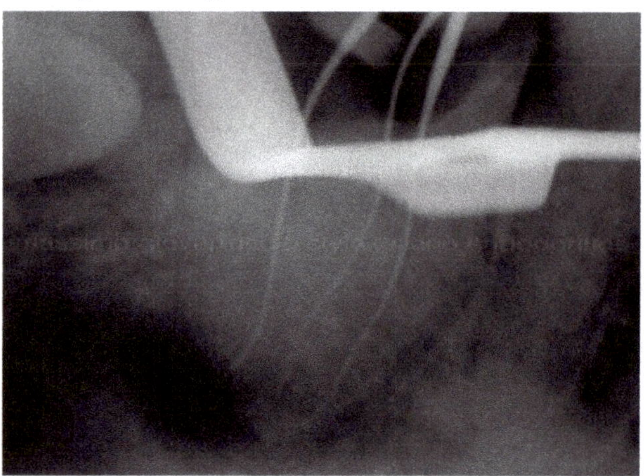

Fig. 9.78:

- With bent files and stop indicators, you should be able to mentally map the canal path around the impediments and thereafter easy dance around them and get the job done.

Removal of radicular restrictive dentin:

Coronal Preflaring

- After access cavity. Preflaring, Canal Scouting and Glyde Path are the first phases of canal instrumentation and it has also been noted that during these phases, the clinician might more frequently encounter procedural difficulties, These problems include instrument fracture, ledge formation, canal zipping or canal straightening, strip perforation, apical perforation, elbow formation and apical blockage. All of these errors can lead to incomplete debridement of the root canal system and contribute to decreased success rates of endodontic therapy, (Fig. 1) Much has been written in the field of endodontics about the importance ofcoronal access. Coronal access needs to be Large enough to allow entry into all canals. While preserving tooth structure for future restoration. The access cavity should be as small as practical.

- The principle of straight-line access into the pulp chamber is generally accepted, straight-line access into the chamber will not ensure straight line access into canals as a triangle of dentin will be present at the orifice, which continues for a few millimeters below the pulpal floor. This dentine triangle needs to be removed and this step of ensuring straight line access into the canal should be accomplished for every tooth even if the pre-operative anatomy seems straightforward.

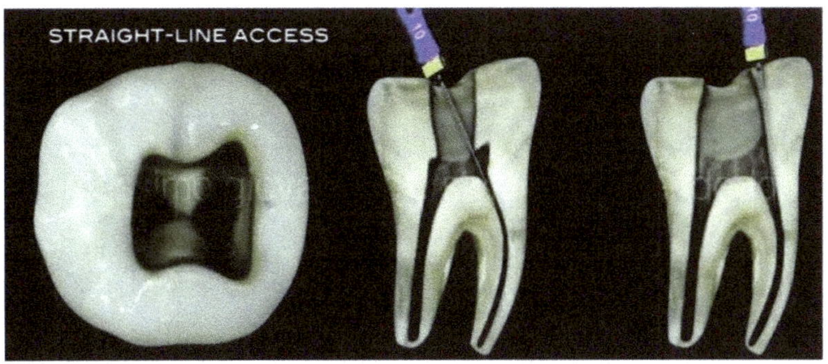

Fig. 9.79 : Coronal preflaring

- Pre-flaring gives the clinician better tactile control when directing small precurved negotiating files into the delicate apical one-third microanatomy. Early coronal two thirds enlargement removes restrictive dentin and reduces significant pressure from the more coronal cutting flutes of any file type.

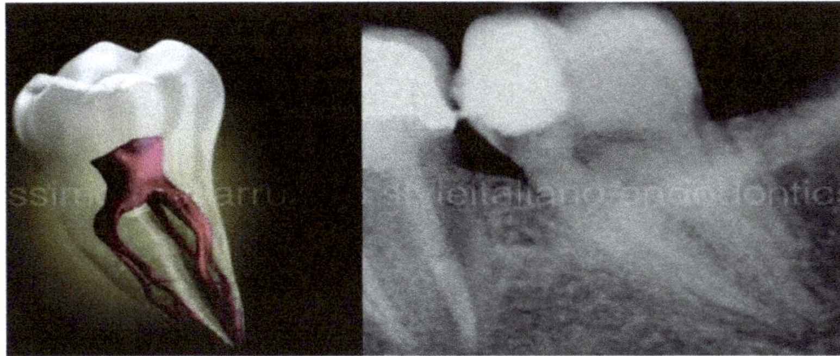

Fig. 9.80 : Coronal preflaring

- Scouting and shaping step become more easy and predictable when the pre enlargement has been performed properly also in the complex root canal system like this second lower molar.

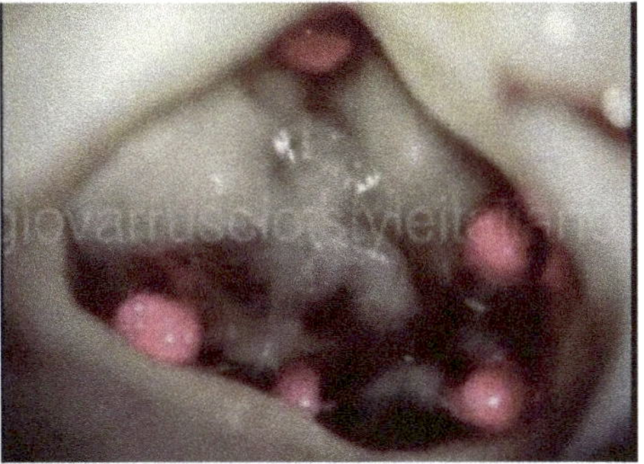

Fig. 9.81 : Coronal preflaring

- Preflaring canals hold a greater and more effective volume of irrigant which serves to enhance cleaning. Narrow, more restrictive preparations are dangerous as files work in virtually dry canals. A preflared canal exhibits shape and holds a greater volume of warm irrigant which accelerates the apical and lateral digestion of pulp.

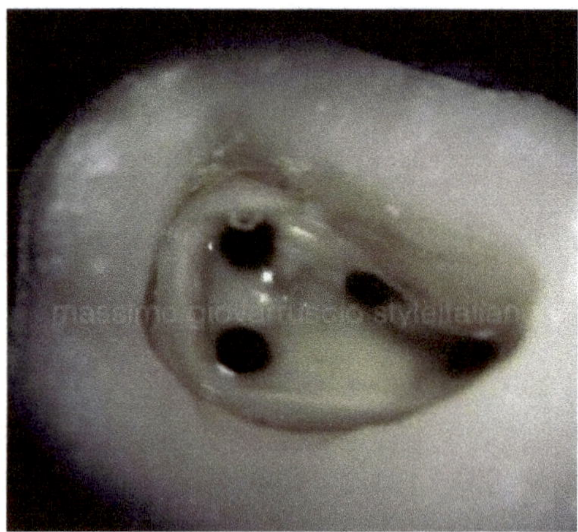
Fig. 9.82 : Coronal preflaring

Preflaring procedures decrease post treatment problems as the bulk of the pulp and, if present, bacteria and related irritants have been removed. Passing files through a cleaned pre-enlarged preparation equates to less debris inadvertently inoculated periapically. Passing files through underprepared canals coronally pushes more irritants periapically and generates more post-operative exacerbations.

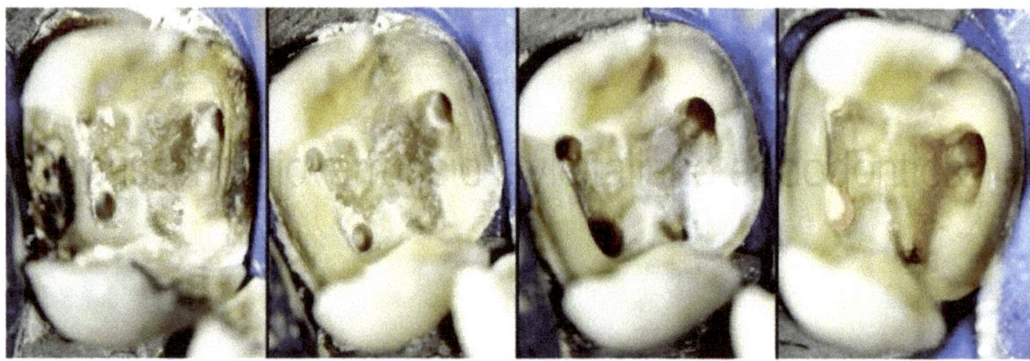
Fig. 9.83 : Coronal preflaring

- Other options for removal of the dentin triangle would include Gates Glidden drills, orifice openers or a series of larger hand files. Gates Glidden drills have the potential to cut to the furcation side of the canal. Over enlargement may result in the thinning of the root wall or a root perforation.

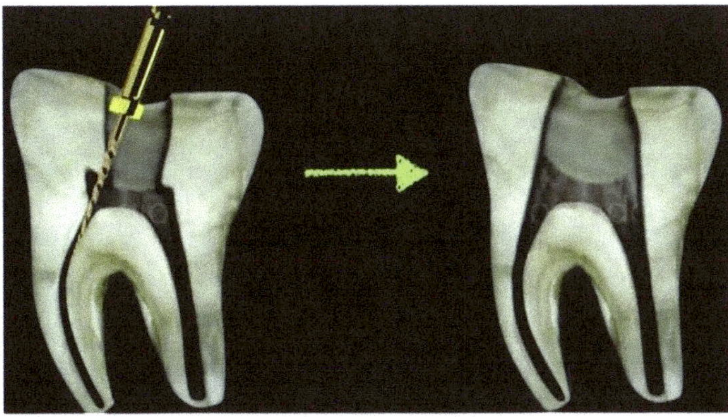

Fig. 9.84:

- Hand files will require more time and are stiff, thereby increasing the risk of altering the natural canal anatomy, but hand instruments can be effective at this level of the canal. Nowadays a Ni-Ti rotary files can be used safely and efficiently.

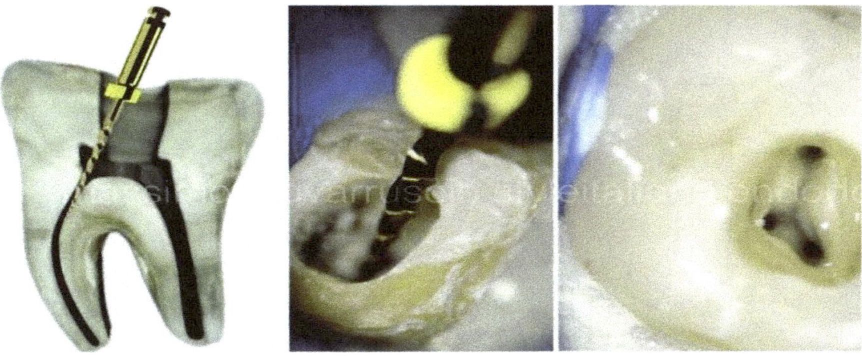

Fig. 9.85:

- Preflaring procedures generally improve diagnostics. A pre-enlarged canal passively accepts a larger file into the apical one third where its terminal extent is easier to visualize radiographically. Electronic apex locators are more accurate when utilized in pre-enlarged canals as instruments are more likely to snug into dentin towards their terminal extents. When the clinician does establish a working length, it will be more accurate as it occurs after a more direct path to the terminus has been established.

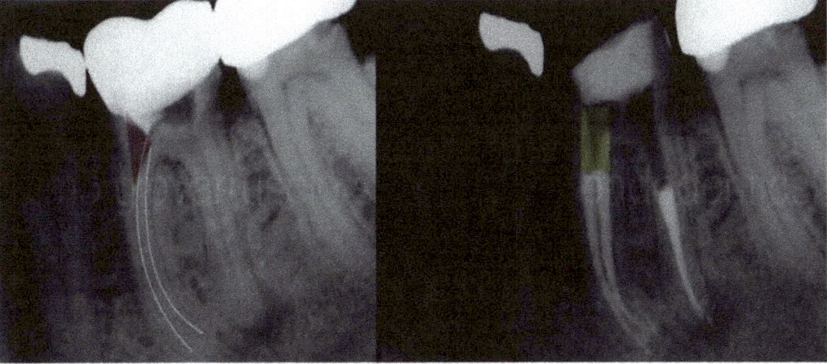

Fig. 9.86:

- A Triangle of Dentine if not removed properly can increase the torsional stress on hands files during working length measurement.

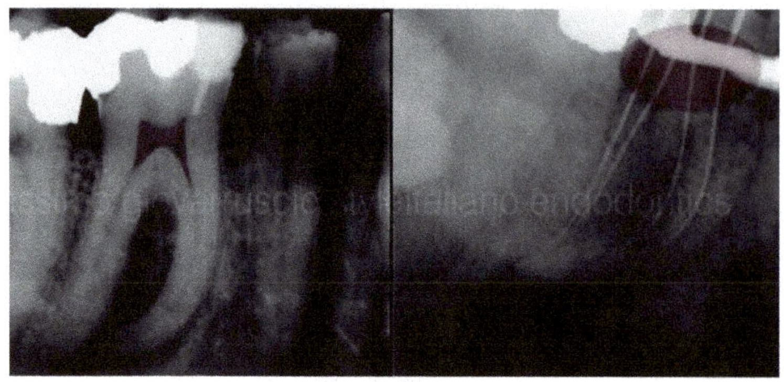

Fig. 9.87:

- The Green Area could be considered a safety area where any rotary instrument is able to work with less torsional stress due to the straight line access.

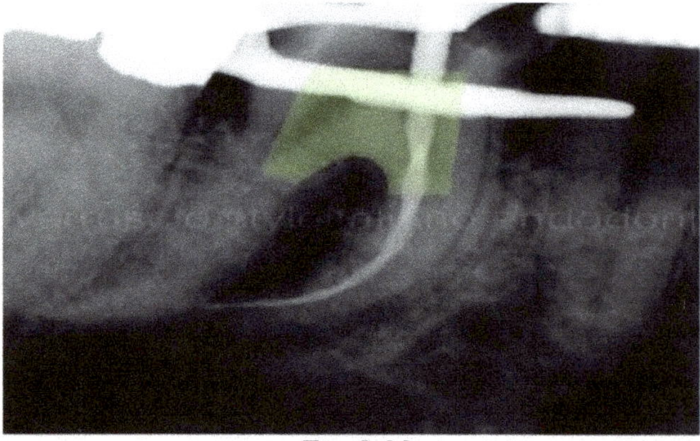

Fig. 9.88:

PROCEDURE TO OBTAIN GLIDE PATH

Insert a selected file into the canal and go all the way till the exact working length. Engage the file into the dentin. Apply lateral pressure, do circumferential filing and withdraw - one cutting cycle is completed. Minimum 2 to 3 cutting cycles, with each size file and at least 2 to 3 sequentially larger files are required to create smooth reproducible glide path.

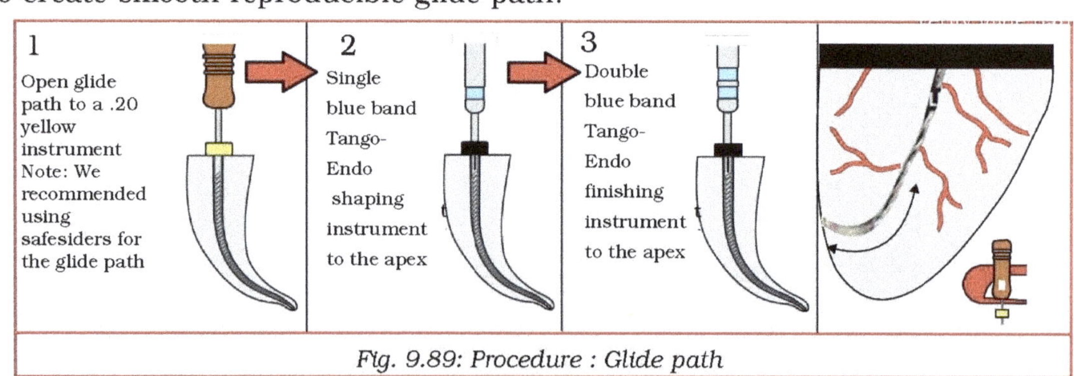

Fig. 9.89: Procedure : Glide path

Glide Path techniques

- The glide path includes four important steps. The first and foremost is locating the canal orifices. To effectively locate the canal orifices, it is mandatory that we know about the normal root canal anatomy and also the possible anatomic variations that are specific to the tooth. The 14 various classifications proposed dictates that the typical root canal system anatomy of a tooth is not specific at all. Hence, with better magnification and illumination, a good knowledge about root canal anatomy and the possible anatomic variations, as well as location of root canal orifices can be determined. The second step is following the canal to the minor apical diameter.

- This can be done using various methods, such as radiographic methods, digital-tactile sense, electronic methods, apical periodontal sensitivity, and paper point measurements. The third step is regarding why the minor apical diameter is a long way off. This may be due to four pos sible reasons :

  1. The canal is clogged or blocked due to necrotic and dentinal debris.
  2. The angle of incidence and angle of access are not the same.
  3. The diameter of the file is wider than the canal.
  4. The shaft of the file is too wide for the canal. The fourth step is the different types of motions employed. The first type of motion is the following motion. The necrotic debris and the calcifications can be removed by using ultrasonics, high-speed burs, and also Mueller burs. Using an irrigating solution, proper agitation techniques, and a gentle slipping and sliding motion, the radiographic terminus can be reached. The second type of motion is the smoothing motion. This is employed only when the radiographic terminus is reached. This makes use of short-amplitude vertical strokes of 1 to 2 mm. Initially with the sun soothing motion, the files are tight, which later may become loose with effective canal enlargement.

- The third type of motion is the envelope motion. The smart and subtle envelope motion will wear away the restrictive dentin in an outward stroke. This is very similar to reverse filing.The fourth type of motion is the balanced force or the Roane technique. This is explained in (Figure 3). In this technique, when the file engages with apical pressure, 1/4 turn should be clockwise followed by, with apical pressure, a 3/4 turn counterclockwise. Progressive instrumentation with larger instruments cuts dentin effectively. Repeat sequence two or three times. Then for the final instance, a 360° turn clockwise (no apical pressure) should be made in order to load onto the file all the dentinal debris collected, and then remove file from canal. When the file is removed from the canal, one can appreciate the presence of dentin on the most apical portion of the file.When properly used, these robust and efficient glide path techniques and motions can negate all of the risks out of rotary shaping.

Glide path preparation using reciprocating handpiece

- The patency of the canal is established using a 10 K file. The tip of the file is precurved and using a watch-wind motion the working length is reached. The same file is then attached to the M4 reciprocating hand piece. With the handpiece activated, the file is withdrawn 0.5 mm from the canal and moved back to its original length. This process is repeated until a glide path preparation is confirmed. A successful glide path is said to be created when the file can travel 5 mm in the root canal without any obstruction.

Glide path and apical extrusion of debris

- It is very well clear that the creation of glide path enhances the performance of Ni-Ti instruments. Glide path preparation allows the preservation of a pathway to the entire working length, thus avoiding excessive binding in the canal and, thus, there is less extrusion of debris. Procedural errors during preparation of root canals, such as apical transportation and irregular foramen widening can lead to poor sealing efficiency with a high rate of extrusion of debris and post operative discomfort. Microhardness values of human dentin may affect extrusion of debris." In teeth with lower hardness, debris may be extruded more readily into the periapical tissues. But, ultimately, the amount of apically extruded debris was decreased when a glide path was created before canal preparation.

Postoperative pain after manual and mechanical glide path preparation

- Pain is a frequent complication associated with endodontic treatment. Mechanical, chemical, or microbial injuries to the periradicular tissues are frequent causes of pain complications. Hence, performing a glide path with hand instrumentation may have a significant impact in reducing the postoperative pain.

Advantages of hand files in preparing glide path

- It aids in initial scouting of canals.
- K-files provide better tactile sensation
- Less potential for separation
- When a small size K-file is removed from the canal the file retains an impression of the canal and also alerts the clinician about the curvature of canal
- The stiffness of stainless steel hand files aids in pathfinding and in negotiating blockages and calcification.
- Lower cost
- No need for a dedicated handpiece

Disadvantages:

- Operator fatigue
- Hand fatigue
- Time required in the preparation of the glide path
- Risk of the introduction of canal aberrations with larger file sizes.
- Greater change to original canal anatomy
- Increased apical extrusion of debris

Conclusion

Every tooth that requires endodontic therapy presents its own set of anatomical challenges to effective instrumentation. Grossman states that the who has not separated an instrument has not done enough root canals. This threat of instrument fracture remains in contemporary endodontics. The preparation of a glide path not only helps to reduce the risk of instrument separation, but also conveys to the clinician an intimate knowledge of the tortuous anatomy of the canal from the orifice to the terminus. The information during glide path preparation enables clinicians to adapt their shaping strategy to the nuances of the canal anatomy of each individual canal. While novel mechanical methods of glide path preparation serve to increase the efficiency of this essential prerequisite of canal shaping, the role of hand instruments should not be overlooked.

J) CROWN DOWN SHAPING TECHNIQUE

Step down technique (top to bottom technique/crown to apex technique/coronal flaring technique)

- It is indicated where ever first binding file (initial file) is not reaching till estimated working length or apex.
- In cases of obstructions, blockages, ledges.
- In cases of severe calcification. In case of dilacerated root. Mesial roots of lower molar.
- Distobuccal/mesio buccal roots of maxillary molars.
- Indicated in Re-root canal cases.

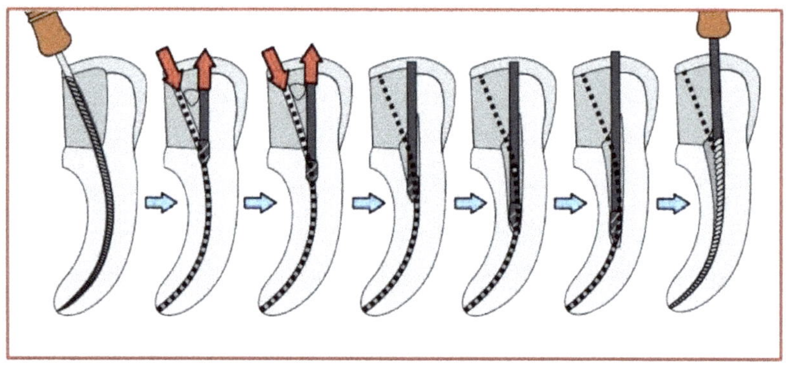

Fig. 9.90: Crown Down

Procedure

Obtaining a glide path for Sx file

Flood the chamber with a viscous chelator (EDTA). Insert the # 6 or # 8 K file in to the canal till the available working length. Engage the file in to the dentin, apply lateral pressure and withdraw the file (one cutting cycle). Insert the next larger file *i.e.* 10 K file, repeat the procedure till the 10 K file becomes super loose. (2-3 cutting cycles with sequentially 2-3 larger size files are required to obtain smooth reproducible glide path). Feed the SX rotary file and brush a follow. After pre flaring is done with Sx files, insert the #6/8 K file all the way till the apex. Feel the apical tug, calculate the exact working length. Once the working length has been calculated, achieve the glide path for the next rotary file.

Obtaining a glide path for S1 S2 F1 F2 file

Pre curving of files is to be done to make the file a smart file. Apical instrumentation with 6, 8 & 10 K file is done till exact working length. Minimum 2-3 cutting cycles.

K) ROTARY SYSTEM

Metallurgy

All rotary files are manufactured from nickel titanium alloy (55% nickel, 45% titanium) because of its shape memory property. The shape memory & super elasticity property is due to phase transition from austinsite to martinsite. Shape memory property means the ability to return to its original shape once the stress is removed. All files are available in austinsitic (mother phase) form. In austinsite stage there is increased resistance to torsional stress and less flexibility. At martinsite phase (weak phase) the files show increase in flexibility, decrease in cutting efficiency, and decreased resistance to torsional stresses. In elastic range all rotary files have shape memory & super elasticity. Beyond the outer limits of elastic range file exhibits plastic range (permanent deformation) Outer limits of plastic range is yield point (breakage).

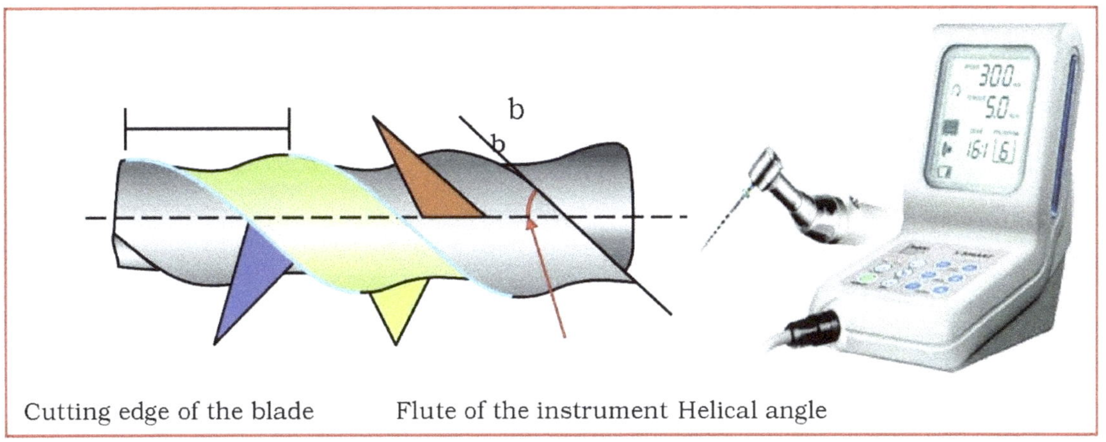

Fig. 9.91: Pitch and Flute

Rotary files

1. Components of files

Taper denotes the per mm increase in the file diameter from the tip towards the file. In 2% taper file diameter increase by 0.02 mm for every 1 mm. In 4% taper file diameter increases by 0.04 mm for every 1 mm. In 6% file, taper diameter increases by 0.06 mm for every 1 mm. Taper helps in preparing canals of wider diameter without enlarging the canals at working length. Taper varies according to size and width of canals, with 2% taper smaller or narrow canals are prepared, with 4% taper medium size canals are prepared and with 6% taper larger diameter canals are prepared. With very larger taper more natural tooth structure gets removed example 8% taper.

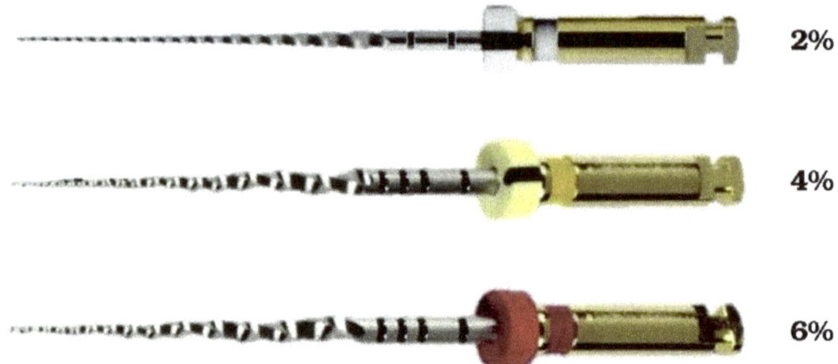

Fig. 9.92: Taper

Flute

Flute is a groove in the working surface is used to collect soft tissue and dentinal chips. The effectiveness of flute depends on its shape, depth and configuration. The shape of flutes in landed files are triple U. The shape of flutes in non-landed files are tringle or convex triangle. The shape of flutes in Hero shaper file is irregular or roughly S shape with positive rake angles.

Radial land

Radial land is a flat cutting surface present between the grooves or flutes. It supports the cutting edge and limits the depth of cut.

It reduces the tendency of the files to screw into the canal. By occupying more space in the canals, it increases cutting efficiency. Maintains the file in the centre of canal and reduces the chances of lateral transportation of the canal.

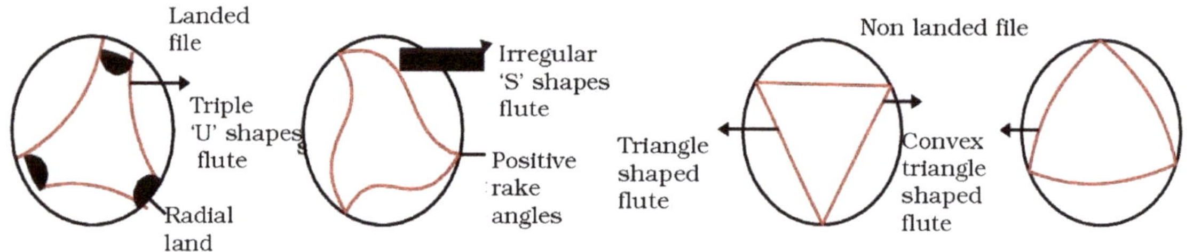

Fig. 9.93: Cross section landed and non landed files

Helix angle

The angle of the cutting-edge forms with the long axis of the file. It determines the file technique to be used, it influences the cutting efficiency. The files with uniform helical angle exhibits less cutting efficacy, files with variable helical angles exhibits more cutting efficacy.

Rake angle

Definition

In perpendicular section the angle formed by the leading edge and radius of the file is called rake angle.

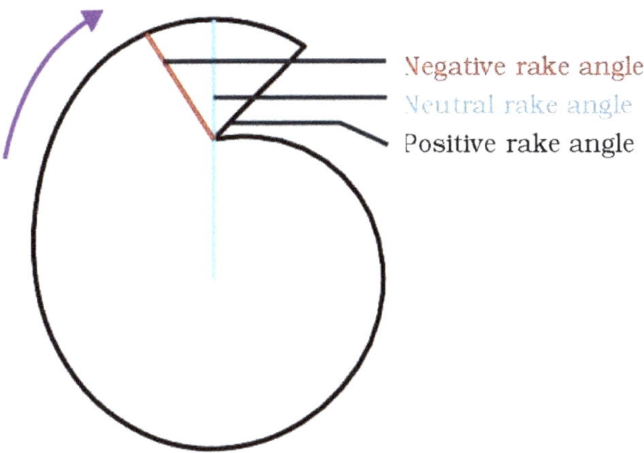

Fig. 9.94: Cross section Rake angle

If the angle formed by the leading edge and surface to be cut is obtuse the angle is said to be positive rake angle which results in cutting action. If the angle formed by the leading edge and surface to be cut is acute, the angle is said to be negative rake angle which results in scraping action. The rake angle should be balanced. Slight increase in positive rake angle increases cutting efficiency. more increase in positive rake angle decreases the cutting efficiency. Hero shaper files have slight positive rake angle so exhibits more cutting efficiency.

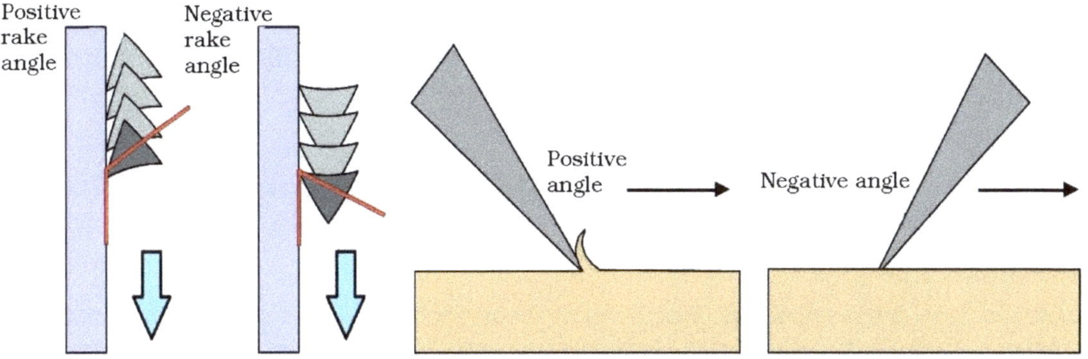

Fig. 9.95: Rake angle

Pitch

Pitch of the file is the distance between the two leading edges. Most files have variable pitch. Pitch vary along the length of file, files with shorter pitch will have more spirals and greater helical angle and greater cutting efficiency. Files with longer pitch will have less spirals and small helical angle and little cutting efficiency.

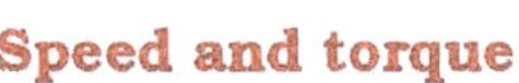
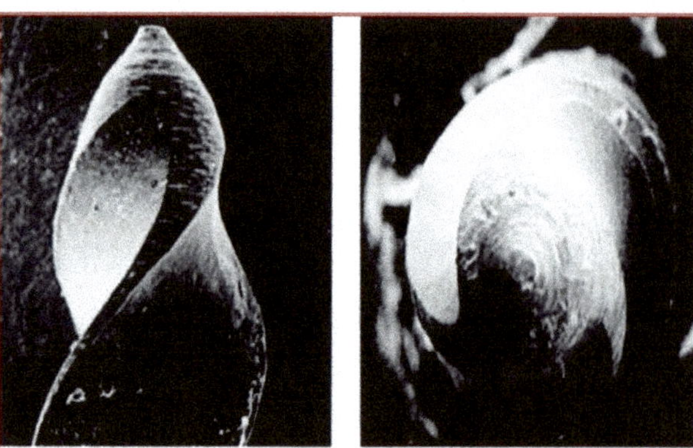

Fig. 9.96:

Tip design

Tip design can affect file control, efficiency and outcome in the shaping of root canal system. When the tip angle is reduced file stays centred within the curved portion of canal and cuts all sides more evenly.

Speed and torque

Speed is from 250 to 500 rpm. The advantages of high speed are more

Fig. 9.97: Flex-R file with modified rounded tip

cutting efficiency. The disadvantages of high speed are loss of tactile sensation, loss of control, more chances of transportation, and more chances of breakage.

Torque 2.5 to 5 N cm. More torque, more instrument progression in the canal. More torque decreases the chances of instrument separation, and instrument blocking. Low torque leads to low progression of instrument in canal. The torque required to rotate a file is determined by surface area of file engagement. More the surface area of engagement, more torque is required.

Kinematics

Kinematics means study of motion of objects. Files can take 2 types of motion Rotation & Reciprocation.

Rotation

Safety is less with rotation. Rotation is motion of file 360 degree in clock wise direction. With Rotation cutting efficiency is more. It pushes the debris coronally. Thereby, decreases the risk of extrusion of debris into the periapical area. The fatigue of file due to intracanal torsional stress is more and the chances of breakage of files are more.

Reciprocation

Safety is more with reciprocation. Reciprocation means both clock wise & anti-clock wise motion. 150 clockwise & 30 anti-clock wise motion. It causes the extrusion of debris into periapical area which leads to post-operative pain. The fatigue of file due to intra canal torsional stress is less so less chances of breakage.

General guidelines

Glide path is must before introducing the rotary files into the canals.

Always use the instrument in sequence.

Never force the instrument.

Use only in well irrigated canals.

Clean and inspect regularly. Avoid over using.

At working length use one file at one time

and at the apex for 0-3 sec.

Use with no apical pressure.

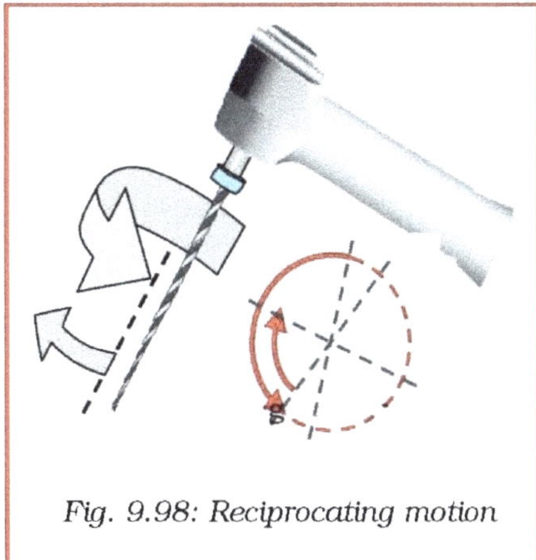

Fig. 9.98: Reciprocating motion

Types of rotary files

There are two main types – Shapers and finishers. Shapers are Sx, S1, S2. Finishers are F1, F2, F3, and F4, F5. Shapers are used to give shape to the canals. Finishers are used to refine the canals.

Sx rotary files

Sx is an axillary file. It is 19 mm in length. Length of working blade is 14 mm. It is used in place of gate Glidden drills. Used as orifice enlarger. It has no identification rings. It is also used in short roots to shape the canal. It is used in removing dentinal triangle and dentinal wedges. Method: paint and follow. D0 is 0.19 mm.

Rules to use Sx o

1. Backstroke brushing motion & Never pushed down in the canal
2. With light pressure
3. Away from furcation
4. Not more than 5mm deep from canal orifice

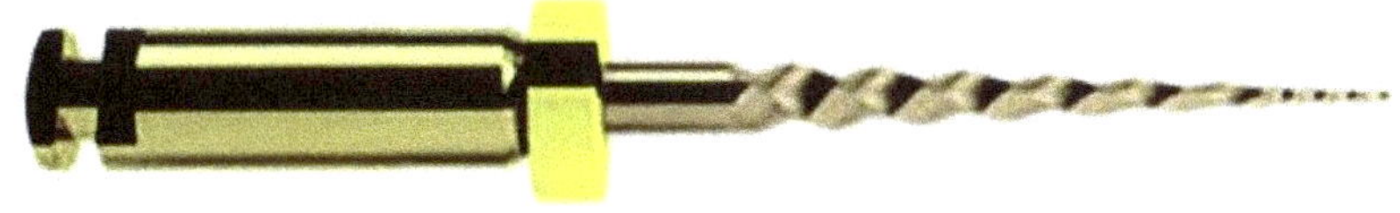

Fig. 9.99: SX

Shaping files
S1 rotary file

Used to shape coronal one third of the canal. It is available in 21 mm 25 mm 31 mm in length. It has purple colour coding. D0 is 0.185.

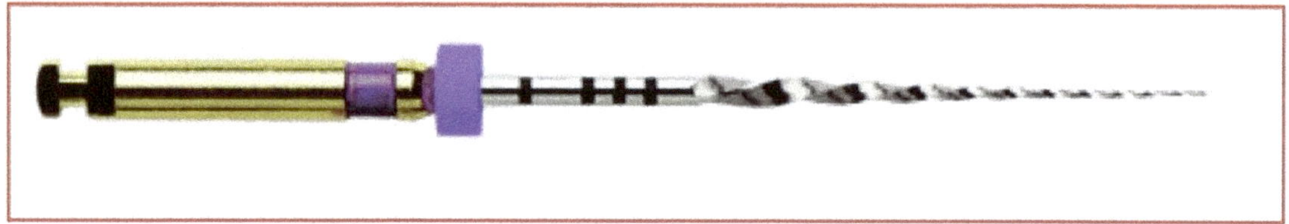

Fig. 9.100: S1

S2 rotary file

It is designed to prepare middle one third.

It is also available in 21 mm, 25 mm, 31 mm. It has white colour coding.

D0 is 0.20.

S1 S2 they do enlarge apical third progressively.

Note: brush and follow.

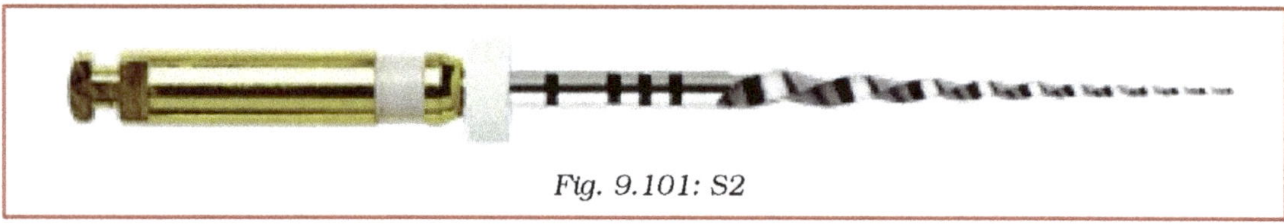

Fig. 9.101: S2

Finishing files

- The three finishing files (F1, F2 & F3) and accessory finishing file (F4 & F5). Finishing files cannot be used for shaping.

- In many cases only one finishing file is required either F1, F2, F3.

- Finishing files F1, F2, F3 have yellow, red, & blue, identification colours respectively on their handles. Diameter is 0.20, 0.25, 0.30 and so on.

- Finishing files should be used for 0-3 sec.

- The number of strokes should be minimum 2-3. Note- watch words (follow and brush).

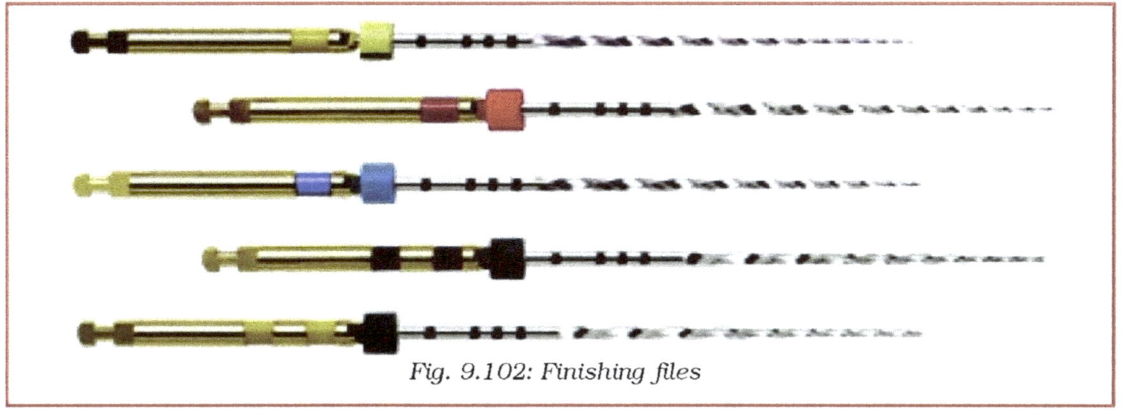

Fig. 9.102: Finishing files

Endosequence

It is determined by the size of glide path. If 10k size file is tightly binding the sequence would be small. If 10k size file is loose the sequence would be medium. If 15k size file is loose the sequence would be large.

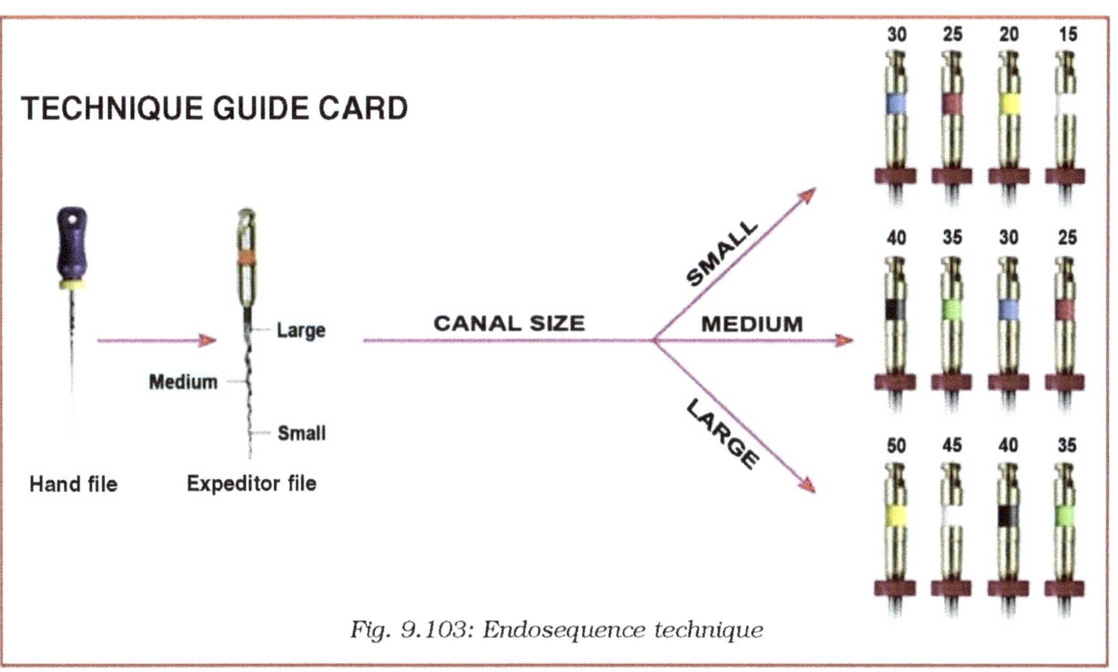

Fig. 9.103: Endosequence technique

Procedure

- Set and adjust all parameters. Feed the file into the canal.
- While using Sx, follow till 1 mm behind the maximum resistance. Brush. While using S1, S2, follow till 1 or 2 mm behind the exact working length and Brush.
- While using finishers, kiss and follow in upward motion.

The WAVEONE single file reciprocating system

- The new wave one NiTi file system is a single use, to shape the root canal completely from start to finish.

- Shaping the root canal to a continuously tapering funnel shape not only fulfils the biological requirements for adequate irrigation to rid the root canal system of all bacteria, bacterial by-products and pulp tissue, but also provides the perfect shape for 3D obturation with gutta percha.

- In most cases, the technique only requires one hand file followed by one hand file followed by one single Wave One file to shape the canal completely.

- The specially designed NiTi files work in a similar but reverse "balanced force" action using a pre-programmed motor to move the files in a back and forth "reciprocal motion".

- The files are manufactured using M-wire technology ,improving strength and resistance to cyclic fatigue by upto nearly four times in comparison with other brands of rotary NiTi files.

- There are many dentist who,for whatever reason, are reluctant to use NiTi rotary instruments to prepare canals, despite the recognised advantages of flexibility, less debris extrusion and maintaining a canal shape, amongst other advantages.

- For them, use of single reciprocating file will be very attractive both in terms of time and cost saving.

- At present, there are three files in the Waveone single-file reciprocating system available in lengths of 21, 25 and 31mm.

- The Waveone small file is used in fine canals. The tip size is ISO 21 with a continuous taper of 6%.

- The Waveone primary file is used in the majority of canals. The tip size is ISO 25 with an apical taper of 8% that reduces towards the coronal end.

- The Waveone large file is used in large canals. The tip size is ISO 40 with an apical taper of 8% that reduces towards the coronal end.

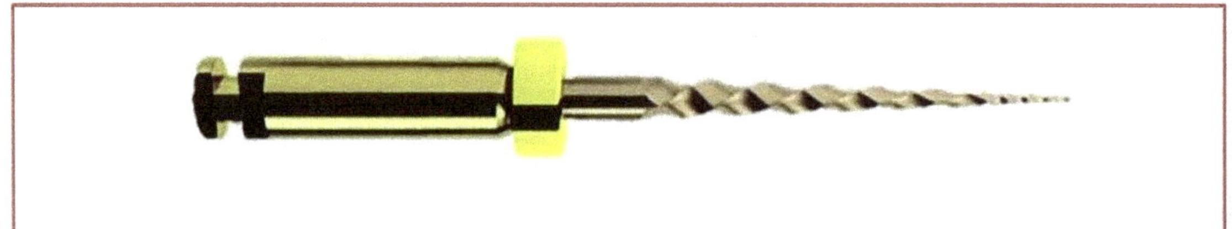

Fig. 9.104: Waveone single file system

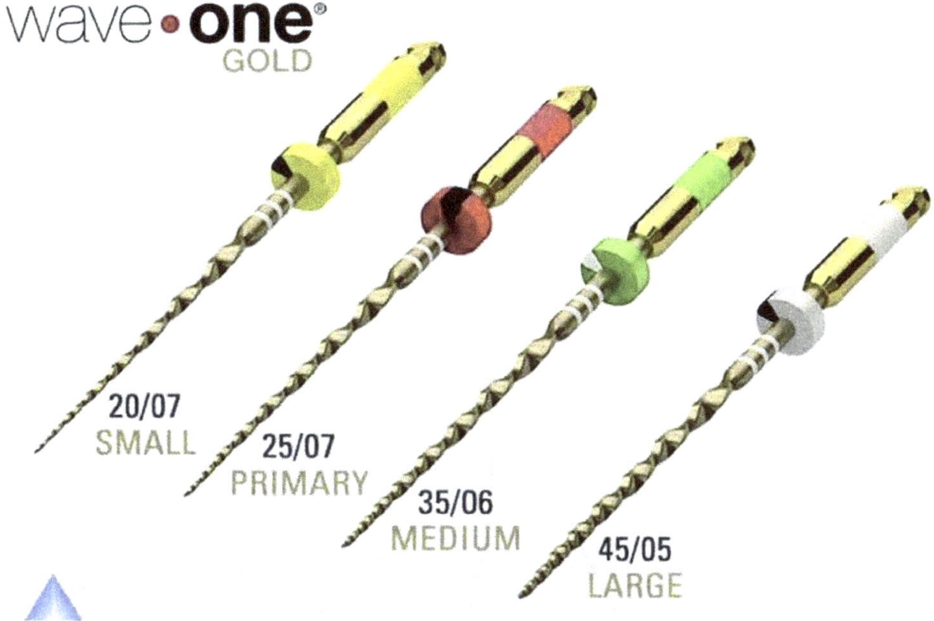

Fig. 9.105:

- The instruments are designed to work with a reverse cutting action.

- All instruments have a modified convex triangular cross section at the tip end and a covex triangular cross section at the coronal end.

- This design improves instrument flexibility overall.

- The tips are modified to follow canal curvature accurately.

- The variable pitch flutes along the length of the instrument considerably improve safety.

- As there is possibility of cross contamination associated with inability to completely clean and sterilise endodontic instruments and the possible presence of prion in human dental pulp tissue, all instruments used inside root canals should be single use.

- Wave one intruments are a new concept in this important standard of care, as they are truly single use.

- The plastic colour coding in the handle becomes deformed once sterilised, preventing the file from being placed back into handpiece.

- The recommandation for single use has added advantage of reducing instrument fatigue which is anyone important consideration with Waveone file, as one file does the work traditionally performed by 3 or more NiTi file.

The Waveone technique involves following stages
1. Straight line access, accepted protocol
2. Wave one file selection
3. Single file shaping
4. Copious irrigation with 5% NaoCl and EDTA before, during and after single file shaping.

File selection and clinical procedure
- Whilst a good preoperative radiograph will give an indication of what to expect before the canal is prepared, number of canals, only the first hand file into the canal will aid in the selection of the WaveOne file as follows:

1) If a 10 k file is very resistant to movement, use Waveone small file.

2) If a 10 k file moves to length easily, is loose or very loose, use Wave One primary file.

3) If a 20 hand file or larger goes to length, use Wave One larger file.

   - Use appropriate WaveOne file to approximately two thirds of canal length.
   - Irrigate copiously
   - Take hand file to length and confirm with an apex locator and radiograph
   - Take Wave One file to length
   - Confirm foramen diameter with hand file the same size as WaveOne file; if snug, preparation is complete;
   - If foramen diameter is larger than WaveOne file, consider the next larger WaveOne file;

Majority of cases will be completed with WaveOne primary file

Guideliness for use:
- Use WaveOne files with a progressive up and down movement no more than three to four times, only little force is required.

- Remove file regularly,wipe clean, irrigate and continue;

- If file does not progress, confirm patent canal and consider using a smaller WaveOne file;

- Whilst glide path management is minimal with WaveOne shaping files,some practitioner will be more comfortable if the glide path is first secured with Pathfiles

- In severely curved canals, complete apical preparation by hand if reproducible glide path is not possible;

- WaveOne files can be used to relocate the canal orifice and expand coronal shape; even in a reciprocating motion use them in a "brushing" action short of length to achieve this.

- Never work in a dry canal and constantly irrigate with sodium hypochloride and later with EDTA.

- As preparation time is short, activate the irrigating solution to enhance their effect, the endo activator is ideal for this.

Wave One obturating solutions:

- Obturation of the root canal system is the final step of the endodontic procedure.

- The WaveOne system includes matching paper points, gutta percha points and Thermafill WaveOne obturators.

- The matching gutta percha points can be used in conjunction with the Calamus Dual 3-D Obturating system.

Advantages of the WaveOne file reciprocating system

- Only one NiTi instrument per root canal and in most cases per tooth

- Lower cost

- Less instrument separation owing to the unique reciprocating movement that will prevent and/or delay the instrument advancing from plastic deformation to its plastic limit;

- Decreases global shaping time, allowing the clinician to spend more time cleaning the root canal system with enhanced irrigation techniques.

- Eliminates procedural errors by using a single instrument rather than using multiple files;

- A new standard of care, eliminating the possibility of prion contamination owing to single use;

- Easy to learn
- Easy to teach

WaveOneresearch

- Canal-centring ability of WaveOne

- Remaining canal wall thickness after instrumentation with WaveOne

- Final shape versus initial shape of canal with Wave ONE

- Canal wall cleanliness with WaveOne.

Other areas of research are flexibility, fatigue and debris extrusion

L) INTRACANAL MEDICAMENTS

Endodontic infection considered to be complex and polymicrobial in nature. In heavily infected roots and more than single visit root canal treatments complete disinfection of root canal system cannot be achieved through BMP and cleaning alone therefore intracanal medication strongly recommended. Although the role of intracanal medication is secondary to cleaning and shaping as a part of controlled asepsis adequate disinfection assisted by intracanal medication reduces the bacterial count, promote periapical healing and enhances endodontic prognosis.

Definition

Temporary placement of biocompatible and stable material into the full length of root canal for the purpose of complete disinfection of root canal system or temporary placement of biocompatible material in to the root canal for the purpose of inhibiting the coronal leakage from gape between cavity walls and filling materials.

Rationale

Although chemo mechanical preparation has an important cleaning effect it cannot eliminate all the bacteria from the root which are harbored in dentinal tubules. The remaining bacteria present in the dentinal tubules may multiple during the period between appointment often reaching the same level that it was at the start of the previous session in case where the canal is not dressed with disinfectants between visits.

Ideal requirements of intracanal antiseptic medicaments

a.   It should be effective germicide and fungicide

b.   It should be non- irrigating

c.   It should remain stable in solution

d.   It should have prolonged antibacterial effect

e.   It should be active in presence of serum and protein derivatives of tissue

f.   It should be capable of penetrating tissues deeply

g.   It should not interfere with repairs of periapical tissues

h.   It should not strain tooth structure

i.   It should be easily introduced into root canal

j.   It should be capable of being inactivated or neutralized in culture medium preven coronal micro leakage and not diffused to the temporary restoration

OBJECTIVES

1) **Elimination of micro-organisms**

   The object is to sterilize (destroy all viable micro- organism) or to disinfect (destroy all pathogens) in the canal space.

2) **Rendering contents of canal inert**

   This represents the attempt usually by chemical means to "mummify or fix" otherwise neutralize tissue or debris left intentionally or unintentionally in the pulp space. If successful this would cause those remnants to become inert and to remain non irritant.

3) **Prevention of control of post treatment pain**

   The objective is to reduce or alter the inflammatory response. Medicament might accomplish this by antimicrobial action or by pharmacologically by alerting the inflammatory response itself. Logically this would reduce the pain that often accompanies inflammation.

4) **Enhancing Anesthesia**

   Agents have been suggested as a means of some how reducing the sensitivity of the inflamed difficult to anthesize pulp. If this were true, the pulp could be removed as subsequent appointment with less anesthetic difficulty.

5) **Control of persistent periapical abscess**

   A continually weeping canal or significant pain or swelling after treatment are signs of an active periapical inflammatory lesion. Medicaments have been suggested as a mean of controlling this difficult situation. The agent in the canal space would have direct access to the preapical lesions. It might by direct action restore a healthy balance

6) **To dry the persistently weeping canals.**

   To remove the microorganism, debris, biofilms and smear layer left after bio mechanical preparation and irrigation.

Indications

❖ **Heavily infected roots in conditions like**
   - Re-root canal cases,
   - Post root canal acute periodontitis
   - Post root canal acute periodontal abscess
   - Chronic periapical abscess
   - Phoenix abscess
   - Active periapical granuloma
   - Infected periapical cyst

❖ **Endodontic lesions of periodontal origin**

In teeth with larger periapical lesion to control passage of periapical exudate in to the canals.

❖ **Poor patient compliance**

If root canal treatment is not completed in a single appointment in patients with poor compliances the risk of aseptic complications increases through a leaky temporary filling.

Classification

1) Essential oils
   - Eugenol

2) Phenolic compounds
   - Phenol
   - Parachlorophenol
   - Camphorated parachlorophenol
   - Cresol
   - Formocresol
   - Creosote
   - Cresatin
   - Cresanol

3) N2

4) Salt of heavy metals
   - Metaphen
   - Merthiolate
   - Mercurophen

5) Halogens
   - Sodium hypochlorite
   - Iodides
   - Chlorhexidine

6) Quaternary ammonium compounds
   - 9-aminoacidine

7) Fatty acids
   - Propionic acid
   - Caproic acid
   - Cuprilyc acid

Calcium hydroxide

Herman introduced calcium hydroxide as a intracanal medicament in 1920. It has acquired a unique position in endodontics because of its uses. It is highly alkaline substance with pH is 12.5 owing to its high alkaline pH only few bacteria can survive.

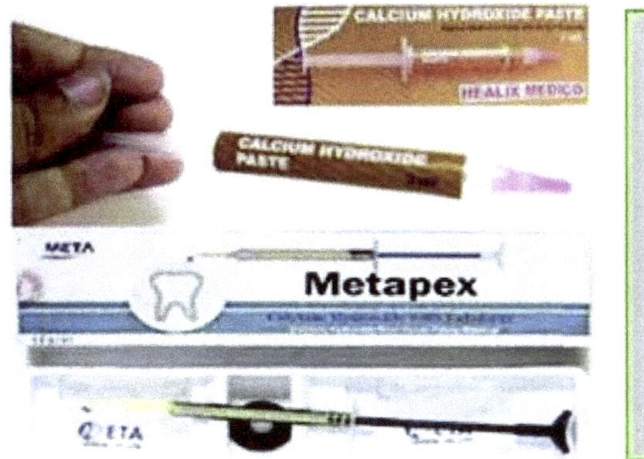

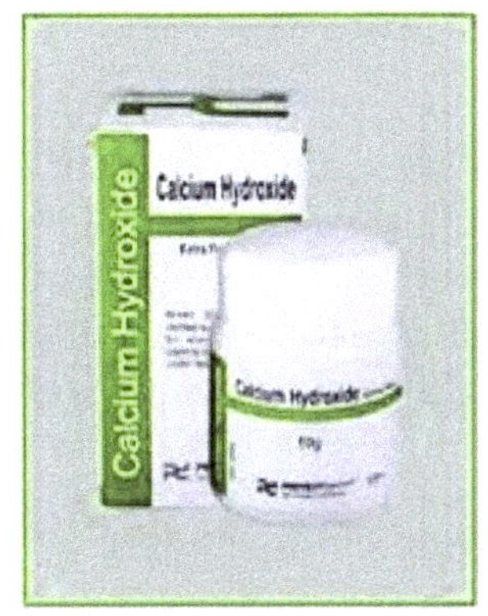

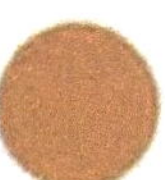

Fig. 9.106:

Mechanism of action

Its antibacterial and the anti-microbial action is due to the release of hydroxylion. The hydroxyl ion act by :

1.   Damaging the cytoplasmic membrane.
2.   Denaturation of bacterial proteins
3.   Damaging the bacterial DNA

It has chelating effect directly or indirectly aid in dissolution of necrotic tissue.

Mode of action

Anti-endotoxin activity

Endotoxin play a fundamental role in the genesis and maintenance of periapical lesions by inducing periapical inflammation and periapical bone resorption. Calcium hydroxide act by inactivating endotoxins.

Anti-fungal activity

Fungal infections appear to occur more often in post root canal apical periodontitis and post root canal acute periodontal abscess. It seems that combination of calcium hydroxide with chlorhexidine have the potential to be used as effective intracanal medicament.

Activity against biofilm

Anti-microbial potential of calcium hydroxide on biofilms have demonstrated inconsistent results further studies are needed to be confirmed.

Availability

- Commercially available in the following farm
- Powder farm powder is mixed with saline or sterile water.
- Single paste or combination with iodoform.
- Non-soluble gel form

Limitations

The handling and proper placement of calcium hydroxide present a challenge to the average clinician and requires skill. Mixing of calcium hydroxide in a proper consistency to be filled root canal and properly carry it to the canal is still a challenge. Though various formulations are available but still its placement in posterior teeth is difficult. Also, the removal of calcium hydroxide is most frequently incomplete result in a residual covering to 20 % to 45% of the canal wall surfaces even after copious irrigation with saline, sodium hypochlorite or EDTA. Residual calcium hydroxide also possess a problem as it shortens the setting time of zinc oxide eugenol based endodontic sealer if used for final obturation.

Methods of removal of calcium hydroxide

- Paste form of calcium hydroxide more difficult to remove compare to powder mixed with distilled water.

- Both 17% EDTA and 10% citric acid were found to remove calcium hydroxide powder mixed with distilled water. 10% citric acid performed better than EDTA in removing an oil based calcium hydroxide paste.

- Hand filling using H files

- Rotary instruments

- Ultrasonic irrigation

- Mixture of sodium hypochlorite and EDTA

Chlorhexidine gluconate

Chlorhexidine digluconate has been recommended both as a root canal irrigant and an intracanal medicament. As a medicament it can be used as 2% CHX gel. Chlorhexidine possess broad spectrum anti-microbial activity and very effective against E. coli and candida species. Also, It exhibits substantivity and low toxicity these properties make well suited for irrigation and intracanal medication, mixture of chlorhexidine and calcium hydroxide may be useful adjuvant in the management of inflammatory resorption. Chlorhexidine mixed with zinc oxide combination highly effective against killing candida albicans.

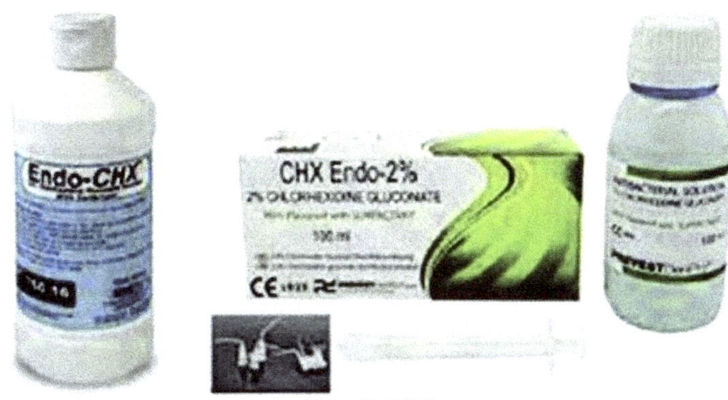

Fig. 9.107:

Antibiotics

Local application of antibiotic may be more effective mode of delivering. infection of root canals is considered to be polymicrobial in nature because of the complexity of root canal infection the use of single antibiotic may not result in effective disinfection of root canal space. A combination of antibiotics may be needed to address the diverse flora encountered. A combination of antibiotics might also decrease the likelihood of development of resistant bacterial strains.

The combination that appears to be most promising as follows:

PBSC paste

-   Penicillin –Effective against gram-positive micro-organisms
-   Bacitracin –Effective against penicillinase resistant micro-organisms
-   Streptomycin- Effective against gram-negative micro-organisms
-   Caprylate sodium–Effective against fungi

Sulfonamide

-   The sulfonamides are chiefly bacteriostatic rather than bactericidal agents which interfere with bacterial metabolism and thereby render micro-organisms more vulnerable to destruction by the defensive mechanism of body.
-   Triple antibiotic paste –ciprofloxacin, metronidazole and minocycline.
-   Modified Triple antibiotic paste –ciprofloxacin, metronidazole and cefaclor
-   Double antibiotic paste - ciprofloxacin and metronidazole

Steroids and antibiotics

-   Ledermix paste is a glucocorticoid antibiotic combination contains
-   Demeclocycline hydrochloride
-   Triamcinolone acetoxide
-   Polyethylene glycol
-   It is recommended for initial dressing particularly if patient presents with endodontic symptoms.

- It can be used as direct and indirect pulp capping agent
- Immediate intracanal placement of ledermix paste after an avulsion injury appears to decreases the resorption and increases favorable healing.

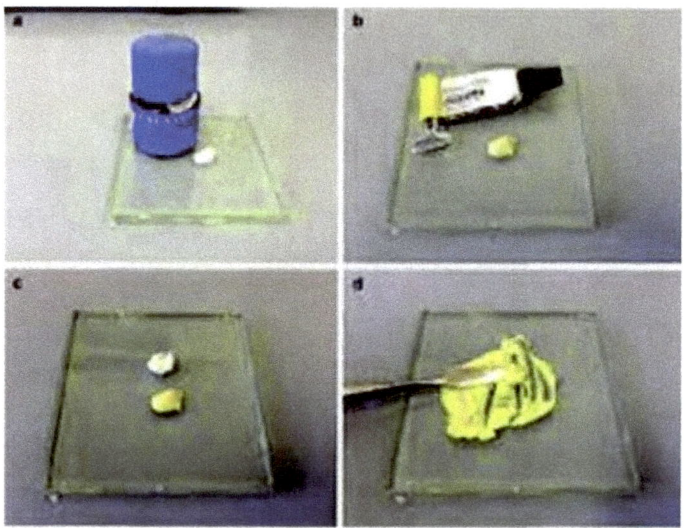

Fig. 9.108:

Recent advances in intracanal medications

- Medicated gutta-percha
- ENDOX
- Bioactive glasses
- PAD

Medicated gutta-percha

There are new gutta percha points in the market that contain calcium hydroxide in a 50% to 51% concentration instead zinc oxide which makes calcium hydroxide placement and removal easy.

Photo activated disinfections:

Photodynamic therapy is based on concept that nontoxic photosensitizer can be preferentially localized in certain tissue and subsequently activated by light of appropriate wavelength to generate oxygen and free radicals that are cytotoxic to cells of target tissue methylene blue is a well-established photosensitizer that has been used in photodynamic therapy for targeting gram negative and gram positive bacteria. Along methylene blue telonium chloride had also been used as a photo sensitizing agent. It is applied in infected area and left in situ for a short period of time. This agent binds the cellular membrane of bacteria which will then rupture when activated by a laser source emitting radiation at an appropriate wave length. Telomium chloride dye is biocompatible and does not stain dental tissue.

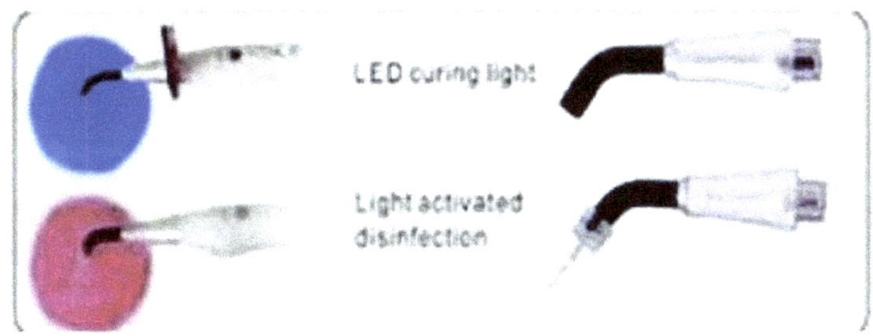

Fig. 9.109:

ENDOX

ENDOX endodontic system has been reported sterilize root canal system by emitting high electric impulses sterilization occurs as result of fulguration and manufacturer claims it is able to both pulp and Bacteria eliminate from the entire root canal system. Recently studies showed that the unit was not able to eliminate pulp tissue from root canal system without mechanical cleaning.

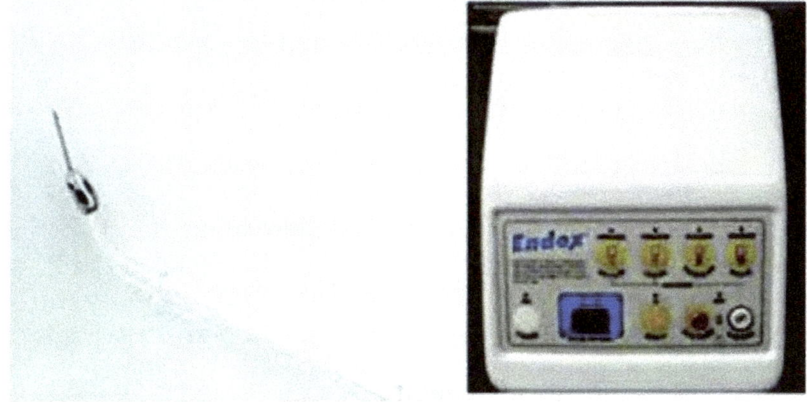

Fig. 9.110:

Recent trends in irrigation of endodontics

1)   MTAD, [Mixture of tetracycline acid and detergent]

2)   Tetraclean

3)   Photo activated disinfections

4)   Electrochemically activated solutions

5)   Ozonated water

6)   Herbal irrigants

MTAD :-

MTAD was enhanced when NAOCL issued as intraconal irrigants before use of MTAD as an final irrigant.

- MTAD does not seem to change structures of dental tubules

- MTAD is effective against removing smear layer along whole length of root canal and in removing organic and inorganic debris and does not produce any signs of erosion or physical changes in dentine.

Electrochemically activated solution – electrochemically activated solution are produced from tap water and salt solutions of lower concentration. Principles of EAC is transferring liquids into metastable state via anode or cathode action by use of an element/element reactor

- The element or reactor is called as FEM i.e flow through electrolyte module.

- The FEM consists of anode and cathode. Anode, a solid titanium cylinder with special coating that fits coaxially inside cathode. These electrodes are seperated by ceramic membrane. FEM is capable of producing solution that have bactericidal and sporicidal activity. They are odourless, safe to human tissue and no corrosive for most metal surfaces. Electrochemically treatment in anode and cathode chambers is anolyte and solution produced in cathode chamber is catholyte

- Anolyte solutions containing mixtures of oxidizing substance demonstrate pronounced microbiocidal effectiveness against bacteria, virus and fungi as well as protozoa.

Tetraclean:-

Like MTAD tetraclean is a mixture of an antibiotic, an acid and a detergent. However, the concentration of antibiotic doxycycline (50 mg / ml), and the type of detergent (polypropylene glycol) differ from those MTAD. Only the NaOCl could disaggregate and remove the biofilm at every time interval tested although treatment with tetraclean caused a high degree of biofilm disaggregation at each time interval when compared with MTAD.

Photo activated disinfections:

Photodynamic therapy is based on concept that nontoxic photosensitizer can be preferentially localized in certain tissue and subsequently activated by light of appropriate wavelength to generate oxygen and free radicals that are cytotoxic to cells of target tissue, methylene blue is a well established photosensitizer that has been used in photodynamic therapy for targeting gram negative and gram positive bacteria. Along methylene blue tolonium chloride had also been used as a photo sensitizing agent. It is applied in infected area and left in situ for a short period of time. This agent binds the cellular membrane of bacteria which will then rupture when activated by a laser source emitting radiation at an appropriate wave length. Tolinomium chloride dye is biocompatible and does not stain dental tissue.

Ozonated water:

Ozone is very powerful bactericide that can kill microorganism effectively. It is an unstable gases capable of oxidizing any biological entity. It was reported that ozone at low concentration, 0.1 ppm, is sufficient to inactivate bacteria cells including their pores. It is present naturally in air and can be easily produced by ozone generator. Although ozonated water is powerful antimicrobial agent against bacteria, fungi, protozoa and virus less attention had been paid to the antibacterial activity of ozonated water in bacterial biofilm and hence in root canal infections.

Herbal: Ayurvedic herbal formulation is know as triphala is a combination of dried and powdered fruits of three medical plants and green tea polyphenols :

-   3 medical plants are terminalia bellerica, terminalia chebula and embelica officinalis.

-   Triphala and green tea polyphenols show similar antibacterial on E Faecalis But triphala shows more patenary on E Faecalis bio film.

Procedure

The canals are finally irrigated with doxycycline or prednisolone and filled with chlorhexidine gluconate gel, or calcium hydroxide. Closed dressing is given with interim cement. Patient is recalled after 7 days to remove the medicament and proceed with obturation.

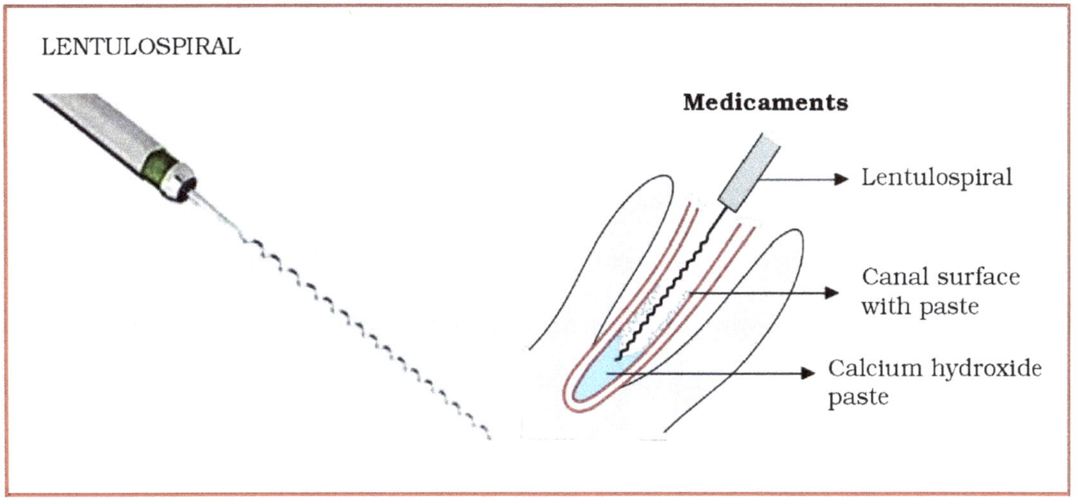

Fig. 9.111: Procedure : Intracanal Medicament placement

M) OBTURATION

THE ONLY THING WORTH RELISHING IS FINISHING.
FINISHING BRINGS GLORY. WITH GLORY
COMES OPPORTUNITY. OPPORTUNITY IS THE
KEY TO PRACTICE.
BE A GOOD FINISHER, BE A GOOD PRACTITIONER.

After shaping and cleaning a well-shaped and totally disinfected root canal system should create the conditions for intact periapical tissues but this unfilled and empty root canal system is inaccessible to the body's immune system therefore it cannot combat coronal leakage accordingly best practices dictates that entire root canal system should be filled completely, as close to cemento-dentinal junction as possible in order to prevent ingress of nutrients and micro-organisms. Carefully and properly achieved obturation will lead to total obliteration of root canal system and formation of three dimensional fluid tight seal which is foundation for long term prognosis of tooth.

Definition

Three-dimensional filling of entire root canal system as close to cemento dentinal junction as possible with biologically acceptable core filling material and very minimal sealer to establish an adequate seal.

Objectives

To prevent re-infection or recurrent infection of the tooth.

After canal preparation and disinfection, the empty space or logical cavity acts as foci of infection so it must be replaced with biologically acceptable stable materials as early as possible to prevent reinfection or recurrent infection by the way of break in the integrity of tooth or through blood circulation (anacoresis).

To restore and re-strengthen the tooth prepared tooth.

Substitution of biologically acceptable and stable filling material in the space previously occupied by the pulp reinforces the endodontically prepared weakened tooth.

To entomb the remaining bacteria

Canal preparation and disinfection cannot eliminate all the bacteria from the root which are harbored in dentinal tubules, residual bacteria after obturation may be denied access to the nutrients and die.

To achieve fluid tight seal

➤ To prevent percolation of periradicular exudate into the pulp space via the apical foramina and or lateral and furcation canals.

➤ To prevent percolation of gingival exudate and microorganisms into the pulp space via lateral canals opening into the gingival sulcus.

➤ To prevent microorganisms left in the canal after preparation from proliferating and escaping into the periradicular tissue via the apical foramina and/or lateral canals.

➤ To seal the pulp chamber and canal system from leakage via the crown in order to prevent passage of microorganisms and/or toxins along the root canal filling and into the periradicular tissue via the apical foramina and/or lateral canals.

Criteria

✓ Tooth must be asymptomatic without the signs and symptoms of periapical periodontitis patient must feel perfectly comfortable with no sensitivity or pain.

✓ Response to percussion test must be negative.

✓ The canals must be clean and free from bacteria, toxins, pus and necrotic plaques. Canals should be inert and dry with no weeping of fluids in the farm of discharge of exudates or bleeding.

✓ No foul odor. Emission of foul odor from canals indicate presence of facultative anaerobic micro-organisms. Intracanal medication with calcium hydroxide is considered before obturation.

✓ If the canals are shaped in previous visit the temporary dressing should not be older than 6 days and should be intact without any distortion in case any distortion has been occurred recontamination of canals due to coronal leakage is suspected. Re-disinfection of canals must be considered before proceeding to obturation.

✓ There should be no signs and symptoms of abscess or fistula if previously present should show signs and symptoms of healing.

✓ Negative culture tests

Confirming the absence of bacteria from anaerobic culture is effective for evaluating periapical lesion resolution process.

Gutta Percha

Introduction

Gutta percha with a unique property of inertness, better sealing abilities and ability to retrieve incase of failure make it is an indispensable material, the preferred choice as a solid core filling material for root canal obturations.

Gutta percha is the preferred choice as a solid, core filling material for canal obturation. It demonstrates minimal toxicity, minimal tissue irritability, and is the least allergenic material available when retained within the canal system. The successful use of the curious material gutta percha seems to have been as insulation for undersea cables. This was in 1848, and patents followed for its use in the manufacture of corks, cement thread, surgical instruments, garments, pipes, and sheathing for ships. Gutta percha golf balls where introduced by the latter part of the 19th century, until 1920, golf balls where called "gutties". In its pure molecular structure, gutta percha is the trans-isomer of polyisoprene and has an approximately 60% crystalline form. The cis-isomer is natural rubber, which has a largely amorphous form. Gutta-percha has three possible phase changes. In the unheated tree or in the cone at room or body temperature, gutta-percha is considered to be in the beta phase. In this phase, gutta-percha is solid, compactible, and elongatible; may become brittle when aged; and does not stick to anything. When heated to temperatures of 42° to 49° "C, gutta-percha undergoes a phase change to the alpha phase. In this phase it is runny, tacky, sticky, noncompactible, and non elongatible. The third, or gamma phase, occurs when heating is raised to 56° to 62 °C, but the properties at this level are not well known and seem to be similar to that of the alpha phase. The significance of these phases, in addition to the changes in physical properties, is that the materials expand when heated from the beta to the alpha or gamma phases, from less than 1% to almost 3%. When cooled down to the beta phase, a shrinkage takes place, of similar percentiles, but the degree of shrinkage almost always is greater than the degree of expansion and may differ by as much as 2%. That means that if gutta-percha is heated above 42° to 49° C (108°-120° F) and then inserted into a prepared canal, a condensation procedure should be applied or some method used to lessen the problem of shrinkage.

Different types of gutta percha availability

Gutta percha points: They have size and shape similar to :

- ISO standardization.

- Greater taper gutta percha: They have taper other than 2%. They are available in 4%, 6%, 8% and 10 % sizes.

- Auxiliary points: They are non-standardized gutta cones.

- They perceive the shape of root canal. Precoated gutta percha: Metallic carriers are coated with gutta percha. Carriers used are stainless steel, titanium, or plastic materials. **Eg:** Thermafill.

- Gutta flow: In these powdered gutta percha is incorporated in resin based sealer. Syringe system: Here low viscosity gutta percha is used.

Eg: Successfil Gutta percha pellets/bars: Available in small pellets and are used for thermoplasticized gutta percha obturation. Eg: Obtura system.

-   Gutta percha sealers: Gutta percha is dissolved in chloroform or eucalyptol to be used in the canal.

-   Medicated gutta percha: calcium hydroxide, iodoform or chlorhexidine containing gutta percha points.

Composition

Gutta percha -percha	matrix	18-22%
Zinc oxide filler	59-76%	
Waxes and resins	plasticizer	1-4%m
Metal sulphates	radio-opaque	1-8%

Advantages

-   Inert (chemically inactive).
-   Dimensionally stable. (does not change its shape and size when subject to temperature and humidity).
-   Semisolid and plasticity.
-   The flexible and semi-solid nature of gutta percha allows it to move in narrow curved canals smoothly.
-   Radio-opacity.
-   Easy to remove.

Disadvantages

-   Lack of adhesion to dentin.
-   Shrinkage on cooling.
-   It has no flow, it does not condense the accessory canals, Lateral canals, multiple foramens and other irregularities.

Note

Gutta percha is sterilized with 5.2% sodium hypochlorite for 1 minute.

N) OBTURATION TECHNIQUES

Each case presents unique situation-a particular method of obturation will not satisfy a single case that requires endodontic treatment, till date no filling or technique has been considered normal having a broad knowledge of options helps the clinician choose the optimal technique for the tooth being treated.

Lateral condensation

It is a traditional simple most commonly thought technique. It has been considered as gold standard to which other techniques have been considered.

Principle

Condensation is best achieved by keeping the sealer, gutta-percha and canal wall interface as thin as possible (To avoid microleakage between sealer and canal wall interface and seepage of oral fluids between gutta percha and sealer). The flexible and semi solid nature of gutta-percha makes it compactable. Compressibility allows gutta percha to adapt excellently to irregularities and contours of the canal by lateral pressure.

Objectives

Fill the canal with gutta percha cones by compacting them laterally against the side of the canal walls.

Procedure

Isolate and dry the canals with paper points. Select the master apical cone that corresponds to the size of master apical file or the last instrument taken into the canal. The master or primary cone is inserted into the canal all the way to the exact working length. Check for the apical fit (tug back). It should fit snuggly and resist removal.

Note

In case of inadequate fit (A) Short of apex – smaller size gutta percha cone or repreparation of canal is considered. (B) Beyond the apex – cut off the gutta percha to exact working length or larger size gutta percha cone is considered.

Select the appropriate master apical cone corresponds in size and taper to the last apical file used, mark and lock the master cone using cotton players based on the final working length check for cone fit as follows.

Visual examination

Master cone should slide easily and completely to the working length.

Reference indentations on the master cone should confirm a seat to the predetermined length.

Tactile sensation

When master cone seated to working the length a definite apical stop and slight resistance to removal should be felt. Master cone should resist displacement.

Radiographs

- In case of:- inadequate fit
- Short of apex – smaller size gutta percha cone or repreparation of canal is considered.
- Beyond the apex – cut off the gutta percha to exact working length or larger size gutta percha cone is considered.
- In case of adequate fit- At working length

Sealer manipulation and application

Sealer is prepared mixing appropriate amount of cement powder within a drop of liquid following manufacturer instructions on a sterile glass slab using sterile spatula. The sealer should be loose and tacky in consistency when pulled with spatula the cement should stretch about an inch above the mixing surface. Final mix should appear smooth, homogeneous and creamy.

The sealer is applied to the canal walls with the help of sterile master apical file with slight downward and upward movements followed by circular motion.

The clean master apical file is dipped in the sealer and carried in to the canal with gentle circular motion, canal walls are coated. The consistency of sealer is critical too thin sealer will not be able to coat the canal may push peri apically. Too thick mix may end up with high cone and short fill. Coat the apical one third of master cone with sealer, carefully insert the cone in to the canal until the beaks of the forceps touches the reference point or indentations on the surface of gutta-percha corresponds to the reference point on the occlusal surface. Once the cone is properly seated to the full working length an appropriate size and type of spreader selected.

Spreader selection

Size of the spreader is determined by the width of prepared canal and lateral fit of the master cone. Smaller the space between canal wall and lateral surface of gutta percha smaller diameter spreader is chosen. Larger the space between grater diameter spreader is chosen. Type of spreader is determined by for straight canals rigid stainless steel spreaders are chosen and for curved flexible nickel titanium spreader is chosen.

Advantages

Better tactile sensation

Less chances of vertical root fracture.

Available in different sizes from 15 to 45. White 15, yellow 20, red 25, blue 30, green 35 and black 40.

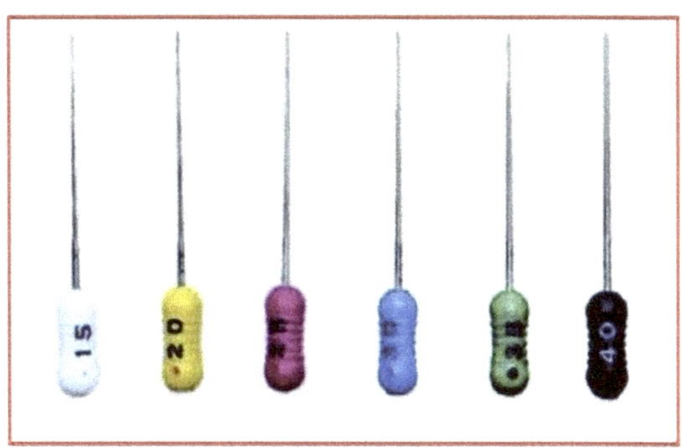

Fig. 9.112: Finger spreaders

Place the stopper on the spreader and adjust it to 1mm short of working length. Prefitted spreader is inserted alongside the master gutta percha cone to a level 1 mm short of the working length. Minimum downward and side to side pressure is applied to the cone apically and laterally, rotate the spreader in clockwise-anticlockwise direction before withdrawal this serve two purposes.

1) Prevents the coronal displacement of master Gutta Percha cone.

2) Aid in compression of gutta percha and sealer against the canal walls.

Place the appropriate size sealer coated accessory cone in the space previously occupied by the spreader reinsert the spreader and condense the accessory cone in the same manner as the master cone keep on using the spreader and keep on adding the accessory cones. Each time spreader should reach 1-2mm short of working length in order to obtain a optimal lateral and apical compaction this confirmed by each accessory cone permitting bit shorter than the previous one adding the accessory cone should be continued until the spreader no longer penetrate the orifice of the canal. Cut off excess gutta-percha with a heated ball burnisher the soften gutta percha is molded and pressed inside the canal so that there should be no gutta percha left in the chamber or on the floor. Gutta percha should be confined to the canals. Final X-ray should be taken in both buccolingual and mesiodistal angulations this will enable the complete visualization of canals. Use cotton or forceful water spray to remove sealer from pulp chamber. Finally the procedure is end by doing transitional or permeant restoration according to the patient and clinician conveniences.

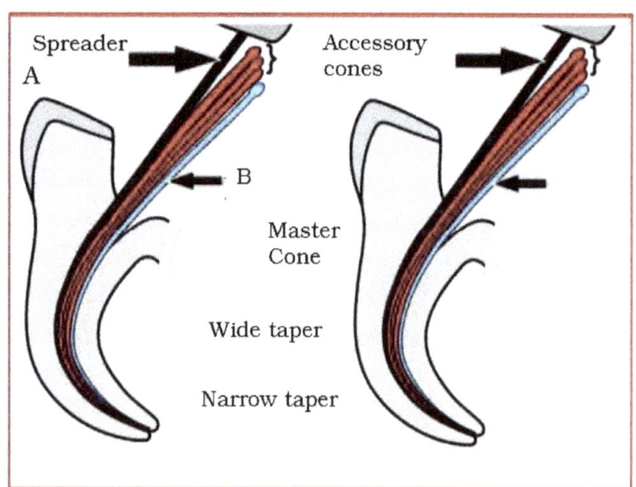

Fig. 9.113:

Advantages

- Simple does not require expensive armamentarium.

- With slight variations and modifications can be used in all clinical situations example can be done in canal with wide open apex or canal with definitive apical stop.

- Excellent length controls less likelihood of carrying the material beyond apex.

- Deep spreader penetration provides excellent apical seal.

- Can be accomplished with any of the sealer.

Disadvantages

- More time consuming.
- Less able to seal the internal defects, lateral canals and complex anatomy of tooth.
- Increased gutta percha and sealer ratio, over the time sealer subject to dissolution and shrinkage......Totally relies upon sealer to fill the internal defects and discrepancies between canal wall and gutta-percha.
- Less homogeneous mass and presence of voids.
- Cracks and fractures of root due to heavy condensing forces.

Warm lateral condensation

The final filling after cold lateral condensation composed of gutta percha cones tightly pressed together joined by frictional grip and sealer lacks homogeneity and has to rely on sealer to fill the voids this would have poor prognosis to overcome this warm lateral condensation technique was introduced.

Definition

An appropriate heat source is introduced during or after cold lateral condensation to soften the gutta percha to enhance its adaptation to internal anatomy of the tooth is called warm lateral condensation.

Principle

Heat results in adhesion of accessory cones to the master gutta percha cone. This fusion of cones produces more homogeneous solid gutta percha mass with less voids.

Indications

- Tooth with internal defects and perforations
- Tooth with C shaped canals
- Tooth with Resorptive defects
- Tooth with Complex internal anatomy of tooth like lateral canals or accessory canals.

Advantages

- More dense filling, more able to fill the internal defects and lateral canals with gutta percha compare to cold lateral condensation.
- Length control advantage over other thermoplastic techniques.
- Less expensive than other thermoplastic techniques.
- Sealer to gutta percha ratio is less compare to cold lateral condensation.
- Less voids and more homogenous mass compare to cold lateral condensation.

Heat sources

- Endotec2, Endo twin, EL down pack
- Endo twin
- Electrically heated vibrating tip –vibration enhances compaction in to the internal defects
- Endotec2
- It is cordless, battery operated thermal condenser with micro-heating element inside the canal tip. There is a fingertip heat control button on the hand piece. The electrical tip or canal tip corresponds to 30 size root canal file.

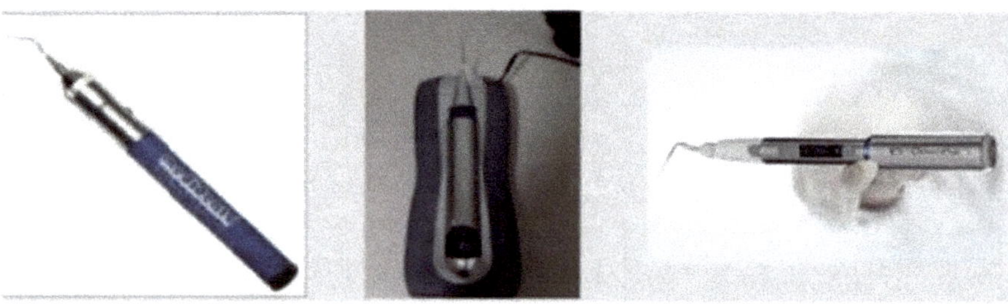

Fig. 9.114:

Procedure

Once the sealer coated master apical gutta percha cone fitted in to the canal to a full working length. Depress the fingertip control heat active button on the endotec2 hand piece to generate heat at the fire end of endotec2 canal tip. The canal tip will reach the controlled temperature within 3-4 seconds and will remain in proper temperature as long as the heat button is depressed, with the heat button depressed place the endotec2 canal tip in to the canal alongside of master gutta-percha cone to a level of 2mm short working length. Fix the metal stopper of the tip for working length control. Press the endotec2 tip apically with mild to moderate pressure avoiding excessive force rotate in a circumferential manner to coat the gutta-percha in all three dimensions. Remove the endotec2 canal tip from the canal in a circular rotary withdrawal motion. Place the cold endotec2 or appropriate size spreader in to the channel has been created now, alongside of the adapted master apical cone and canal walls apply slight lateral and apical pressure to condense the gutta percha apically and laterally. Withdraw the spreader from the canal place the accessory cone in the space previously occupied by the spreader, again insert the heated canal tip deep in to the canal it will not penetrate as deep as before. Apply mild to moderate apical rotary motion to further spread and condense accessory cones of gutta percha in to dense homogeneous mass. Continue add accessory gutta percha cones and heat condense with each repetition the condenser will penetrate 2-3mm shorter than the previous depth. Repeat the procedure until the canal tip no longer penetrate the orifice of canal. Soften gutta percha is molded and pressed inside the canal so that there should be no gutta percha left in the chamber or on the floor. Gutta percha should be confined to the canals. Use forceful water sprayor to remove sealer from pulp chamber. Finally the procedure is end by doing transitional or permeant restoration according to the patient and clinician conveniences.

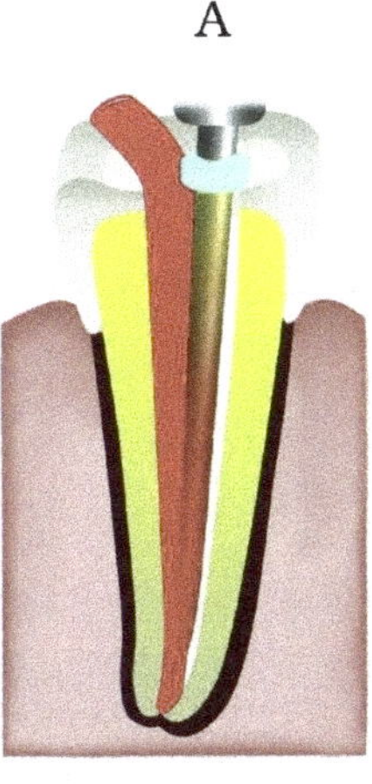

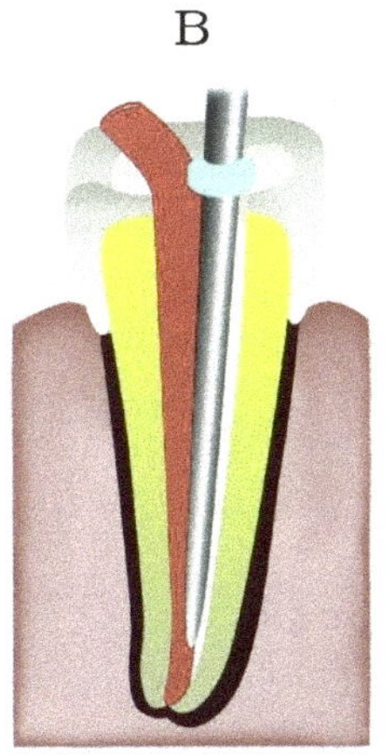

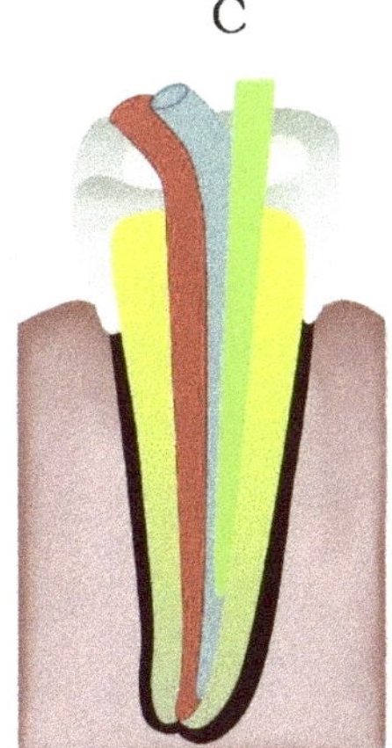

A	B	C
Endotech2 canal tip 2mm short of working length	Spreader along the side of master cone 2mm short of working length	Additional cones

Fig. 9.115:

Warm vertical condensation

In 1967 Herb Schilder introduced warm vertical compaction technique to improve the obturation quality in root canal irregularities. He used heat soften gutta percha and different types of pluggers to pack it since then this technique forms the basis for many other techniques such as sectional, thermo soften, continuous wave..etc.

Principle

The thermo-soften gutta percha has compaction potential it adapts to the irregularities and flow in to the lateral canals within the root canal system.

Definition

It is a three-dimensional filling technique done by applying pressure in vertical direction to the thermo-soften gutta percha and thereby forcing it flow and fill in the entire root canal system.

Prerequisite

- A continuous tapered funnel should be present from orifice to the apex decreasing in cross sectional area every millimeter apically.

- Preparation should flow with the natural curvature of the canal.

- Apical constriction should be kept as narrow as possible to prevent the extrusion of sealer and gutta-percha through the apex.

- Original shape of apical foramina should not be changed

- The natural position of apical foramina should not be moved.

Procedure

Plugger selection

- Choose a largest diameter plugger which fits loosely over a range of few millimeter in coronal one third of the canal.
- Select a smaller diameter plugger that will work freely in the middle third without obstruction.
- Finally select smaller diameter plugger that can fit passively within 4-5mm full working length.

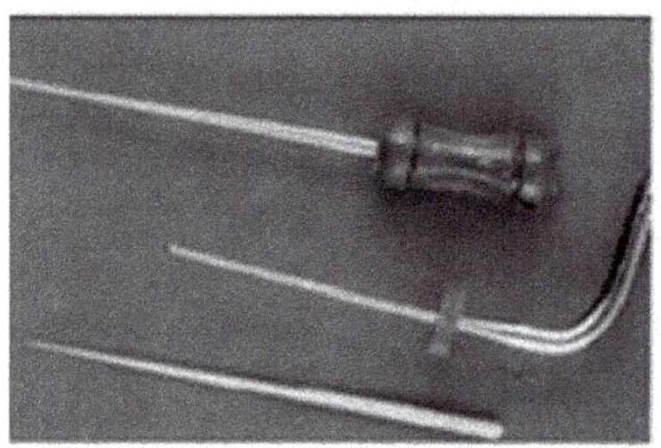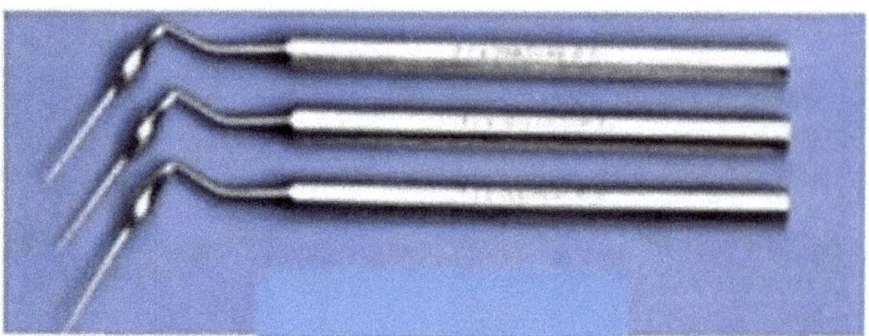

Fig. 9.116:

Down fill

First wave of condensation

Use appropriate heat source to sear off excess gutta-percha as deep as possible from the orifice of the canal. Insert the heat carrier instrument in to the dense mass of gutta percha a few millimeters of heat wave moves through the dense mass of gutta percha soften the gutta percha thermo-soften gutta percha has compaction potential using larger diameter plugger soften gutta-percha molded and adapted. The sharp end of plugger is used to compact the gutta-percha laterally and the blunt end of plugger is used to compact the gutta percha vertically with slight vertical strokes if the plugger is smaller than canal width series of strokes are applied finally a sustained press against gutta percha mass for 5 -10 seconds forces the gutta percha sideways and downwards the movement of gutta-percha mass laterally and vertically in depth over a range of few millimeter is called wave of condensation.

Second wave of condensation

Insert the heat carrier instrument, activate and plunge, plunge in to the 3-4mm of coronal aspect of gutta percha. A 4-5mm of heat wave passes through, softening dense mass of gutta percha. Deactivate the cuff let the instrument cool about 3-4mm of gutta percha bit is removed upon withdrawal of cooling instrument, insert the prefit smaller diameter plugger in to the space created after the removal of gutta percha. Mold, adapt and compact the soften gutta percha. Sustained press against gutta percha mass for 5 -10 seconds forces the gutta percha sideways and downwards; this movement of gutta-percha mass laterally and vertically in depth over a range of few millimeter completes second wave of condensation.

Third wave of condensation

Heat carrier instrument reintroduced, activate and plunge. Plunge in to the most coronal aspect of gutta percha mass. About 4-5mm of heat wave pass through the apical portion of gutta percha mass till its apical end. Deactivate the cuff let the instrument cool upon removal of cooling instrument a bit of about 3-4mm of gutta percha mass removed leaving behind the apical gutta percha mass in the main canal and lateral canal. Insert the smallest plugger in to the space created by the removal of gutta percha with slight vertical strokes the gutta percha adopted and condensed to plug the apical one third of the canal this completes third wave of condensation.

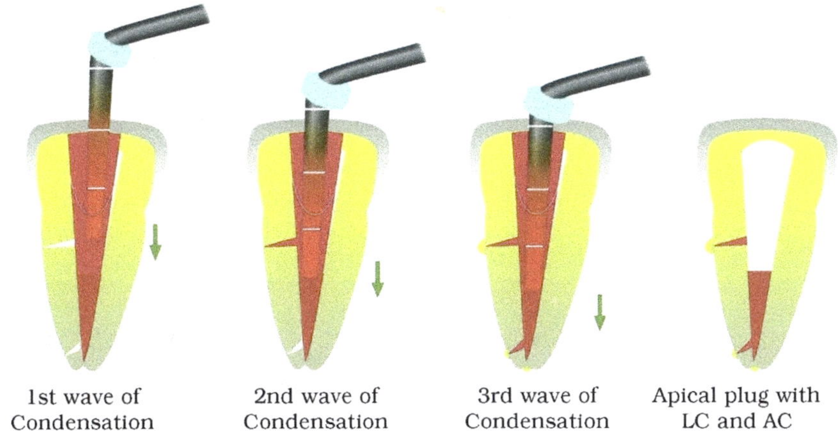

Fig. 9.117:

Back fill

Upon the completion of down pack of the canal, the back fill of the canal can be accomplished coronally by injecting small segments of gutta percha 2-3mm in to the canal and vertically compacting with pluggers up to the orifice of canal or to a shorter point if post is advised. It comprises filling the 5-7mm of body of canal this area is quite wide can accept the passive placement of syringes between the gauges 18-25mm.

Canal walls are coated with thin layer of sealer, small amount of gutta percha should be extruded to warm the needle and discorded the warm needle quickly introduced in to the canal and hold it for 5 seconds. To thermo-soften the top 2mm of already established apical of gutta percha this facilitates the fusion and cohesion of both parts of gutta percha and avoids the formation of voids between two parts of gutta percha. Be sure the surface of apical plug of gutta percha must be flat before starting back filling to avoid void formation. Press and hold the activator cuff on the hand piece to begin the flow of gutta percha from the needle tip, allow the flow to gently push the hand piece few millimeter coronally. Depress the activator cuff to stop the flow, remove the needle from the canal. Use the prefit plugger to adapt and compact the material. Each time after compacting the segment keep load on the cooling material to offset the shrinkage. Reinsert the needle in to the canal space against the compacted material again press and hold the activation cuff to restart the flow until a few millimeters of canal has been filled release the activator cuff to stop the flow. Remove the needle another larger diameter plugger is used to compact and condense the material. Repeat this dispensing and condensing procedure until canal is filled to desired level.

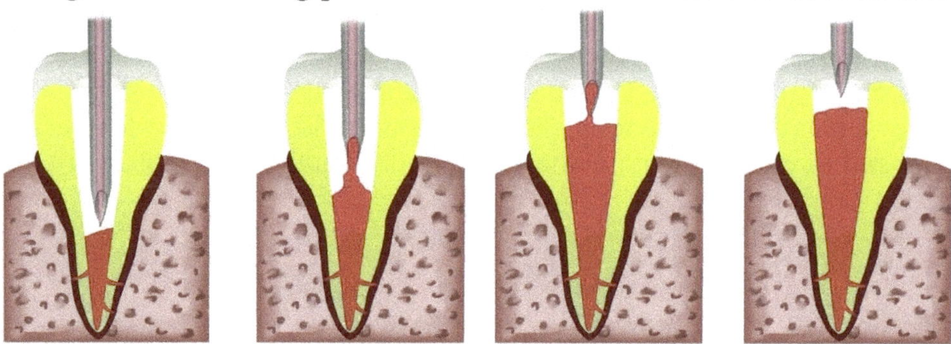

Warm needle in contact with apical plug of GP

Filling the body of canal with thermoplasticized Gutta Percha

Fig. 9.118:

Advantage

-   Fill the lateral canals and accessory canals effectively more dense filling in lateral canals compared to lateral condensation technique.
-   Excellent apical and latera seal, higher healing rate with previous apical periodontitis.
-   Better flow and adaption of gutta percha in root canal irregularities, minor discrepancies, isthmuses, fins and webs.
-   Low risk of void formation and more homogeneous filing.
-   The resultant obturation composed of more gutta percha and less sealer leading to better long term prognosis.
-   Higher healing rate with previous apical periodontitis.

Disadvantages

-   More time consuming, technique sensitive and difficult to master.
-   Costly equipment and armamentarium
-   Less length control and risk of apical extrusion of sealer and gutta percha in to the periapical area which cannot be retrieved through the canals.
-   Risk of vertical root fracture due to undue stresses.
-   Thermal damage to periodontal ligament if temperature guide lines are exceeded.

Limitations

-   Difficulty in curved canals rigid pluggers are unable to penetrate to the necessary depth.
-   Excessive dentin removal to accommodate appropriate plugger weaken the tooth.

Continuous wave condensation

Warm vertical compaction is the gold standard for three-dimensional filling of prepared root canals but as it utilizes multiple steps and multiple pluggers for down packing it is time consuming, technique sensitive and difficult to master. The difficulties of Schilders technique are lessened with the advent of electronic 3D obturation devices. Continuous wave technique evolved by combining the functions of Schilders pluggers and Masreleiz's electronic heat carrier in to single heat carrier. Continuous wave technique utilizes single tapered pluggers to soften the gutta percha at the same time condense it. Compare to warm vertical compaction it has the advantage of enhanced application and fast packing.

Continuous wave heat pluggers

The CWHP pluggers evolved by combining the functions of Schildre's pluggers and masreleiz's electronic heat carrier. The design of CWHP closely approximates shape of tapered root canal preparations and resembles the tapers of non-standardized master cones. Made of dead soft stainless-steel body with an electronic copper wire inside fairly flexible can be bent in order to down pack closer to the desired depth in small canals.

Available in 5 different sizes

Size		Tip Diameter	Use
Extra-fine	.04	0.3mm	minimally invasive endodontic shapes
Fine	.06	0.5mm	small shapes
Fine medium	08	0.5mm	medium shapes
Medium	10	0.5mm	large shapes
Medium large	12	0.5mm	very large shapes

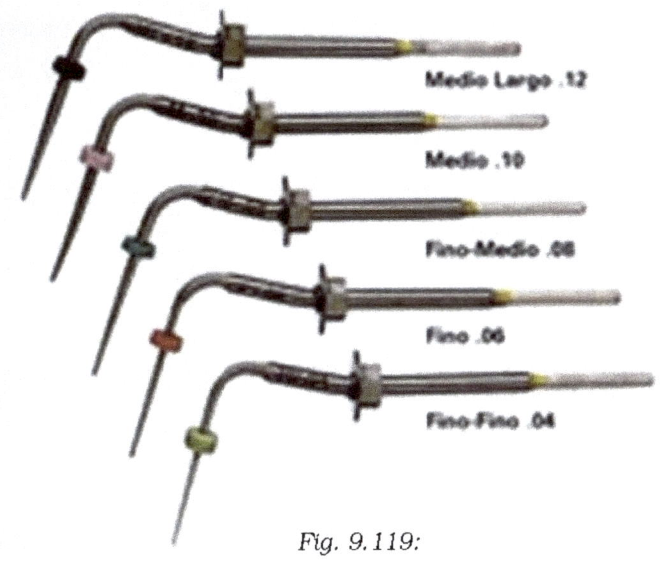

Fig. 9.119:

System B heat source

System B heat source can monitor the temperature at the tip of its heat carrier device delivering a precise amount of heat for a longer period of time. B system has a temperature setting of up to 60°C. physical properties of gutta percha need temperature close to 20°C. higher temperature up to 35°C for shorter period of time will not cause irreversible periodontal damage.

The temperature setting on the display and the temperature at the tip of the plugger must be correct. Incorrect setting may lead to the following.

Excess temperature	Inadequate temperature
Periodontal damage	Poor adaptation
Void formation	Poor flow
Poor quality condensation	Void formation

Different heat sources systems have different settings 25°C on display receives high temperature 2mm from tip 16°C. Endotwin has advantage of vibrations along with warm vertical compaction temperature setting between 17°C and 22°C.

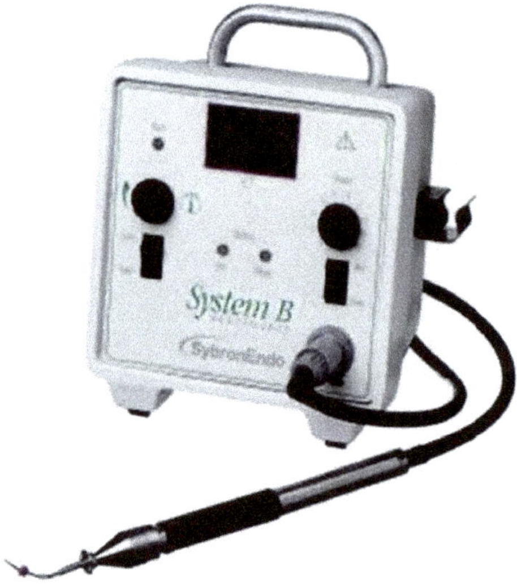

Fig. 9.120:

Cone fit

The master cone is cut 0.5 to 1mm short of working length to accommodate vertical movements from compaction.

Plugger fit

Choose the system B plugger that matches the shape of prepared canal and master gutta percha cone prefit the plugger in the root canal to binding point. Adjust the stopper on the plugger occlusal reference point.

Procedure

Apical condensation

Turn the system B heat source on to the use and place it in the touch mode, set the heat at 20°C. press the heat button on, the preheated plugger is drive down smoothly through the gutta percha. Heat is kept on the plugger is pressed further and further deep in to the dense mass of gutta percha mass until the stopper on the plugger is 2mm above the occlusal reference or plugger is 2mm short of binding point at this point, depress the heat button off while keeping the downward pressure on the cooling carrier. This downward apical pressure forces the gutta percha and cement in to the lateral complex anatomy of tooth, as the plugger reaches its ultimate depth that is binding point apply sustained press on the cooling apical mass of gutta percha for 10 seconds to prevent cooling shrinkage. While maintaining the apical pressure press the heat button on again for 1 second, depress the button off and wait for 1 second as the plugger begin cooling rock it side to side in the canal space, this motion separates gutta-percha mass in to segment apical to heat plugger and segment coronal to heat plugger. When the carrier is withdrawn the segment coronal to the plugger comes out along with plugger leaving apical mass of gutta percha and sealed lateral and accessory canals this is called separation burst.

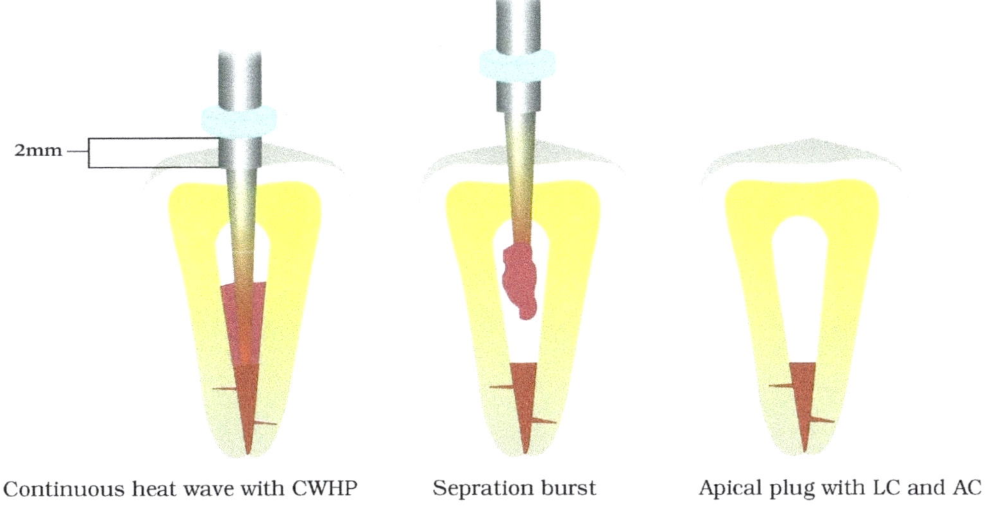

Continuous heat wave with CWHP   Sepration burst   Apical plug with LC and AC

Fig. 9.121:

Back fill

Upon the completion of down pack of canal the back fill can and accomplished coronally by injecting small segments of gutta percha 2-3mm in to the canal and vertically compacting with pluggers up to the orifice of canal or to a shorter point if post is advised. It comprises filling the 5-7mm of body of canal this area is quite wide can accept the passive placement of syringes between the gauges 18-25mm.

Canal walls are coated with thin layer of sealer, small amount of gutta percha should be extruded to warm the needle and discorded the warm needle quickly introduced in to the canal and hold it for 5 seconds. To thermo-soften the top 2mm of already established apical of gutta percha this facilitates the fusion and cohesion of both parts of gutta percha and avoids the formation of voids between two parts of gutta percha. Be sure the surface of apical plug of gutta percha must be flat before starting back filling to avoid void formation. Press and hold the activator cuff on the hand piece to begin the flow of gutta percha from the needle tip, allow the flow to gently push the hand piece few millimeter coronally. Depress the activator cuff to stop the flow, remove the needle from the canal. Use the prefit plugger to adapt and compact the material. Each time after compacting the segment keep load on the cooling material to offset the shrinkage. Reinsert the needle in to the canal space against the compacted material again press and hold the activation cuff to restart the flow until a few millimeters of canal has been filled release the activator cuff to stop the flow. Remove the needle another larger diameter plugger is used to compact and condense the material. Repeat this dispensing and condensing procedure until canal is filled to desired level.

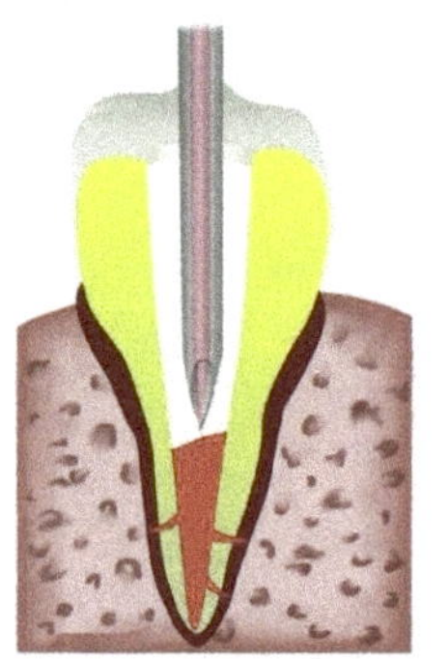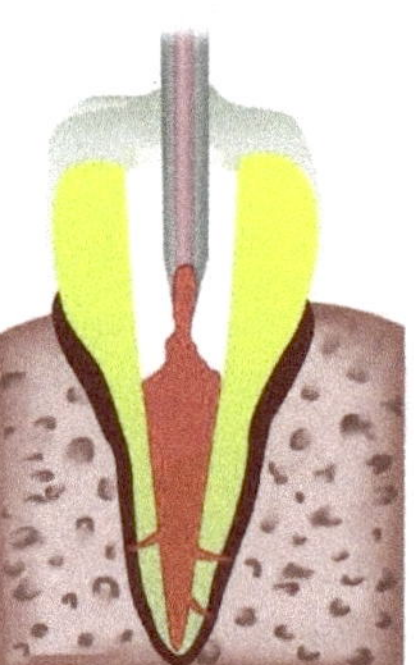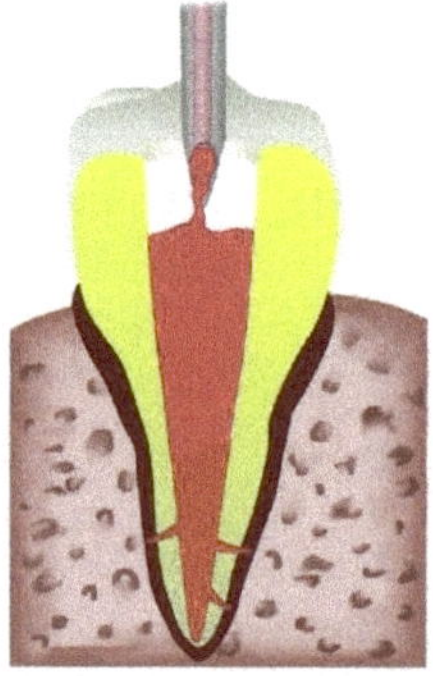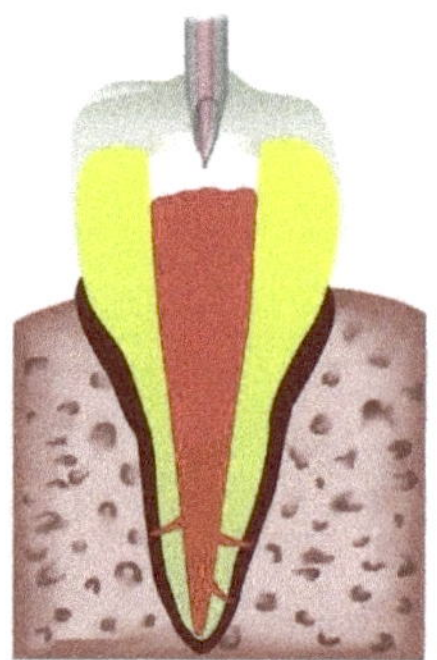

Warm needle in contact with apical plug of GP   Filling the body of canal with thermoplasticized Gutta Percha

Fig. 9.122:

Modified continuous wave condensation

In continuous wave condensation after separation burst cleaning of remaining gutta-percha at the orifice and coronal area before back packing is difficult and time consuming, for the purpose of simplification and acceleration obturation modified continuous wave is designed, this technique does not require removal of coronal gutta percha from the canal walls after down packing. It is simple, effective technique because adaptation gutta-percha and sealer with fewer voids this technique is mor effective in wide and medium sized canals where back packing can be done by single cone that matches the taper and shape of plugger.

Procedure

Turn the B system source on to the use and place it in the touch mode. Set the heat at 20°C. Press the heat button on. The preheated plugger is drive down through gutta percha keeping the heat button on. The plugger is pressed further and further deep in to the gutta percha mass until the stopper is 2mm above the occlusal reference point or plugger is 2mm short of binding point at this point, depress the heat button off while maintaining the apical pressure on the cooling plugger, the plugger is pushed downward until the stopper on the plugger touches the occlusal surface. Once the plugger reaches its ultimate depth that is binding point apply sustained press on the cooling apical mass of gutta percha for 10 seconds to prevent cooling shrinkage. Instead of doing separation burst wait for 10 seconds let the plugger cold down and detach from gutta-percha. Push apically and rotate to break it loose, finally tease it out, we left with the space the exact shape of plugger and then we can match with that back-fill cone has same diameter and taper.

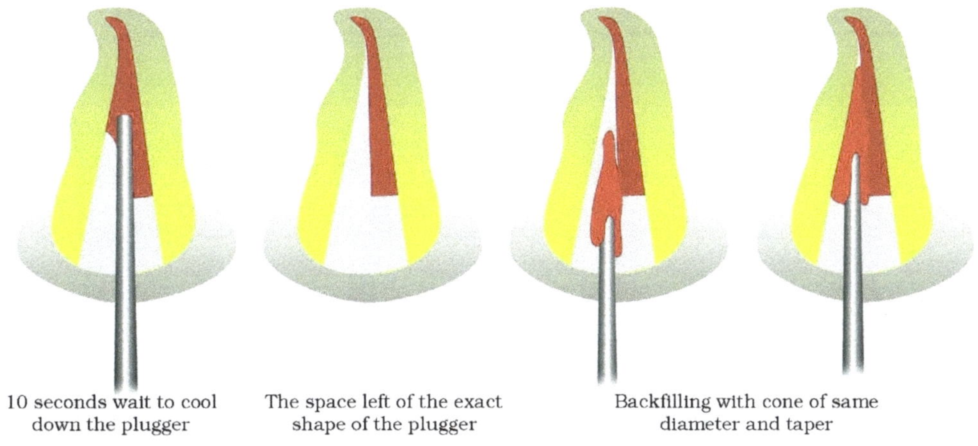

Fig. 9.123:

Thermal hydraulic condensation

The traditional continuous wave condensation technique utilizes high temperature 20°C which melts up the gutta percha quickly like a hot knife a red hot knife cut the butter. Provides no adequate time for the gutta percha to flow along pressure which results in incomplete obturation of lateral canals to compensate this thermal hydraulic condensation was developed. Thermal hydraulic condensation generates improved hydraulic pressure needed.

Orifice plug creation

Set the obtura two system on to the use, place the heated tip at the orifice and sear off the coronal portion of cone while injecting the thermo-plasticized gutta percha in to the canal. Choose the smaller diameter plugger than the diameter of orifice to condense thermo-soften gutta percha, this will create orifice plug that will create maximize hydraulic forces of condensation.

Apical condensation

Turn the B system heat source on the use. Place it in touch mode. Keeping the heat button on, the plugger is pressed further and further deep in to the dense gutta percha mass until the stopper on the plugger is above 3-4 mm from reference point. This downward press creates enough hydraulic and forces the gutta percha and sealer in to the lateral canals. As the plugger approaches the binding point resistance to apical pressure will be felt or tip may even stop, at this point have your assistant to raise the temperature to 30°C. Apply apical pressure to push the plugger to binding point then quickly with draw the plugger this separation burst will take 2 seconds the heat is turned up to 30°C to plasticize gutta percha in most apical portion of canal. Using dovgan plugger that fits within 3-5mm of working length apply up-down tapping motion and condense gutta percha for a few seconds. As the material cools stop condensing and apply apical pressure for about 10 seconds to prevent cooling shrinkage.

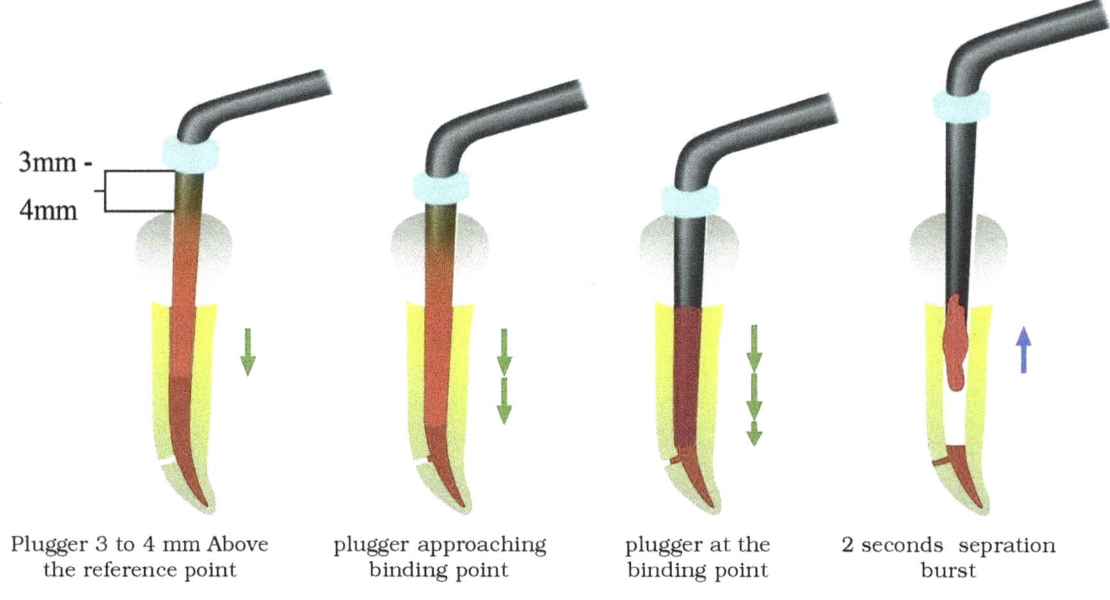

| Plugger 3 to 4 mm Above the reference point | plugger approaching binding point | plugger at the binding point | 2 seconds sepration burst |

Fig. 9.124:

Back filling

Upon the completion of down pack of canal the back fill of the canal can be accomplished coronally by injecting small segments of gutta percha of 2-3mm into the canal and vertically compacting with pluggers up to the orifice of canal or to a shorter point if post is advised .it comprises filling the 5-7mm of body of canal this area is quite wide can accept the passive placement of syringes between the gauges 18-25mm.

Canal walls are coated with thin layer of sealer , small amount of gutta percha should be extruded to warm the needle and discorded the warm needle quickly introduced in to the canal and hold it for 5 seconds. to thermo-soften the top 2mm of already established apical of gutta percha this facilitates the fusion and cohesion of both parts of gutta percha and avoids the formation of voids between two parts of gutta percha. Be sure the surface of apical plug of gutta percha must be flat before starting back filling to avoid void formation. Press and hold the activator cuff on the hand piece to begin the flow of gutta percha from the needle tip, allow the flow to gently push the hand piece few millimeter coronally. Depress the activator cuff to stop the flow, remove the needle from the canal. Use the prefit plugger to adapt and compact the material. Each time after compacting the segment keep load on the cooling material to offset the shrinkage. Reinsert the needle in to the canal space against the compacted material again press and hold the activation cuff to restart the flow until a few millimeters of canal has been filled release the activator cuff to stop the flow. remove the needle another larger diameter plugger is use to compact and condense the material. Repeat this dispensing and condensing procedure until canal is filled to desired level.

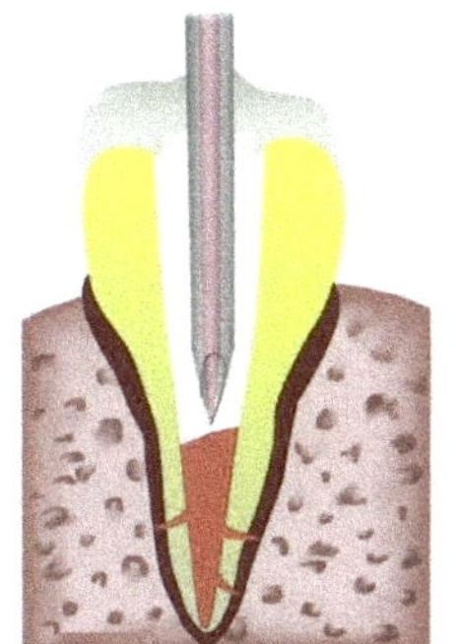
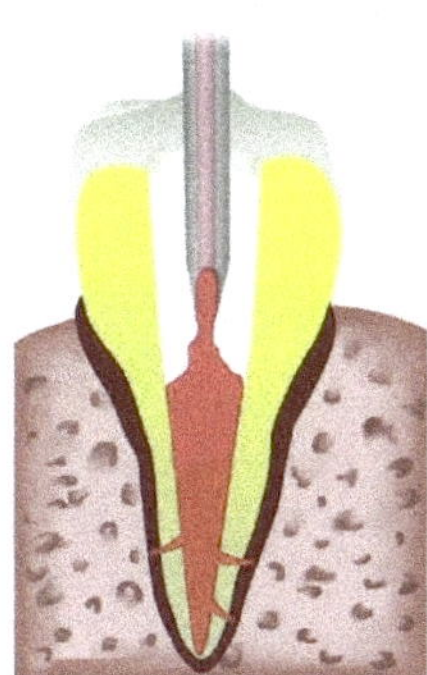
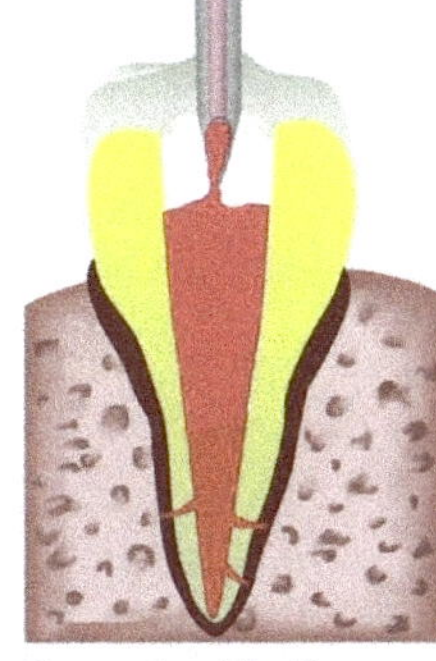
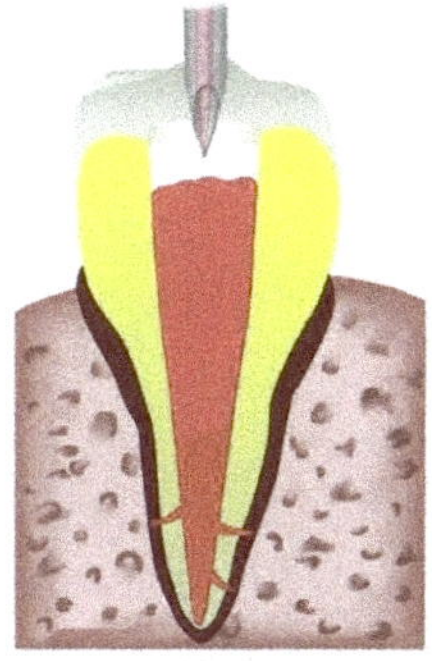

Warm needle in contact with apical plug of GP   Filling the body of canal with thermoplasticized Gutta Percha

Fig. 9.125:

Hydraulic Condensation

This technique is based on hydraulic fluid pressure. Bio ceramic sealer is used for this technique. This is sealer-based condensation. In this technique sealer acts as a filler. Bio ceramic sealer is highly biocompatible, does not get dissolved by oral fluids.

Composition of bio ceramic sealer

1. Alumina
2. Zirconia
3. Active bioglass
4. Hydroxy appetite
5. Calcium phosphate.

Advantages of bio-ceramic filler over gutta percha

It does not shrink after cooling.

It has anti-microbial properties

 It bonds to the dentin

It expands slightly while setting

It exhibits more flow.

It is non-resorbable, and stays in canal for long time.

The main advantages are it fills lateral canals, accessory canals multiple foramen perfectly due to its flow.

Simple hydraulic Condensation (Procedure)

Final irrigation with EDTA increases the antimicrobial properties of sealer. Isolate and dry the canals. An appropriate size cone is selected corresponds in size and taper to the last apical file used, mark and lock the master cone using cotton players based on the final working length check for cone fit as follows.

Visual examination:

Master cone should slide easily and completely to the working length.

Reference indentations on the master cone should confirm a seat to the predetermined length.

Tactile sensation

When master cone seated to working the length a definite apical stop and slight resistance to removal should be felt. Master cone should resist displacement.

Radiographs

Short of apex – smaller size gutta percha cone or repreparation of canal is considered.

Beyond the apex – cut off the gutta percha to exact working length or larger size gutta percha cone is considered.

In case of adequate fit - At working length

Sealer application

-   Dispense small amount of sealer in to the dispensing tip or on to the mixing pad from bio-ceramic sealer syringe. Clean master apical file dipped in to the sealer to coat the canal walls uniformly with slight pumping actions followed by clockwise and counter-clockwise circular motions.

-   Master cone coated with sealer insert in to the canal and check for final adaption and fit. If enough space exists between canal wall and master gutta percha cone the cone is additionally coated with sealer. If lot of space exits additional cones are placed.

-   The sealer coated master cone slowly inserted in to the canal and gently proceeds towards working length as you proceed downwards and forwards master cone will make up the bulk of canal and generates the sufficient hydraulic forces which pushes the sealer out in to the fine complex anatomy of canals. Near apical stop rotate the master gutta percha cone clockwise and counter clockwise to a positive seat at working length. Sear off the master cone at the canal orifice with the appropriate heat sources as far as down possible. Use the appropriate size plugger to condense the master cone and bio-ceramic sealer filling apically and laterally. Use forceful water spray or to remove sealer from pulp chamber. Finally, the procedure is end by doing transitional or permeant restoration according to the patient and clinician conveniences.

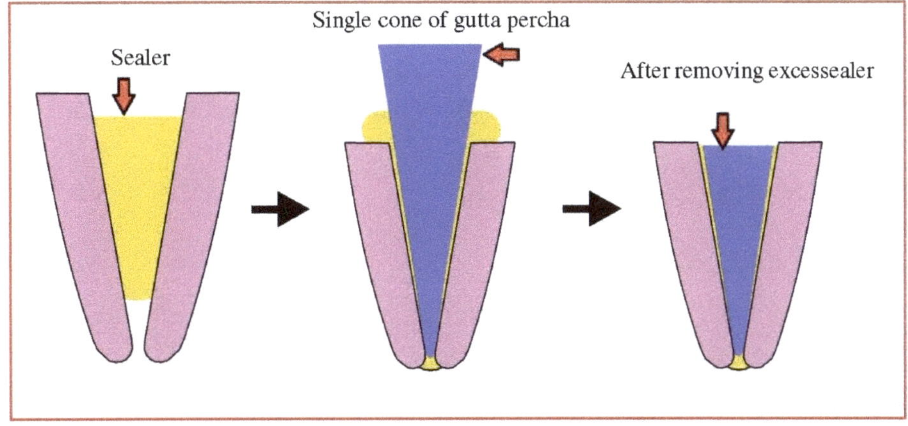

Fig. 9.126: Simple hydraulic condensation

Advanced hydraulic condensation technique

In this technique sealer is directly injected in to the canal from the BC sealer syringe then BC sealer coated cone is cemented in to place to full length having a high magnification or microscope for direct visualization of how much sealer being injected in to canal is must if you dispense more sealer your master cone may hang up high and ends with short fill. If you inject less sealer it may not be suffice the purpose so requires high magnification or microscope.

In this technique BC sealer coated cone is used the BC sealer coated cone can enhance the bonding between sealer and gutta percha thereby minimizes the microleakage between gutta-percha and sealer interface. The leakage occurs more readily between gutta-percha and sealer interface rather than sealer and canal wall interface so it is important have a good bond between sealer and gutta percha interface. BC sealer coated surface is hydrophilic and non-BC sealer coated cone surface is hydrophobic. Bio ceramic sealer is hydrophilic therefore BC sealer coated cones are recommended for hydraulic condensation.

Sealer is injected directly in to the canal from the BC sealer syringe then BC sealer coated cone is cemented in to place to full length having a high magnification or microscope for direct visualization of how sealer being injected in to canal is must, if you dispense more sealer your master cone may hang up high and ends with short fill.

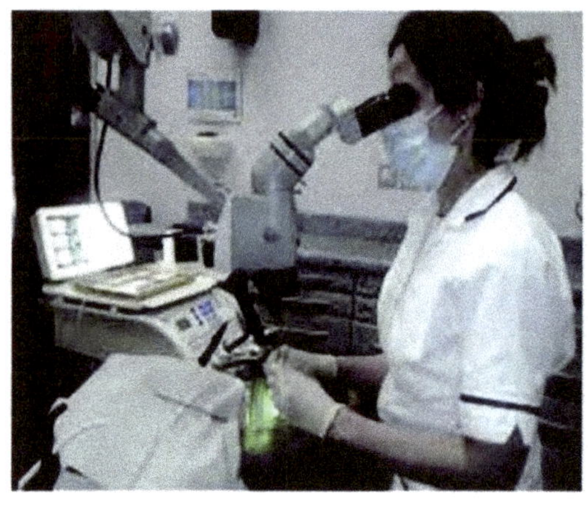

Direct visualization with microscope

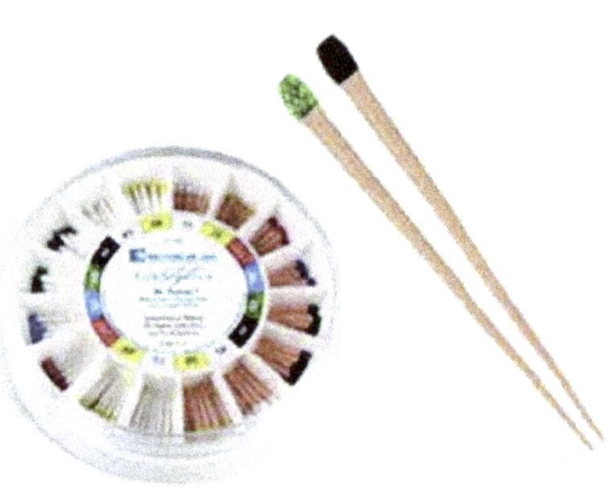

BC sealer coated cone

Fig. 9.127:

The role of gutta percha in this technique

Acts as carrier for sealer

It helps in controlling the working length.

It provides the path for re-treatment

Obturation By Stainless Steel Cones Or Titanium Cones

It is done in very narrow, fine, tortuous canal that can't be filled properly with gutta percha.

Example:

In third molars.

In mesio angular impactions.

In patients with reduced mouth opening.

Due to its rigid nature it easily fits in the narrow curved tortuous canals.

Due its rigidity the length control is excellent.

It is useful in bypassing ledges and blocks. It is dimensionally stable material.

Resin-based sealer or bio ceramic sealer are more appropriate in obturation of stainless steel cones or titanium cones.

Thermomechanical condensation

It is a three-dimensional obturation technique approximates the thermal condensation as regards quality of obturation and with respect to approach it is comparable to lateral condensation. It was introduced by McSpadden in 1979 also called as McSpadden compaction. This technique based on the use of special condenser called McSpadden compactor or gutta condenser.

McSpadden compactor

It is supplies in different sizes and shapes as an engine driven hand powered Ni-Ti instrument. In its structure it is similar to head storm file its threads are however oriented in opposite direction, the threads are directed in apical direction. It fits in to the contra-angled hand piece rotates at 5000 to 15000 RPM and generates frictional heat.

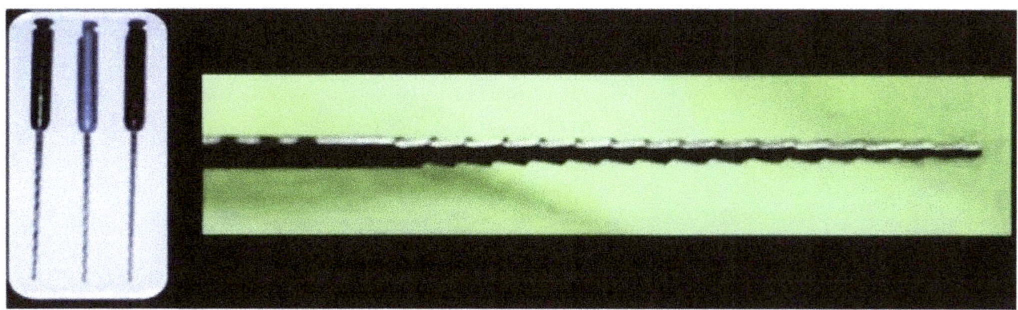

Fig. 9.128: Compactor Blade

Principle

Frictional heat from the compacter decreases the viscosity of gutta percha and thereby increases its plasticity. The thermo-plasticized gutta percha has compaction potential the apically directed compacter threads drive the thermo-soften material into the intricacies of the canal under pressure.

Indication

Straight wide prepared canals of non-rounded or oval cross section.

Prerequisite

- Preparation should have solid apical stop apical stop to prevent apical extrusion.

- Preparation should have higher taper ratio to accommodate compacter.

- The canals should be enlarged at least 45 sized instrument with step back technique and at least 0.4 taper with step down technique.

- Canal preparation should be straight to avoid instrument breakage

Procedure

A compacter is selected according to width and length of canal and precoated it with a layer of gutta percha. Precoating the compacter with gutta percha serves two purposes.

Prevents gauzing of dentinal walls.

Owing to its fluid state and friction prevents the displacement of master gutta percha by adapting to it.

A master cone coated with a sealer fitted to a working length and condensed with spreader as described in lateral condensation. With a preadjusted stopper on the compacter, the compacter gently guided into the canal with in 1.5mm short of apex along the side of gutta-percha and rotated at 8000 to 15000 RPM at this speed heat generated by friction softens the gutta percha the softened material forced downward apically and sideways laterlly by the threads of compacter.

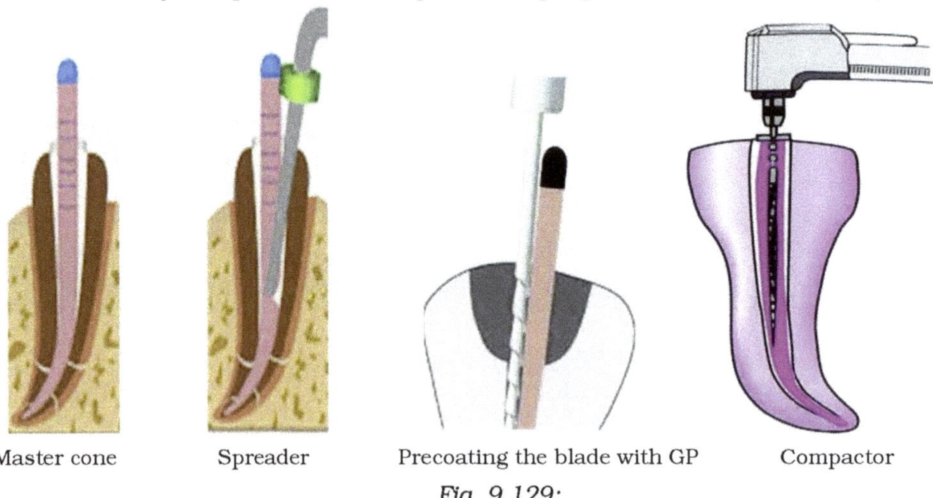

Fig. 9.129:

Chemo-plasticized compaction

- There is still a place for customization of gutta-percha points to improve the apical fit of gutta percha in the following conditions
- In large open apex
- Large root end resorptions
- Occurrence of apical deltas
- Commonly used gutta percha solvents chloroform, eucalyptol, halothane and xylitol

Procedure

The tip of master cone is soften by dipping it in gutta-percha solvent for 30 second, gently carry the cone in to the canal with a locking player adjusted to the working length, bind or tamp the soften cone in the canal until the beaks of player touches the reference point. It will form the custom impression of apical region .

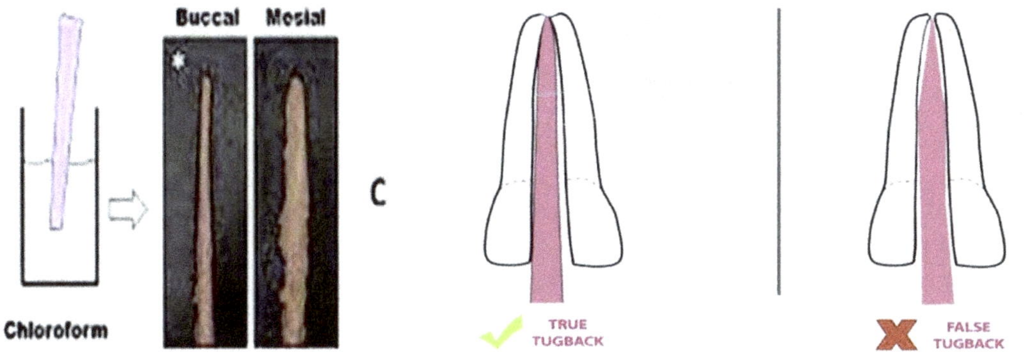

Fig. 9.130:

Custom cone technique

Occasionally the apical sizes of the prepared root canals may be larger where traditional master gutta percha cones cannot be adapted in these cases gutta-percha customized to achieve a tug back. A single master cone of increased diameter is created which is then sized with in the canal until a tug back is achieved.

By joining soften multiple gutta percha cones from bottom to tip a single giant master cone of increased diameter is prepared then sized with in the canal until a tug back is achieved.

Procedure

Select an appropriate size master cone soften it with one or more accessory cones by carry over heat flame and rolled together with two glass slab until a single giant master cone of larger diameter is created.

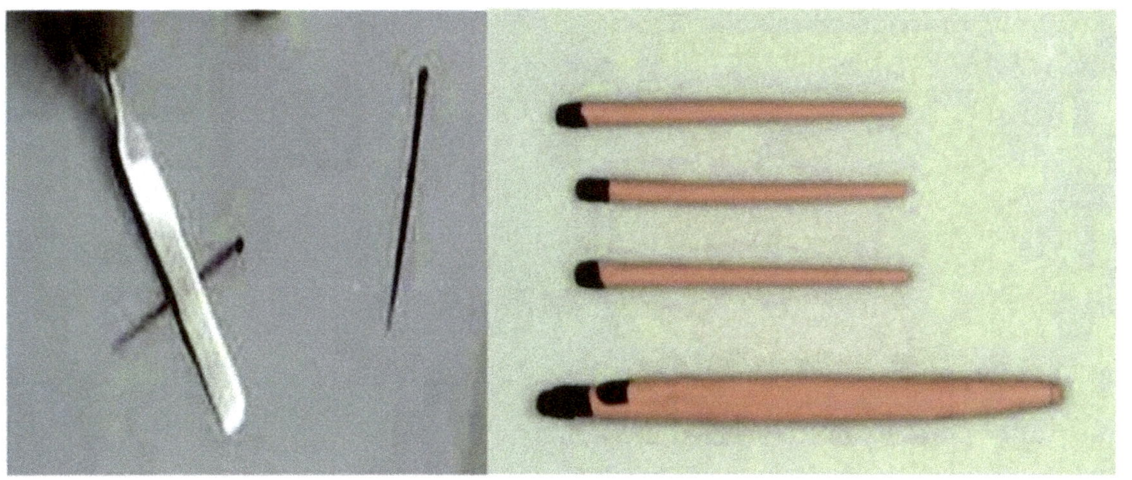

Fig. 131: Custom cone technique

Single cone obturation

Historically the idea of using single gutta percha cone for obturation was rejected because this method would depend too heavily on sealers that were subject to dissolution and shrinkage over the time and influences the long-term prognosis of tooth. With the advancement in specific rotary instrumentation system the canals are prepared with pro-tapered instruments and filled with size matched pro-tapered gutta percha cones and also with the introduction of newer class of filling materials gutta flow and sealers like bio-ceramics the interest has been renewed in single cone obturation technique.

Definition

It refers to use of a size matched greater tapered cone to fit the preparation of canal precisely.

Indications

Use of the single cone technique relies on the ability to create a tapered circular preparation or existing natural circular canal preparation.

Round smaller diameter canals would require lesser preparation hence recommended.

Contraindications

Oval shaped larger diameter canals would require excessive preparation hence not recommended.

Canals with complex anatomy is not suitable.

Gutta flow

Canals with simple anatomy are suitable.

It is the first cold flowable injectable gutta-percha sealer combination in silicon polymer matrix. Used in conjunction with master gutta percha cone in single cone obturation technique without the need of compaction.

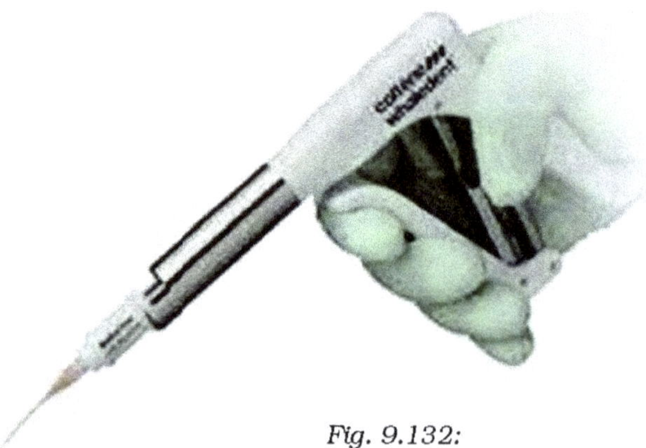

Fig. 9.132:

Procedure

An appropriate size cone is selected corresponds in size and taper to the last apical file used, mark and lock the master cone using cotton players based on the final working length check for cone fit as follows.

Visual examination

- Master cone should slide easily and completely to the working length.
- Reference indentations on the master cone should confirm a seat to the predetermined length.

Tactile sensation

When master cone seated to working the length a definite apical stop and slight resistance to removal should be felt. Master cone should resist displacement.

Radiographs

- In case of: - Inadequate fit
- Short of apex – smaller size gutta percha cone or repreparation of canal is considered.
- Beyond the apex – cut off the gutta percha to exact working length or larger size gutta percha cone is considered.
- In case of adequate fit - At working length.

Gutta flow filling

It is a unique mixture of finely grounded gutta percha powder with particle size less than 30 microns. Roekoseal root canal sealer and preservative nano silver.

Gutta flow packed in individual use capsule that provides a safe, simple hygienic delivery. Single dose capsules are triturated following manufacturer instructions canal tip placed on the capsule in to the dispensing gun. Small amount of the gutta flow mix dispensed on to a pad to confirm that color is pink ensuring complete mix.

Gutta flow can be placed directly in to the root canal using dispensing gun and canal tip. The canal tip must always sit loosely in the root canal, place the canal tip in to the root canal to the predetermined filling depth. Set the rubber stopper gently dispense a small amount of gutta flow in the canal it should be seen rising up around the canal tip inject small amount required when you see gutta flow rising in the canal stop dispensing.

Selected master cone is coated with additional gutta flow by dipping it in a dispensing tip or in to the material on a pad. Slowly inset the master cone and gently proceed towards working length as you proceed downwards and forwards master cone will make up the bulk of canal and generates the sufficient forces which pushes the gutta flow material out in to the fine complex anatomy of canals.

Near apical stop rotate the master gutta percha cone clockwise and counter clockwise to a positive seat at working length. Sear off the master cone at the canal orifice with the appropriate heat sources as far as down possible. Use the appropriate size plugger to condense the master cone. Use forceful water spray to remove sealer from pulp chamber. Finally, the procedure is end by doing transitional or permeant restoration according to the patient and clinician conveniences.

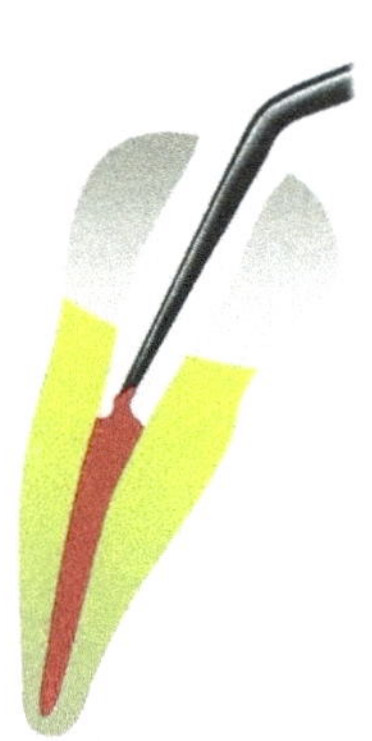
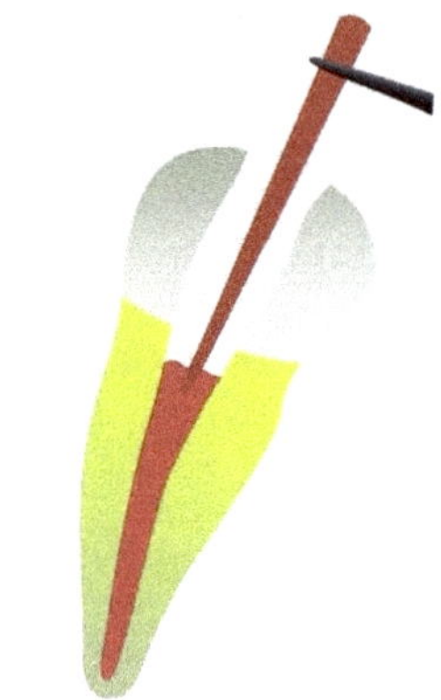

Injecting GF with canal tip   *Master cone with additional GF*

Fig. 9.133:

Carrier based gutta percha technique

Carrier based obturation simultaneously deliver and compact the warm gutta percha to the full working length of the canals that have sharp curvature.

Indications

Long narrow curved canals

Canals that have sharp curvatures at coronal or middle one third.

Therma fill

It is three-dimensional filling technique introduced by W Benson IN 1978 it comprises.

Flexible metal carriers like stainless steel or titanium or plastic carriers coated with alpha phase gutta-percha. They are available in ISO standard sizes as well as variable tapered sizes.

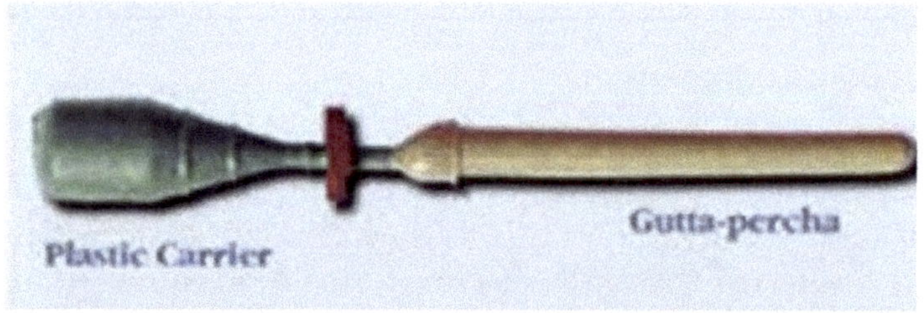

Fig. 9.134:

Prerequisite

Roots with good apical constriction

Preparations of root canals with an apical taper at least 0.04.

Not recommended

Difficult reach posterior teeth

Limited buccal opening

Procedure

Originally obturators are stainless steel k files covered with a uniform alpha phase gutta percha. Obturators then heated in a Therma prep oven for 15 -20 seconds and placed in a canal already coated with sealer with firm apical pressure to the marked working length. Note (the operator has approximately 10 seconds to retrieve the obturator from the oven and place in to the canal.) Verify the fit of obturation taking radiograph when found correct while stabilizing the carrier with index finger sectioned at the level of the pulpal floor. Final obturation characterized by the presence of a stainless steel instrument surrounded by gutta percha and sealer when the use of post indicated it is very difficult remove the stainless instrument to overcome this k file replaced by a grooved plastic carrier made from a biocompatible radio opaque plastic. Groove increases flexibility and poly sulfone present in plastic carrier dissolve in most of the solvents used in dentistry facilitate retreatment. Plastic material can be more easily sectioned at the level of the pulpal floor after being placed in a canal with a safe end cutting bur.

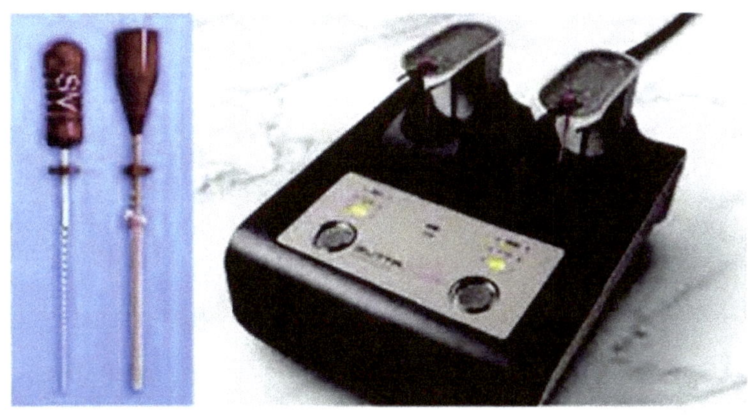

GP with metal carrier   *Therma prep oven*

Fig. 9.135:

Gutta core

Recently plastic carrier was replaced with gutta percha carrier obturator now called gutta core. Carrier is made from a cross linked gutta percha that is intimately adhere to surrounding gutta percha.

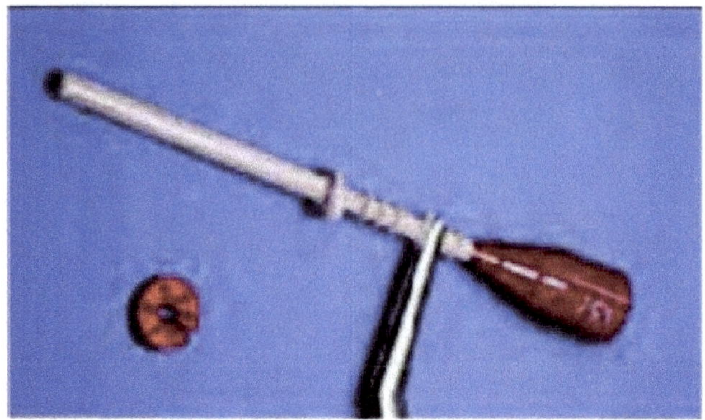

GP with gutta percha carrier

Fig. 9.136:

Advantages

- Post space created readily
- Easy to remove in the retreatment situation
- Eliminates the existing gape between carrier and gutta percha.
- Easy to break off the handle
- Marks are used to define working length
- Moves the gutta percha to full working length

Disadvantages

- Expensive
- Technically difficult
- Difficult in curved canals

Technique

- For gutta core obturators only metal verifiers are used
- Verifiers are used to check the size of the canal and available space for the carrier and the plasticized gutta percha .
- Verifiers are inserted to full working length and their position should be confirmed with X-ray even apex locators can be used for the same purpose.
- The size of the correct metal verifier should correspond to last apical file used obturators then heated in a Therma prep oven for 15 -20 seconds and placed in a canal already coated with sealer with firm apical pressure to the marked working length.

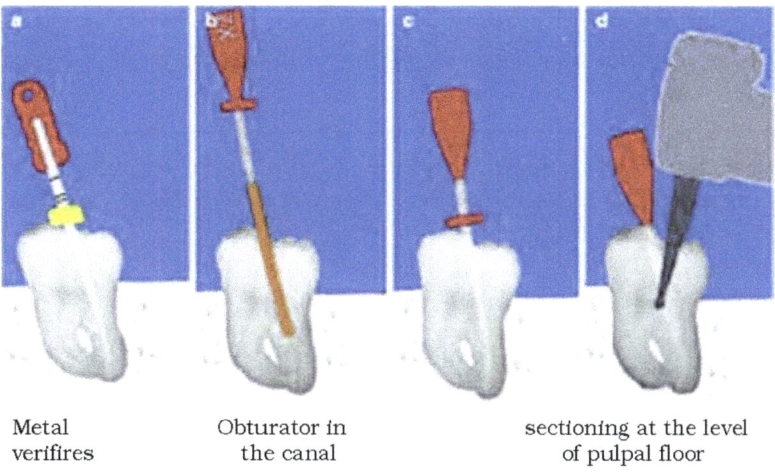

Fig. 9.137:

NOTE:

The operator has approximately 10 seconds to retrieve the obturator from the oven and place in to the canal.) verify the fit of obturation taking radiograph when found correct while stabilizing the carrier with index finger sectioned at the level of the pulpal floor.

Simple fill

It is a carrier based sectional obturation technique used in conjunction with specially designed light speed rotary instruments carriers with 5mm apical plug of gutta percha attached which performs cold condensation carrier chosen according to the diameter of the file.

Technique

The carrier with 5mm apical plug of gutta percha attached inserted in a canal already coated with sealer with firm apical pressure to the marked working length. The handle of the carrier is rotated quickly in clockwise and counter clockwise direction two and more times to disengage the apical plug of gutta percha from the carrier. The remaining body of the can be back filled with lateral compaction or thermo-plasticized gutta percha techniques.

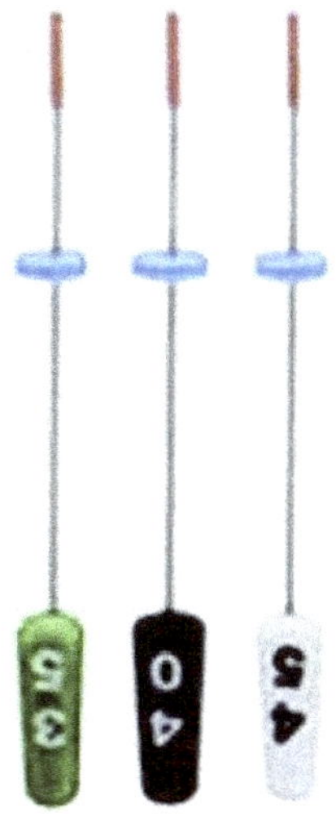

Fig. 9.138: Carrier with 5mm apical plug

Thermo-plasticized gutta percha techniques

Instead of placing the gutta percha inside the canals and applying heat to cause it to flow gutta percha heated and soften outside the tooth and inject the thermo-soften material in to the tooth the injected material flow apically with minimal compacting pressure fill the canal system in all three dimensions. If minimal compacting pressure not applied there will be poor adaptation of material to the canal walls and results in void formation.

Principal

An electric unit with pistol grip syringe to which silver needles ranging from 18 - 25-gauge size attached to deliver the thermoplastic material to the canal. Exertion of pressure on the trigger activates the piston that presses gutta-percha toward the tip of instrument. Control unit allows the operator to adjust the temperature and thus the viscosity of gutta percha. The plunger is designed to prevent the back flow of gutta percha.

Prerequisite

- Should have continuous tapering funnel for smooth flow of soften gutta percha.
- Should have a good apical barrier to avoid extrusion of excessive material in the periodontium.

Indications

- After down filling to back fill the body of canals
- For obturation of root with internal resorption and perforations.
- After closure and maturation of the root following apexification.
- After obtaining apical barrier with MTA
- Portions of the canal that had remained unnegotiable to endodontic instruments.

Advantages

- Better seal between canal walls and gutta-percha interface.
- Results in flow of gutta percha in the fine intricacies of root canal system.
- Results in moment of gutta percha and sealer in to dentinal tubules.

Disadvantages

- Lack good predictable apical control during obturation may lead peri apical extrusion.
- Clinician does not have precise control on either the pressure that is exerted or the amount of gutta percha being introduced in to canal.
- Possibility of heat damage to periodontium if temperature guidelines are neglected

Drawbacks

- High temperature that gutta percha reaches with in syringe before being introduced in to the canal may lead poor quality condensation.

- Voids may be formed if gun is withdrawn out of canal too quickly or insufficient heat to soften the gutta percha.

Obtura system

Obtura system consists of a handheld gun that contains a chamber surrounded by a heating element in to which pellets of gutta percha are loaded and heated and syringe to which silver needles are attached to deliver the therma -plasticized material to the canal.the control unit allows the operator to adjust the temperature and thus the viscosity of gutta percha.the plunger is designed to prevent the back flow of gutta percha the selection of needles ranges from 18 to 25 gauge size obtura sysem heats the gutta percha -160C TO 200c.

- Obtura II Introduced in Harvard institute. It consists of electrical unit with pistol grip syringe and specially designed gutta percha pellets which are heated to approximately 360 to 390 F for obturation.

- Obtura III consists of a handheld gun that contains a chamber surrounded by a heating element in to which pellets of gutta percha are loaded and heated.

- Silver needles are attached to deliver the therma-plasticized material to the canal and gutta percha then compacted using appropriate size pluggers obtura system III heats the gutta percha -160C TO 200c.

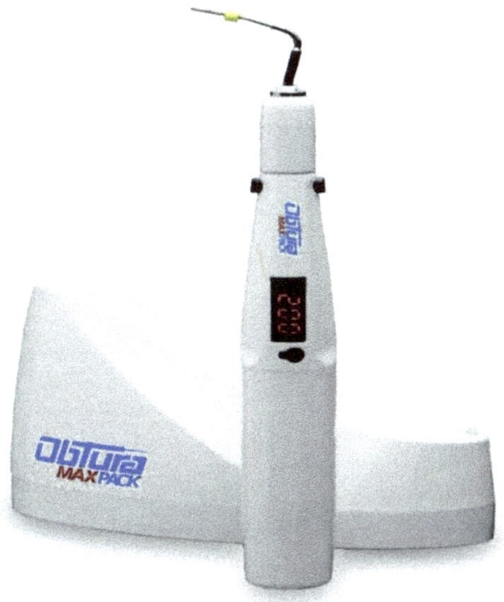

Fig. 9.139:

Technique

- Prefit a cold plugger and a silver needle to 4 -6mm from the apical terminus.

- Apply sealer in the canal.

- Insert the needle passively in to the canal and hold it properly in a predetermined position avoiding apical pressure gently inject the soften gutta-percha, in 2 to 3 second it fills the apical segment and begin to lift the needle out of the tooth.

- Nowuse the prefit cold pluggers dipped in isopropyl alcohol to compact the material apically then back filling of the remainder canal done.

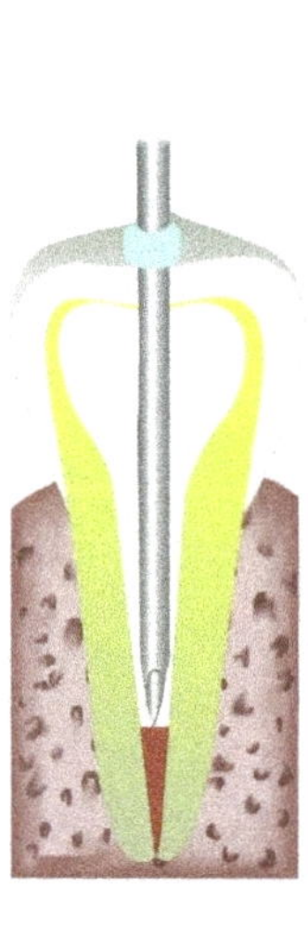

Needle in
to the canal

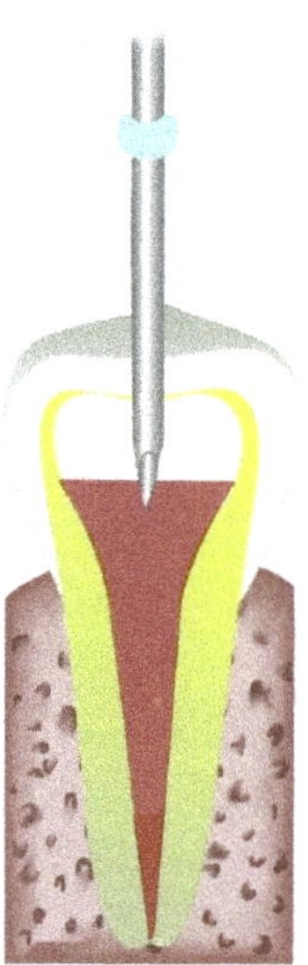

Lifting out of
needle

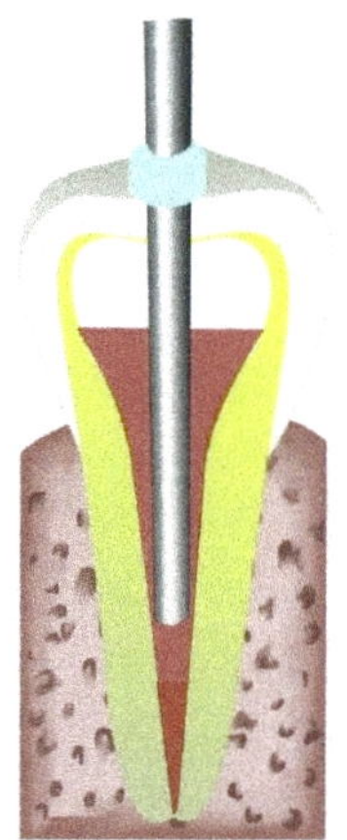

Prefit plugger to
compact material apically

Fig. 9.140:

Ultrafil 3D

This system utilizes alpha phase gutta percha heats the gutta percha to 90C
Ultrafil 3D technique involves heating unit, cannulas and injection syringes
There are three types of gutta percha cannulas

Regular set	low viscosity	30min	setting time
Firm set	low viscosity	4min	setting time
Endo set	higher viscosity	2min	setting time

The manufacturer recommends compaction after the initial set with both materials. Endo set has a higher viscosity and does not flow as well it is recommended for techniques employing compaction and set in 2 minutes.

Technique

Cannula is placed 6 to 7 mm from the apex and confirmed. It is placed in heater for minimum 15 minutes before use.

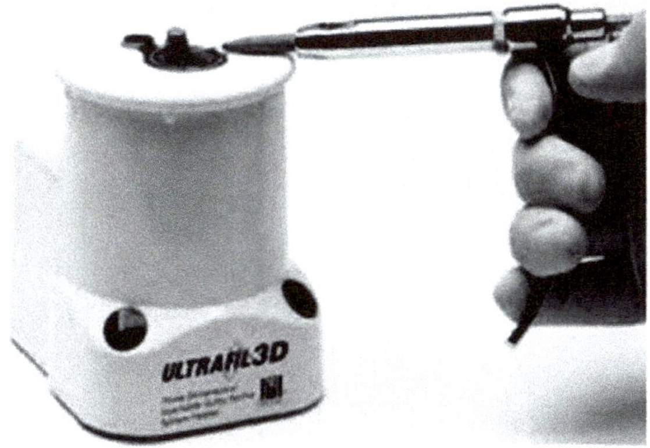

Fig. 9.141:

Insert the needle passively in to the canal and hold it properly in a predetermined position avoiding apical pressure gently inject the soften gutta-percha material as the warm gutta-percha fills the canal its back pressure pushes the needle out the canal, within 10-15 seconds it fills canal.

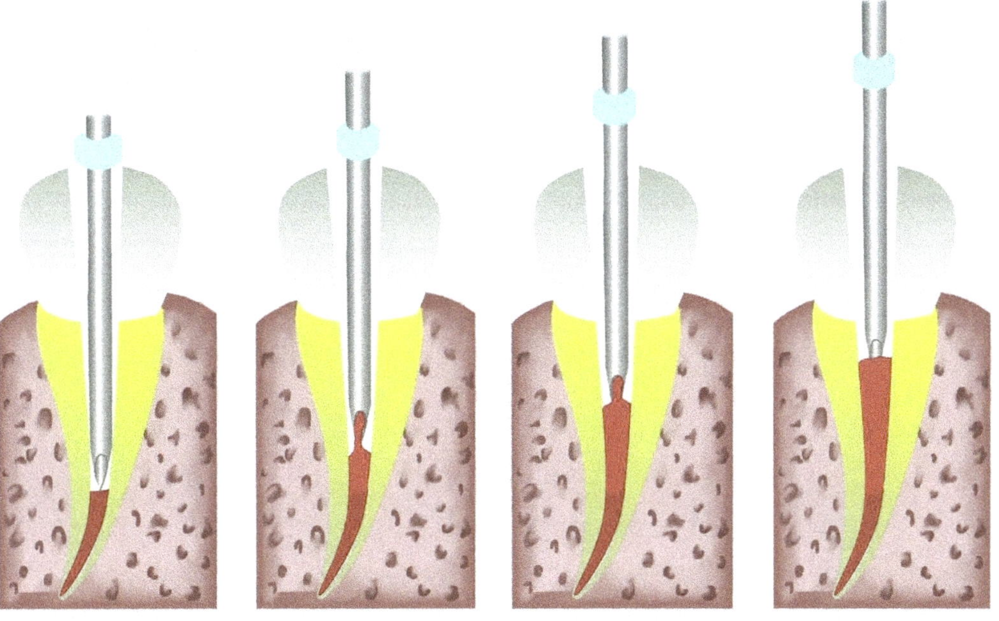

Cannula is placed 6 to 7 mm from the apex   *Fills the canal in segments within 10 to 15 seconds*

Fig. 9.142:

O) ROOT CANAL SEALERS

Three-dimensional fluid tight sealing of root canal system is ultimate goal of endodontic treatment to prevent the reinfection of the canals and for preserving the health of periapical tissues as the gutta percha has no adhesive qualities to the dentin regardless of the obturation technique used sealers play major role in achieving three dimensional fluid tight seal by filling spaces, voids and minor discrepancies exit between gutta-percha and canal walls.

Definition

Materials used to establish adequate three-dimensional fluid tight seal between gutta-percha and root canal walls.

Functions

- Establish adequate seal between core filling material and canal walls, prevents reinfection and preserves the health of periapical tissues.
- Seals the spaces, voids and minor discrepancies that exist between gutta-percha and canal walls perfectly and enhances the attainment of impervious seal.
- Fills and serves as a filler for lateral canals, accessory canals, Isthmuses, fins, webs and multiple foramens.
- Acts as an anti-microbial agent can assist in microbial control.
- Acts as a lubricant while condensation.
- Radio-opaque allows the visualization in the radiographs for the assignment of quality of seal and also discloses the presence of lateral canals, accessory canals and multiple foramina's.

Ideal requirements of root canal sealers

- Should be tacky in consistency when mixed.
- Should provide good adhesion between the canal's walls and obturating material.
- Should have minimum shrinkage. Should be radiopaque.
- Should not be irritating to periapical tissues.
- Should not stain the dentine or tooth.
- Should be bactericidal.
- Should be insoluble with tissue fluids.
- Should have adequate working time.
- Should be easy to remove.(when necessary)
- Should not have mutagenic or carcinogenic properties.
- Should not provoke any immune reaction.

Classification

1) Zinc oxide eugenol-based sealers
   - Grossmans formula
   - Roth's 801
   - Tubliseal
2) Calcium hydroxide-based sealers
   - Sealapex
   - Apexit
3) Glass ionomer based sealers
4) Resins based sealers
   - Ah plus
   - Ah 26
   - Epiphany
   - Diaket
5) Bio-ceramic sealers
6) MTA sealers

Zinc oxide eugenol cement-based sealers

These are supplied as Grossman's sealer, Tuli sealer, Roth sealer, Watch's sealers. These are the most advocated and widely used sealers provides good seal

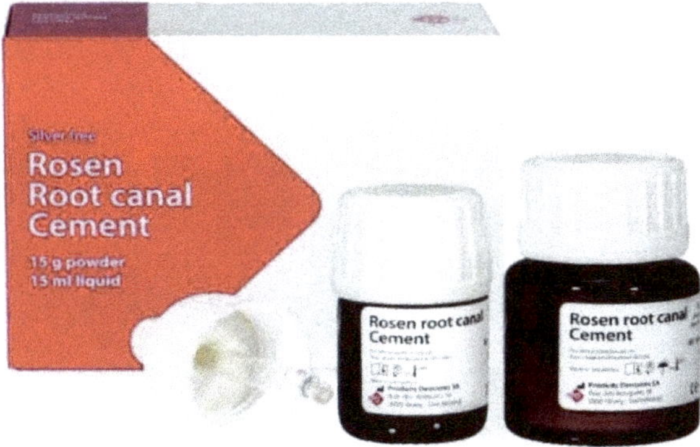

Fig. 9.143:

Properties

- Zinc oxide eugenol cements modified for endodontic use. Mixing vehicle is mostly eugenol.
- Slow setting time Setting time adjusted for adequate working time.
- Increased plasticity even after set and flow under load.

Advantages

- Exhibits desensitizing effect on exposed dentin
- Poses antimicrobial properties, bactericidal discourages bacterial growth
- If accidentally extrudes in to the periapical area easily gets resorbed.
- Radio opacity 4-5mm of aluminium

Functions

- Fill the lateral canals and accessory canals very effectively.
- Fill the irregular spaces and discrepancies between the canal walls and the core filling material.

Disadvantages

It shrinks after setting.

Dimensionally weak due to continuous loss of eugenol make it weak and unstable

Calcium hydroxide-based sealers

- These are supplied as it is supplied as seal apex, apex seal, vita pex, dycal.

- It has been used in endodontics as a filling material, medicament and sealer mainly because of its antimicrobial properties and osteogenic potential.

- The setting reactions are complex even though the surface of sealer becomes hard inner mass remain soft for an extended period.

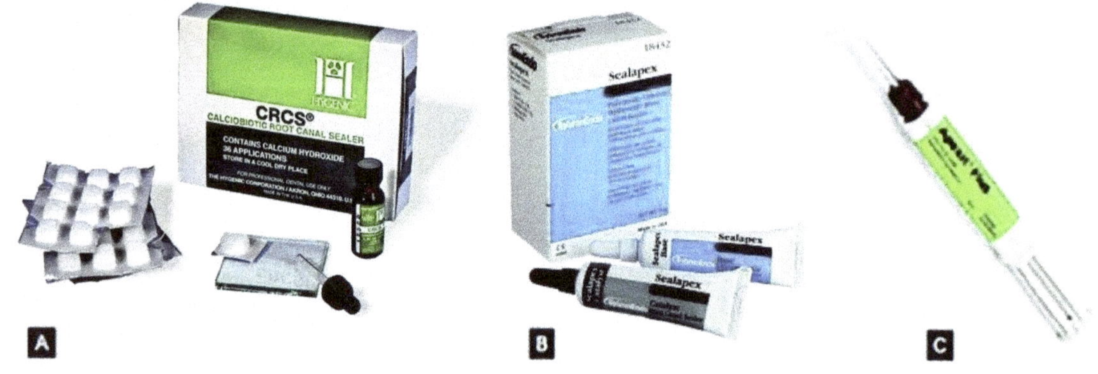

Fig. 9.144:

Advantages

- Exhibits sustained anti-microbial property.
- Induces repair and stimulates hard tissue formation.
- Biocompatibility within an acceptable range compare to other sealers.
- Flow is close to AH plus and tubliseal.

Uses

- Used in immaturely formed root apex.
- Used in open apex or root end resorptive defects.
- Used in cases of repairable transportations and perforations.
- Setting time - less than 2 hours.
- <u>PH -</u> 11 to 12.5.

Limitations

- Exhibits high water sorption dimensionally weak.
- In terms of leakage not superior to other type of sealers.
- Because of their solubility don't fulfil the criteria of ideal sealer.

Epoxy resin-based sealers

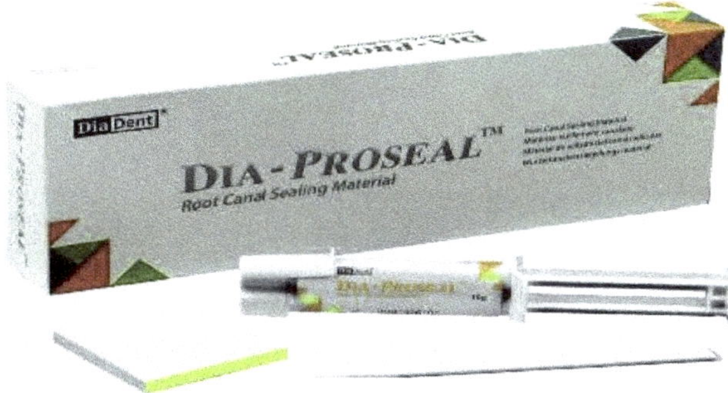

Fig. 9.145:

AH-plus sealer is supplied as two paste system

Tube 1 Resin paste	Tube 2 Amin paste
Epoxy resin Calcium tungstate Zirconium oxide Iron oxide	Adamethas amine NN d-5-o diamine Zirconium oxide AerosolSilicone oil

Advantages

- Reduced solubility
- High dimensional stability
- Better apical seal
- Slightly expands during setting
- Micro retention to canal wall surface

Working time = 4 hours

Setting time = 8 hours

AH 26

Epoxy resin characterized by reactive epoxide ring polymerized by the breaking of this ring.

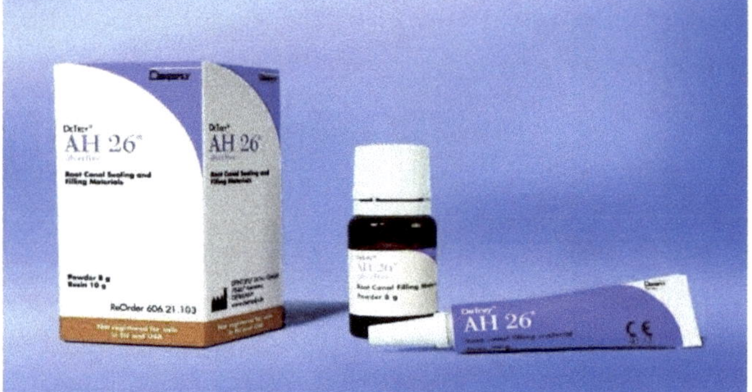

Fig. 9.146:

Properties

* Good adhesive property
* Good flow
* Antibacterial
* Contracts slightly while hardening
* Low toxicity

Addition of hardener makes cured resin chemically and biologically inert.

Consist of yellow powder and viscous resin liquid mixed to thick creamy consistency.

Slow setting 36- 48 hrs at body temperature and 5-7 days at room temperature.

Long setting time and material fluidity.

No cracking or separation from dentinal walls.

It releases formaldehyde during setting.

Silicon based sealers

Diaket

It is a polyvinyl resin, and reinforced chelate formed between zinc oxide and diketone.

It hardens rapidly about 6-8 minutes on glass slab even more rapidly on root canal.

Known for its resistance to absorption superior to other sealers in tensile strength and resistance to permeability.

Mild inflammatory reaction occurs when overfilled.

Commonly used to cement endosseous implants.

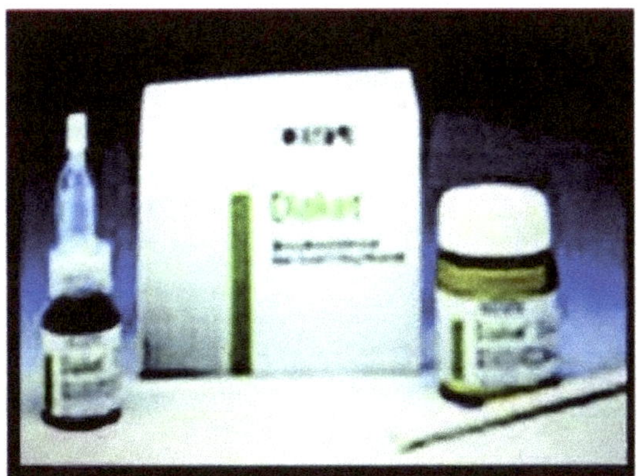

Fig. 9.147:

Endo fill

It is a injectable resin sealer used in combination with core material or as a sole filling material. Injected in to the canal space with pressure syringes.

Advantages

- Exhibit good adaption to the tooth structure and fills internal anatomy.
- Non-resorbable material.
- Low toxicity.
- High radio-opaque.
- Low viscosity.

Disadvantages

- Difficult remove from canal for retreatment.
- Can not use in presence of moisture canals must be dry.
- Exhibit shrinkage upon setting.
- Setting time –8 to 9 minutes.
- Ease of preparation used within 20 minutes for better results.

Roeko seal

The main ingredient polymethyl siloxane main advantage it shows 0.2% expansion instead of shrinkage

Extremely low film thickness allows the sealer to flow in the fine intricacies of canal.

Excellent flow properties

Excellent biocompatibility well tolerated by tissues

Dimensionally stable, zero solubility

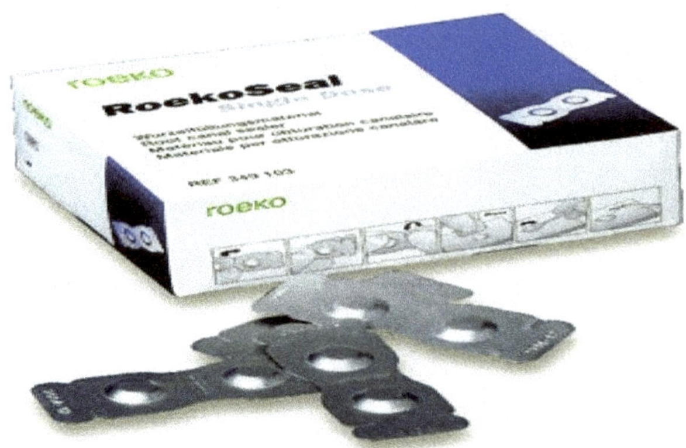

Fig. 9.148:

Calcium phosphate-based sealers

It is well known that calcium phosphate sealers have a high biocompatibility because of their composition almost identical to that of tooth and bone material. Recently new calcium phosphate-based sealers are developed.

Apatite root I II III.

Bio-seal.

Cap-seal I.

Cap-seal II.

Apatite composed of hydroxyapatite and tricalcium phosphates.

Favorable tissue resorption.

Acceptable biocompatibility.

Good sealing ability.

Bio-seal hydroxy apatite containing eugenol sealers mainly used for vertical condensation.

Glass ionomer cements

Because of its adhesive qualities and fast set often used in combination with a single cone obturation technique.

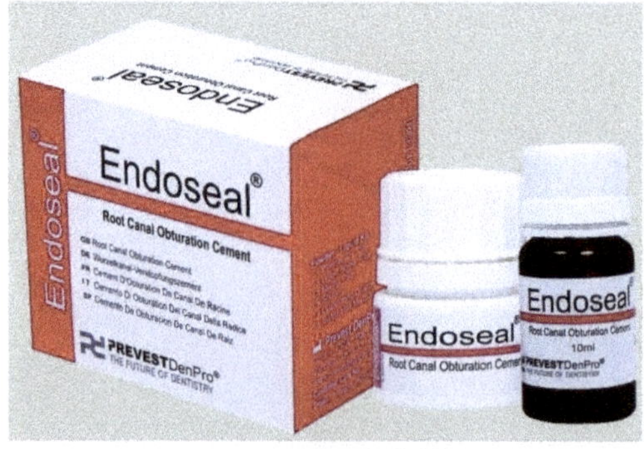

Fig. 9.149:

Composition

Supply as powder and liquid

Powder	Liquid
Calcium fluoro-aluminosilicate glass Calcium volframate Silicic acid	Polycarbonic acid and maleic acid Copolymers Tartaric acid Water

Advantages

- Chemically bond to the dentin provides physical support for fracture reinforces the root
- Optimal flow properties
- Ability provide more stable apical seal
- Biocompatible
- Non toxic

Disadvantages

- Short working time
- Fast set
- Difficulty in removing the sealer from canal walls in case of retreatment

Bio-ceramic sealers

- It is a calcium phosphate silicate-based cement which is premixed, injectable and hydrophilic supplied as
- I Root SP
- Endo sequence BC sealer

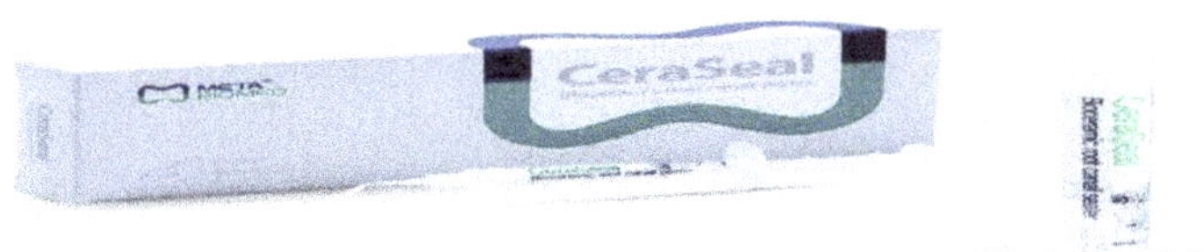

Fig. 9.150:

Composition of bio ceramic sealer

1. Alumina
2. Zirconia and zirconium oxide
3. Active bio glass tricalcium silicate, dicalcium silicate and colloidal silica
4. Hydroxy apatite
5. Calcium phosphate and calcium hydroxide

pH: of BC sealer during setting process higher which increases bactericidal property.

Setting rection.

Uses moisture that remains with in the dentinal tubules after irrigation to initiate complex setting reactions and slightly expands slightly while setting.

Advantages
- Biocompatible.
- Non toxic.
- Bond strength similar to AH plus sealers.

Advantages of bio-ceramic filler over gutta percha
- It does not shrink after cooling.
- It has anti-microbial properties.
- It bonds to the dentin.
- It expands slightly while setting.
- It exhibits more flow.
- It is non-resorbable, and stays in canal for long time.
- The main advantages are it fills lateral canals, accessory canals, multiple foramen perfectly due to its flow.

MTA based sealers

It is a white Portland cement highly biocompatible and stimulate mineralization. Its bioactive nature induces dentinogenesis and cementogensis, supplied as Pro Root Endo sealer and Fill apex, MTA obtura ,CPM Sealer.

Composition
- CaO2 – 75%.
- SiO2– 25%.
- Zirconium oxide.
- Calcium chloride.
- pH = 12.5.
- Setting time = 3 hours.
- Working time= less than 4 minutes.

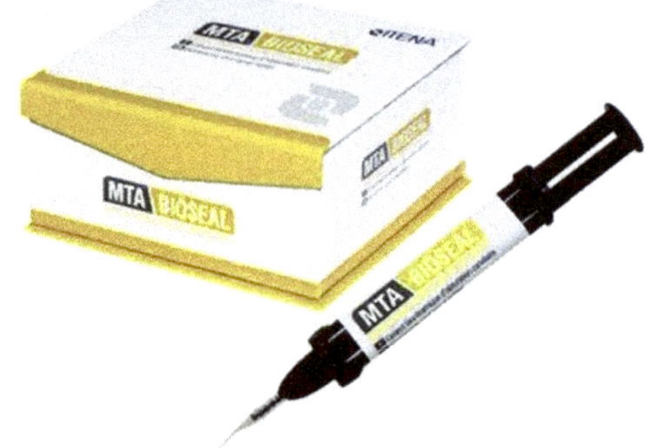

Fig. 9.151:

Properties
- ❖ Flow –high flow rate and low film thickness enhances the penetration of sealer into the fine intricacies of root canal system.
- ❖ More strength than CaOH (calcium hydroxide).
- ❖ Radio-opaque - radiographic diagnosis is easy.

Advantages

- Highly Biocompatible.
- No shrinkage on setting.
- Hydrophilic – sets in presence of moisture.
- Exhibits dentin bonding properties.
- Exhibits antimicrobial properties.
- It slightly expands while setting.

Disadvantages

- Compressive strength is inadequate.
- Long setting time.
- Less working time.
- Improper handling properties.
- Difficult to remove from the canals during re root canal treatment.
- May cause discoloration due to release of ferrous ion.

Sealer application

- Determine the working length.
- Complete drying of canals.
- Application using paper points or master gutta percha cones or master apical files.
- Excessive sealer is removed.
- Applying excessive sealer results in inadequate flow of gutta percha.
- Lack of gutta percha at the apical extent of canal.
- An unacceptable seal.
- Applying insufficient sealer results in poor seal between the core filling material and canal walls.
- Inadequate filling of accessory canals, lateral canals, multiple foramina's...etc
- An unacceptable seal.

Note

- All the filling materials should be confined to the root canal system because.
- If the material is extruded in to the peri radicular tissue it can be highly irritating and may reduce the probability of healing by 25%.
- Zinc oxide eugenol-based sealers probably irritating because of eugenol.
- Epoxy resin based sealers are more biocompatible.

10
Mishaps in Endodontics

> *IGNORANCE BREEDS FEAR.*
> *FEAR IS AN OPEN INVITATION TO MISHAPS.*
> *KNOWING BREEDS ATTENTION.*
> *ATTENTION IS AN OPEN INVITATION TO SUCCESS.*
> *BE A KNOWER, BE ATTENTIVE, AVOID MISHAPS.*

LEDGES

Unintentional notching or grooving in the dentin leading to under mining of tooth.

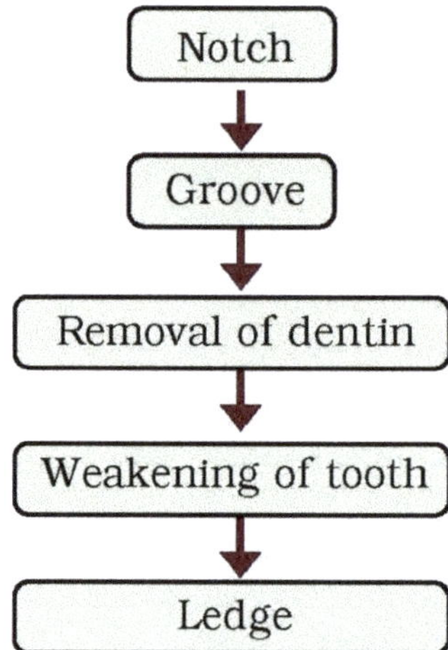

Types

- Coronal ledges
- Radicular ledges

CORONAL LEDGE

The ledge occurs in the coronal portion of the tooth during access cavity preparation.

Cause

Using large round burs and inverted cone burs.

RADICULAR LEDGE

- Occurs in root portion of tooth during shaping.

- Occurs due to using stiff stainless-steel files in narrow curved canals. Stainless steel files regain their shape memory and do not remain centred in the canals, this creates ledges and leads to transportation of files.

Causes

a. Severe calcification

b. Severe sclerosis.

c. Use of rigid files in curved cannels.

d. Use of large files in narrow cannels.

Prevention

- Flooding the chamber with viscous chelating agents to dissolve the inorganic content of smear layer.

- Doing copious irrigation with sodium hypochlorite to dissolve the organic content of smear layer.

- Precurving the apical 3 mm of file.

- Performing regular recapitulation.

- Carrying the initial file to the exact working length. Selecting the size and type of file wisely.

Management

- Early detection is better most of the time as small ledges go unnoticed and undetected, they get filled during filling and obturation.

- Be attentive to the alteration in finger tactile sensation against resistance. Finger tactile sense develops with practice, more the practice greater is the finger tactile sense.

- Sudden change in the path of files.

- Loss of Working length if the ledge is large.

ADVERSE SEQUEL OF LEDGES

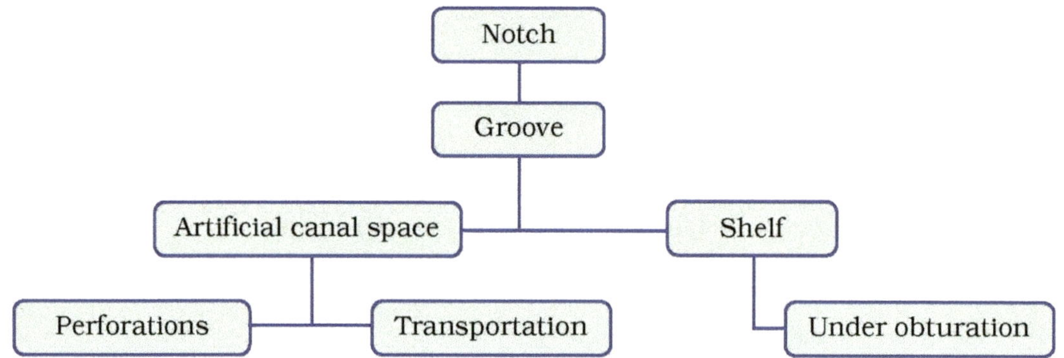

Procedure

Bypassing the ledge

Cervical 1/3rd preflaring is done with Sx file. Flood the chamber with viscous chelators.

In narrow canals precurved flexible no 6 k or 8 k or 10 k file abraded at its tip to make it sharp is selected.

In large wider canals no 15 or 20 or 25 k file cut at its working edge obliquely to make it sharp is selected. Introduce the selected file in to the canal.

Slide the file slowly away from the ledge with low intensity up and down strokes until the file makes its way and slips through the narrow curvature of canal to the exact working length. The procedure is repeated with sequentially larger files until the ledge fades away.

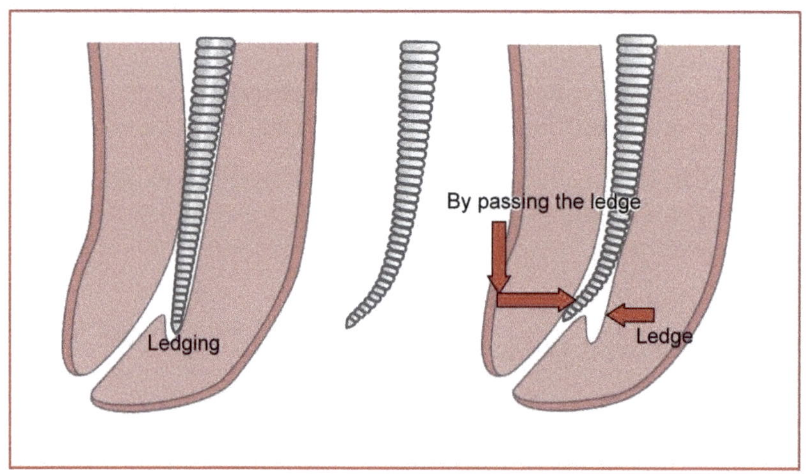

Fig. 10.1. By passing the Ledge

PERFORATION

Definition

It is an accidental unpleasant dentist induced communication between the pulp cavity & periodontium.

Types of perforations

1) Coronal perforations:

2) Root perforations:
    i.   Furcal/cervical
    ii. Lateral
    iii. Apical
    iv. Strip perforation
    v.   Zipping
    vi. Transportation

Adverse sequel of perforations

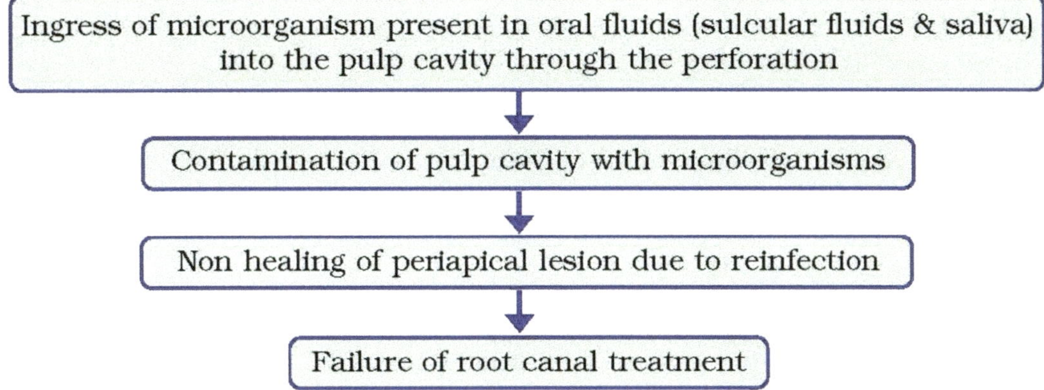

CORONAL PERFORATION

Occurs in the crown portion of the tooth during access cavity preparation.

Causes

Poor knowledge of anatomy of tooth.

Failure to understand the root crown angulations especially in mandibular and maxillary premolars and upper and lower anteriors.

Neglecting the laws of access cavity preparation.

Failure to maintain the long axis of the bur to the long axis of tooth. Failure to Penetrate at the centre of the crown at the level of the CEJ.

Common sites are labial surface of anteriors & labial surface of premolars.

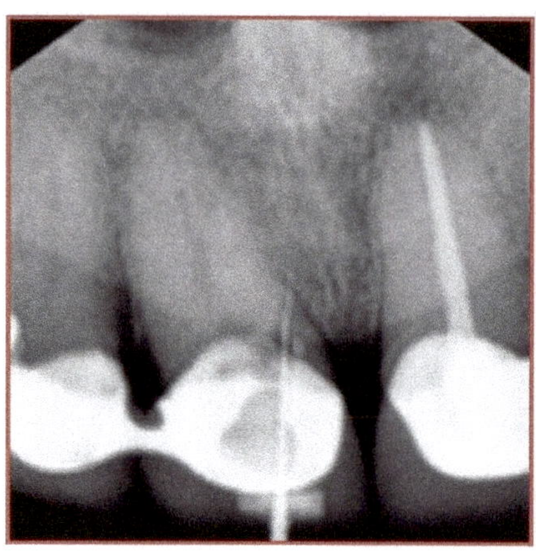

Fig.10.2 : Coronal Perforation

MTA (MINERAL TRIOXIDE AGGREGATE)

Composition

- CaO_2 – 75%
- SiO_2 – 25%
- pH   = 12.5
- Setting time = 3 hours.

Properties

- Radio-opaque.
- Highly Biocompatible.
- No shrinkage on setting.
- More strength than CaOH (calcium hydroxide).
- Hydrophilic – sets in presence of moisture.
- Exhibits dentin bonding properties.
- Antimicrobial properties.
- It slightly expands while setting

Adverse sequence of coronal perforation

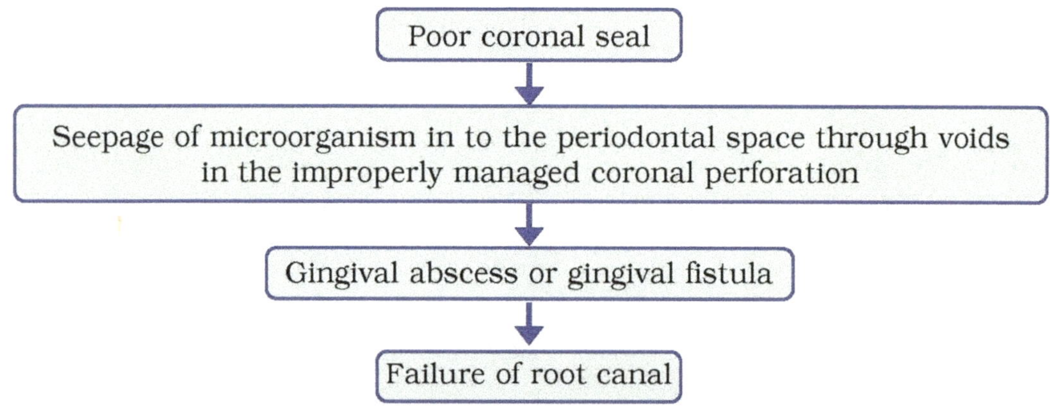

Management

Act immediately and aseptically. Stop bleeding with haemostatic agents– apply mild to moderate pressure with sterile cotton pellet soaked in Adrenaline or Ethamsylate against the perforated site for 1 or 2 minutes. Once the bleeding stops, the perforated site is disinfected with highly diluted sodium hypochlorite. Sterile cotton pellet soaked in highly diluted sodium hypochlorite is pressed against the perforated site with mild pressure.

Isolate and dry the perforated site.

Mix the MTA in sterile water on a sterile glass slab to a proper consistency. Place the MTA over the perforated site with help of a carrier and do not apply pressure.

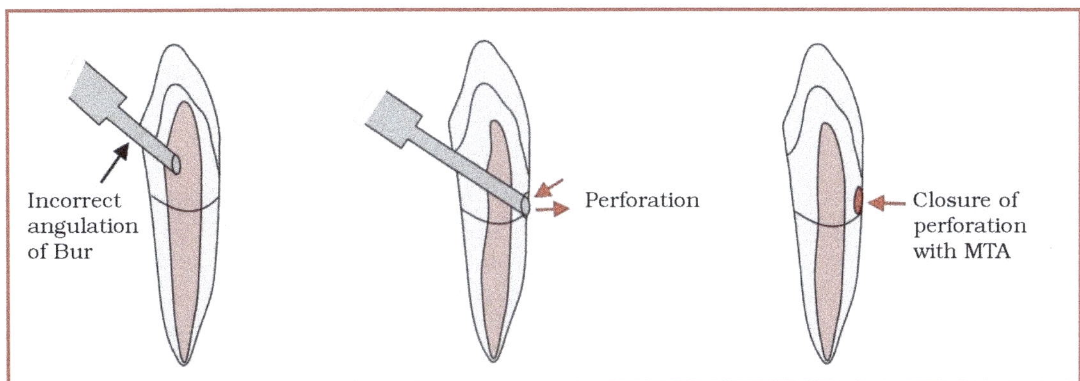

Fig. 10.3 : Management of Coronal perforation

Root perforation

Types of root perforation

1. Furcal
2. Cervical
3. Lateral
4. Apical

FURCAL PERFORATION

It occurs through the pulpal floor below the furcation in multirooted teeth.

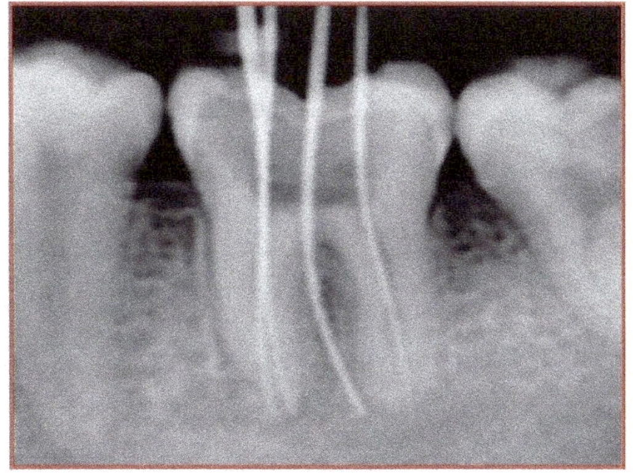

Fig. 10.4: Furcal perforation

Causes

-   Working under poor illumination.
-   Inadequate extension of access cavity.
-   Severe calcification and sclerosis of pulp chamber.

CERVICAL PERFORATION

- Occurs in the cervical portion of tooth. More apical the perforation occurs better would be the prognosis.

- Occurs while searching the canals.

- Occurs through the paracervical dentin around orifice of canals.

Causes

Working under poor illumination. Inadequate extension of access cavity. Severe calcification and sclerosis of pulp chamber.

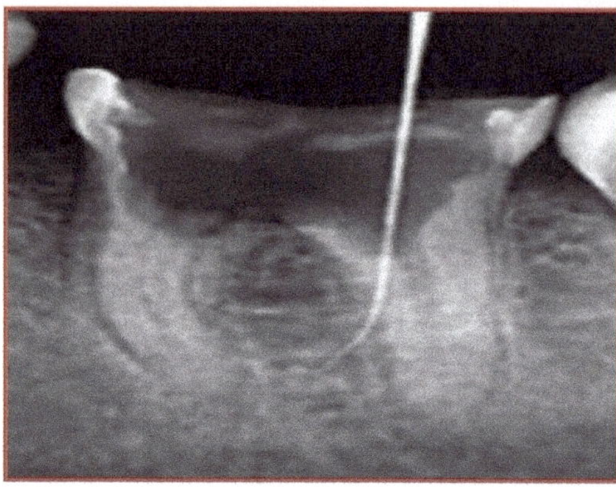

Fig. 10.5: Cervical perforation

LATERAL PERFORATION

Occurs through the body of root. (cervical 1/3rd and middle 1/3rd of root) Commonly occurs in curved and narrow roots. *e.g.* Buccal roots of maxillary molars, Mesial roots of mandibular molars, Roots of multirooted molars.

Causes

- Failure to pre-curve the file.
- Using nonflexible rigid files
- Using large files in narrow canals.

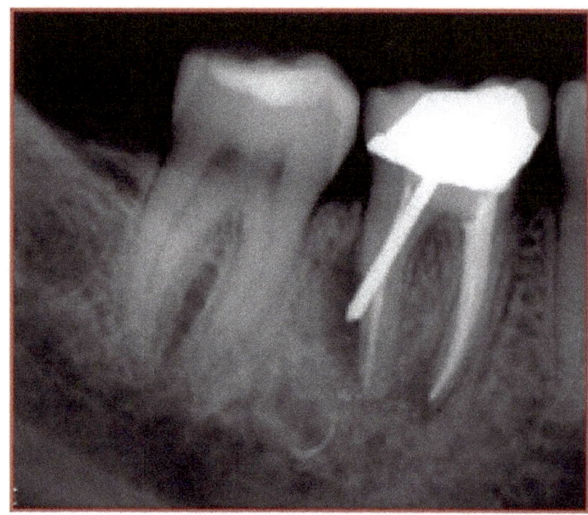

Fig. 10.6: Lateral perforation

Mode of Occurrence

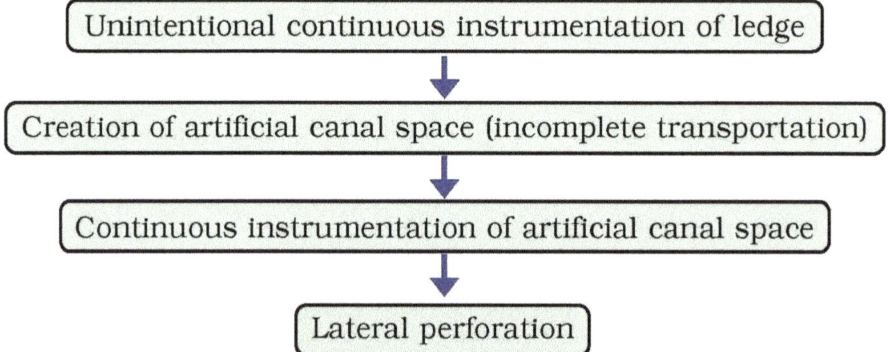

Apical perforation

It occurs through the apical foramen due to over instrumentation beyond the apical constriction. It gets filled during obturation. Use CaOH (calcium hydroxide) as sealer while obturation. Does not influence the long-term prognosis if obturation is densely compacted without voids.

STRIP FORMATION

Occurs mostly in mesial roots of mandibular molars below the furcation area.

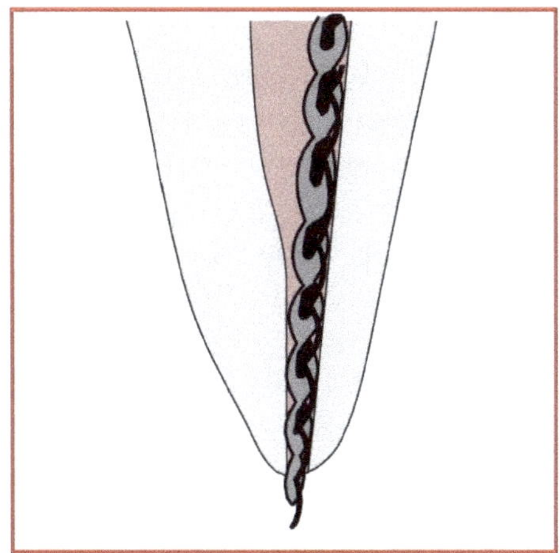

Fig. 10.7: Apical perforation

Causes

1) During pre-flaring of cervical 1/3rd with SX file in crown down technique of shaping.

2) During preparation of post space with Gates Glidden drill.

3) During retrieval of separated instruments.

Note :

Concave depression on the distal surface of mesial roots of mandibular molars is more prone to strip perforation. Convex mesial surface away from the furcation is thick and not prone to stripping.

If it does not get sealed properly, it affects the long-term prognosis of tooth.

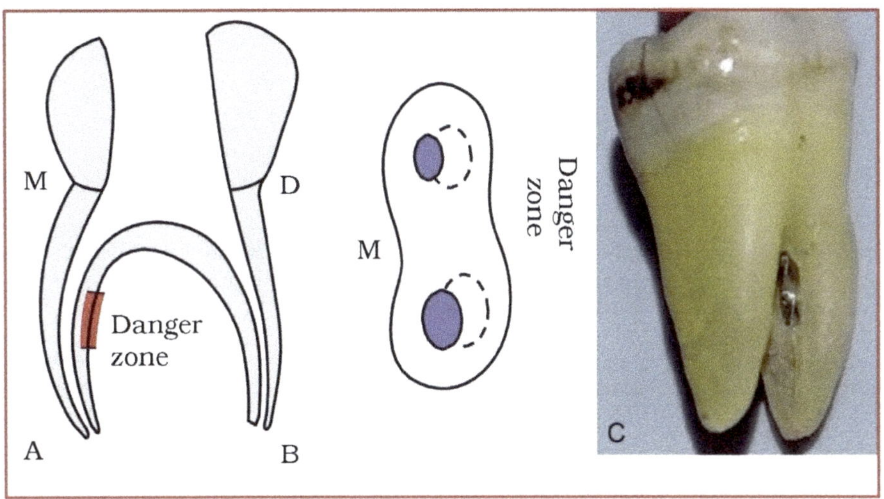

Fig. 10.8: Strip perforation

TRANSPORTATION

Unintentional continuous instrumen- tation of ledge leads to creation of a new artificial foramen and is called transportation. Apical transportation- occurs through the apical 1/3 of root. Lateral transportation-occurs through the body of root. Can't get filled during obturation and leads to very poor prognosis of tooth and failure of root canal treatment. Re root canal treatment is contraindicated if the root canal treatment has failed due to transportation.

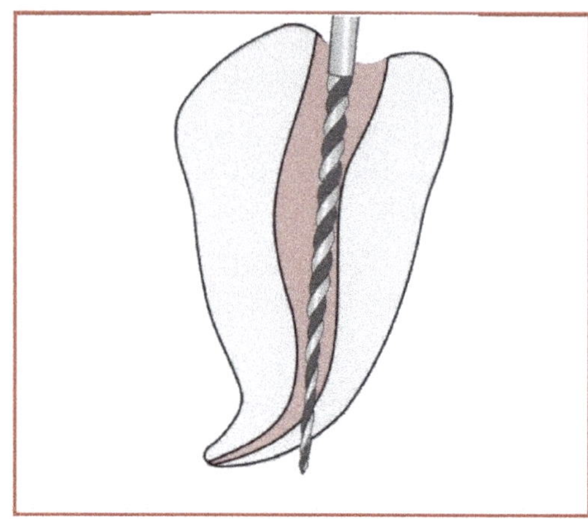

Fig. 10.9 : Apical perforation

Zipping

Transportation through the apical foramen is called zipping. Due to zipping, cleaning and shaping of the natural anatomic foramen is left behind leading to failure of root canal.

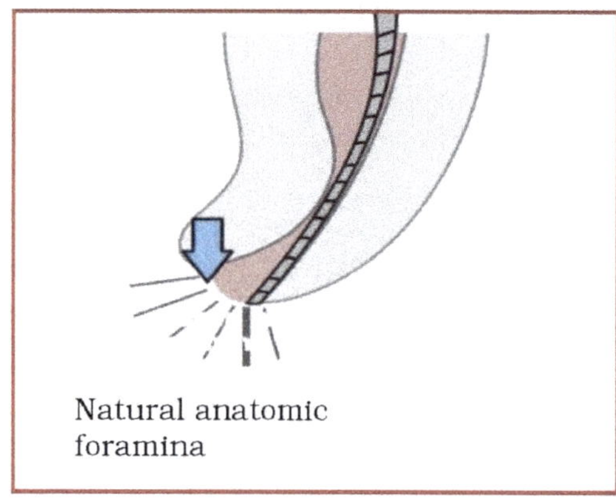

Fig. 10.10 : Zipping

Adverse sequel of radicular perforations

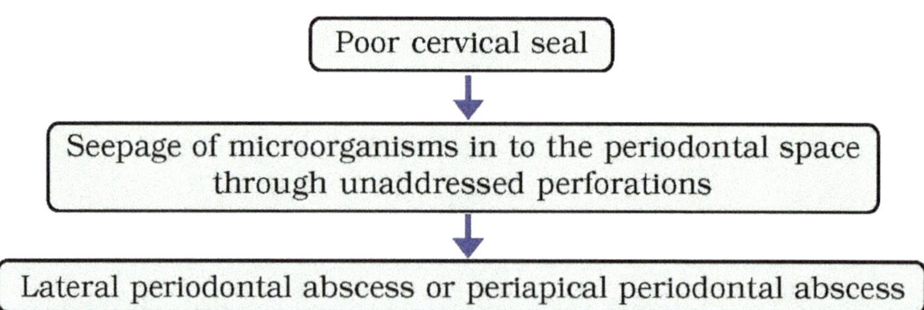

APICAL BLOCKAGE

Blockage of apical constriction with smear layer leading to loss of apical patency and working length. Maintenance of apical patency and working length throughout the procedure is critical for endodontic success.

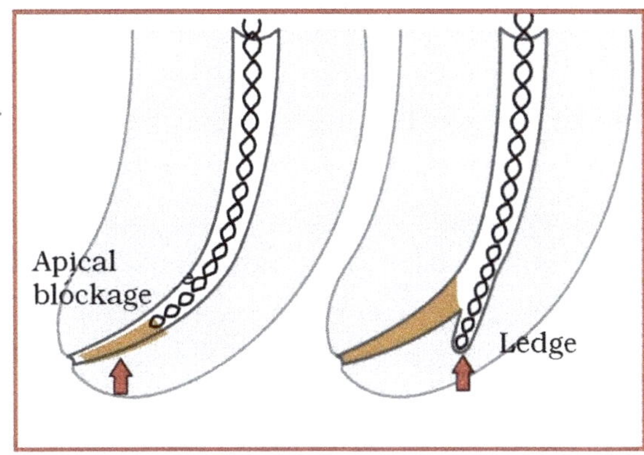

Fig. 10.11 : Apical blockage

Prevention

- Thorough irrigation with sodium hypochlorite.

- Flooding the chamber with viscous chelators like EDTA.

- Carrying the initial file to exact working length.

- Selecting the size and type of initial file wisely. In curved canals use flex-R files.

- In narrow canals use flexor-files.

- In wider canals 10 or 15 k files should be used. In narrow canals 6 or 8 k files should be used. Precurving the apical 3 mm of the file.

- Recapitulation and skipping to smaller size files regularly.

Adverse sequel of apical blockage

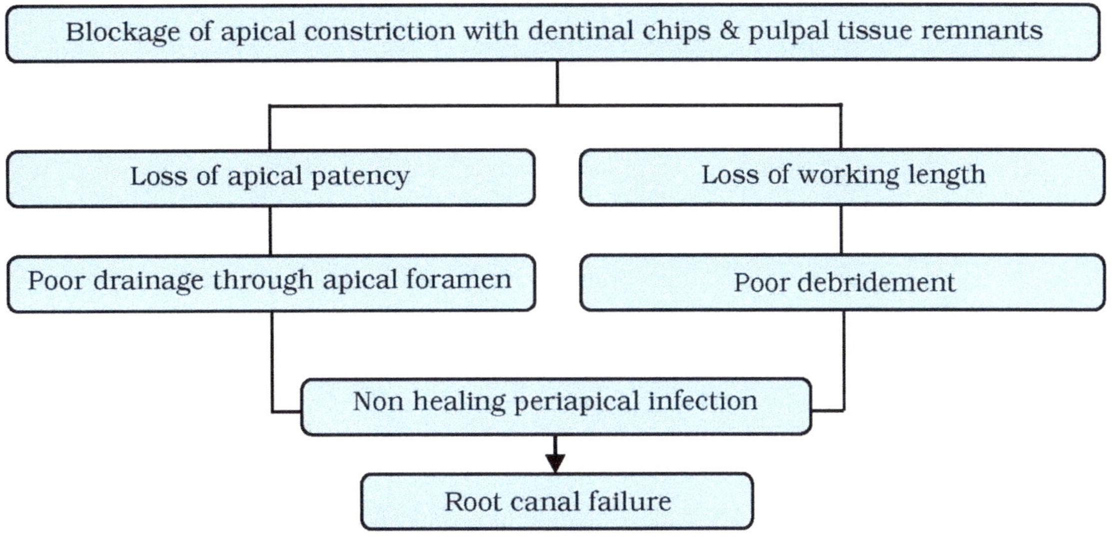

Concepts to prevent blockages

- Establishing and maintaining apical patency throughout the cleaning and shaping procedure is mandatory in preventing apical blockage.
- Initial file selection is crucial in preventing blockages.
- In distal roots of lower molars, palatal roots of upper molars, mandibular canines and maxillary anteriors the initial file is 15 k size file.
- In mandibular incisors, multirooted premolars, and mesial roots of mandibular molars the initial file is 10k size file.
- In mesial roots of third molars, mandibular lateral incisors, buccal roots of upper molars initial files used are 6 or 8 k file.

OVER OBTURATION

Causes

- Apical perforation through the foramen.
- Wide open apex.
- Excessive condensation forces during obturation.

Treatment

- If the tooth was vital without periapical lesion during the treatment and Patient is asymptomatic - No treatment is required.
- If tooth was non vital with periapical lesion during the treatment and patient is asymptomatic - Wait and watch.
- If the tooth was non vital with periapical lesion and patient is symptomatic then - Re root canal treatment is suggested, Apicectomy in anterior teeth. Root resection in upper molars and Hemi section in lower molars are the other treatments of choice.

Note: Mild discomfort and pain due to irritation of overextended gutta percha is managed by prescribing low doses of steroids for shorter duration.

ROOT FRACTURES

Horizontal root fractures

Horizontal apical 1/3 Root fracture

Causes

1) Excessive condensation forces during obturation.

2) Using hand pluggers instead of finger pluggers in lateral condensation technique.

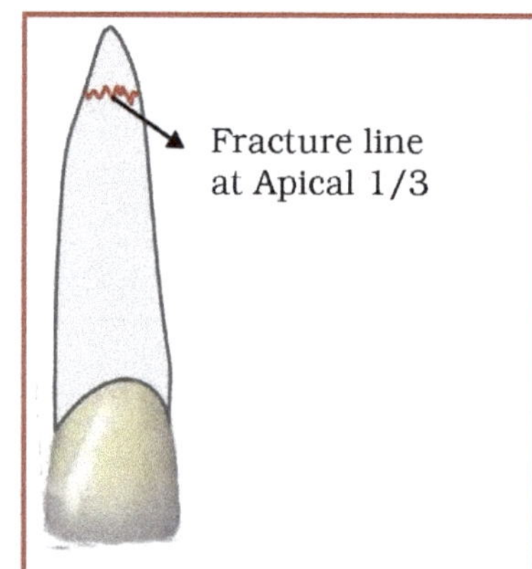

Fig. 10.12: Horizontal apical 1/3 Root fracture

Common sites

Distal roots of mandibular molars, Palatal roots of maxillary molars, Roots of anterior teeth.

Treatment

No treatment is required.

Horizontal cervical 1/3 fracture

Causes

1. Trauma
2. Deep bite
3. Decreased overjet

Common sites

Upper and lower anteriors

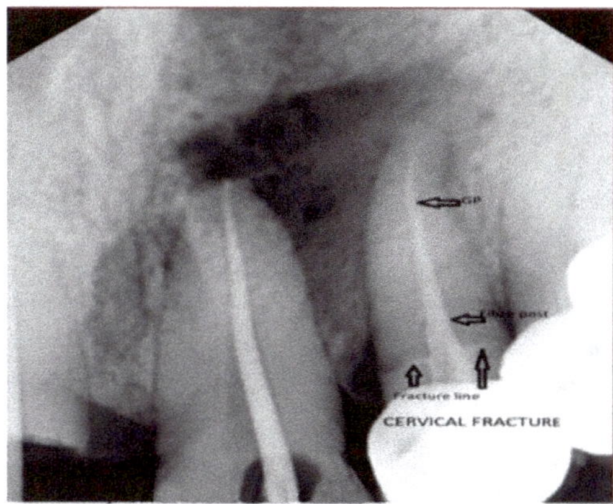

Fig. 10.13: Horizontal cervial 1/3 fracture

Treatment

By stabilising the undisplaced fragments with ligature wire root canal treatment is performed followed by retention and reinforcement of tooth with flowable composite.

Horizontal middle 1/3 root fracture

Common sites

Maxillary central and lateral incisors

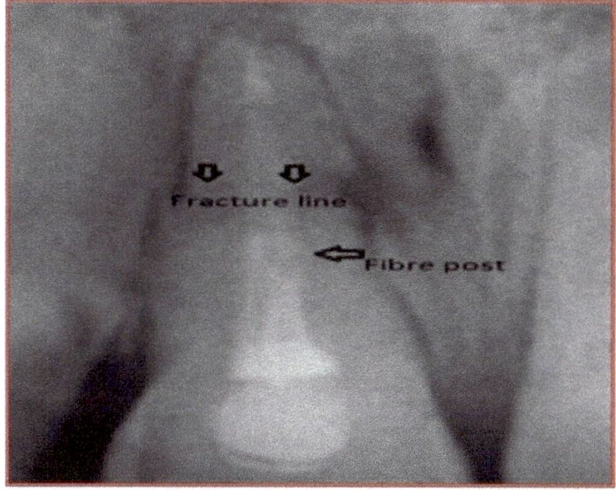

Fig. 10.14: Horizontal middle 1/3 root fracture

Treatment

Fracture segments are stabilized and retained with fibre post in conjunction with flowable composite.

VERTICAL ROOT FRACTURE

Causes

Excessive removal of root dentin during

a) Preflaring of cervical 1/3 of root in crown down technique
b) Removal of separated instruments
c) Post space creation
d) Stripping and perforations.

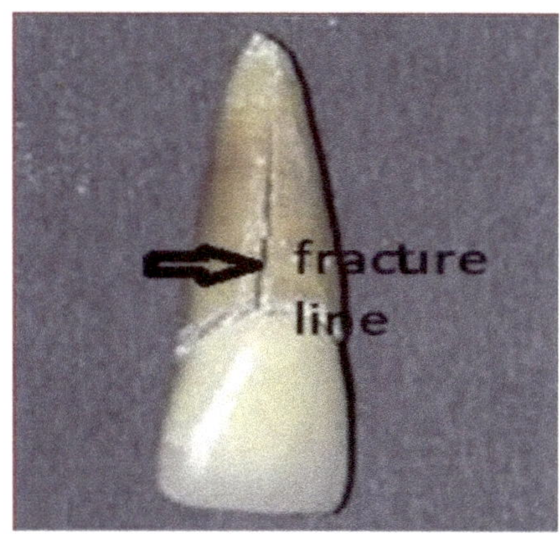

Fig. 10.15: Vertical root fracture

Other causes

Failure to give 2 mm occlusal clearance before access opening especially in patients with deep bite, decreased overjet and decreased vertical dimension of occlusion.

When to suspect a vertical fracture!!!

- Snappy sound during procedure
- Mobility of fragments
- J-shaped radiolucency on radiograph
- Multiple sinuses
- Deep periodontal pocket.

Treatment

Stabilisation of fractured fragments with molar bands, Completion of root canal treatment.

Retention and reinforcement of fractured fragments with fibre posts in conjunction with flowable composite.

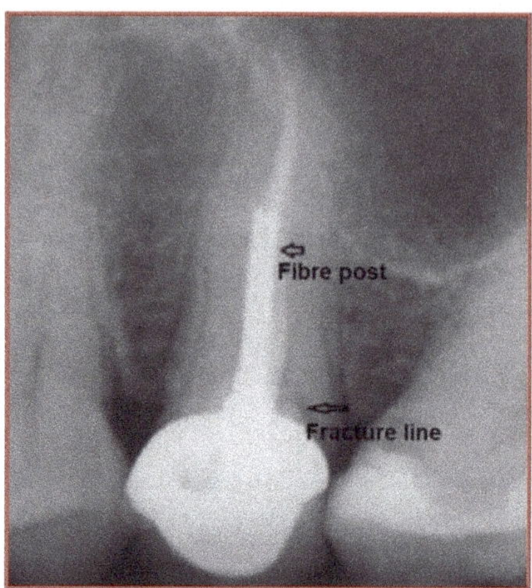

Fig.9.16: Post treatment radiograph

EXTRUSION OF SEALERS IN TO THE PERIAPICAL AREA

Causes

- Perforation through apical foramen.
- Over instrumentation beyond the apical constriction.
- Wide open apex.
- Excessive condensation forces during obturation.
- Too thin consistency of sealers

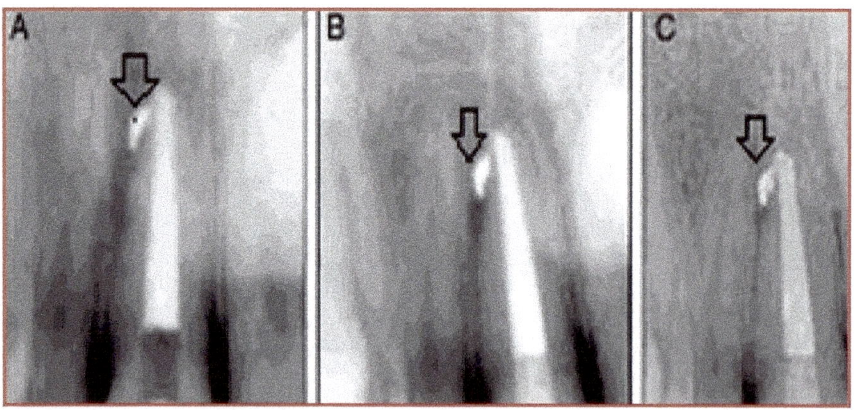

Fig. 10.17: Sealer in periodontal area

Treatment

Pain and discomfort are managed with steroids and antihistaminic drugs. Resorbable sealers like zinc oxide and calcium-based sealers do not cause significant problems. Non resorbable sealers like bio ceramic sealers in excessive quantity may cause root canal failure.

BROKEN FILES & SEPARATED INSTRUMENT:

Mainly occurs due to Failure to inspect & discard the files regularly. Commonly occurs in buccal roots of maxillary molars and mesial roots of lower molars due to their curvature. Occasionally occurs in multirooted premolars and mandibular lateral incisors due to their narrow canal diameter and curvatures. Rarely occurs in straight rooted teeth unless there are manufacturer defects in the file.

Aetiology

Breakage of hand files

- Failure to do precurving (bending the apical 3 mm of file) while using in curved narrow canals.

- Failure to do recapitulation and skipping to previous size file regularly. Not using flexible files in narrow curved canals.

- Forcing files through narrow curvatures especially in double curved canals.

Separation of rotary file

- Not using the files in sequential order.
- Inadequate straight-line axis in double curved canals.
- Inadequate glide path preparation with hand files before introducing rotary files.
- Working in dry environment not using irrigation and lubrication.

Concepts

We have to have the knowledge of some concepts to avoid file breakage:

- Main disadvantage of nickel titanium rotary files are they do not show signs of fatigue before separation.

- In plastic stage they exhibit more flexibility which makes the operator more curious and greedier to use the file continuously without discarding.

- In parent state (austinsite phase) file exhibits more cutting efficiency and less elasticity. After undergoing stress (after its usage in 6 to 8 canals) it gets transformed to martensitic phase in which the file exhibits more elasticity and less cutting efficiency.

- Beyond the outer limits of elastic range the file exhibits plastic range. Beyond the outer limits of plastic range files exhibit yield point and separate.

- Elastic range $\longrightarrow$ plastic range $\longrightarrow$ yield point $\longrightarrow$ separation

- So wider the plastic range lesser is the separation.

- Rotating files are subject to two types of stresses.

- In straight canals-intracanal torsional stresses.

- Occurs due to repeated twisting or bending of files owing to blockages and obstructions.

- In curved canals-cyclic fatigue.

- Files rotating in curvature are subjected to elongating forces from inside and compressing forces from outside repeatedly in a cyclic manner which makes files weak and liable to separation.

- So, in curved canals flexibility of file is mandatory to avoid separation.

- In straight canals cutting efficiency is mandatory to avoid separation.

Prevention

Using heat treated files

- Heat treated files have more flexibility and more fatigue resistance
- Separate less.

Using twisted files

- Twisted files have more cutting efficacy and surface hardness more resistant to separation.

Using files with radial lands

- Files with lands occupy more space in the canal and have less tendency to screw in to the dentin and separate.

- Preparing doubly curved canals and apical 1/3 with stainless steel hand files as much as possible.

Torque

- Increasing the torque in case of blockages, calcifications and obstructions
- More torque more progression of instrument
- Less chances of separation.

Speed: Working in optimum speed reduces the chances of separation while working in very high speed or very low speed increases the chances of separations.

Time: Too long engagement of the file in the canal increases the chances of separation of the file in to the dentin.

Shapers 10 to 20 sec. Finishers 0.3 to 0.6 sec.

Management

No need to be panic. A separated file can be effectively managed by considering the following factors and knowing some concepts - Knowledge of anatomy of the tooth, Features of instrument separated, Time of separation, Status of the tooth at the time of treatment. Site of separation.

Anatomy of tooth

Curvature starts from the apical 1/3, from cervix till middle 1/3 almost all roots are straight so when any separation occurs in body of canal straight line axis is possible - retrieval is possible. When separation occurs in apical 1/3 straight line access to the separated fragment is not possible, thus retrieval is not possible.

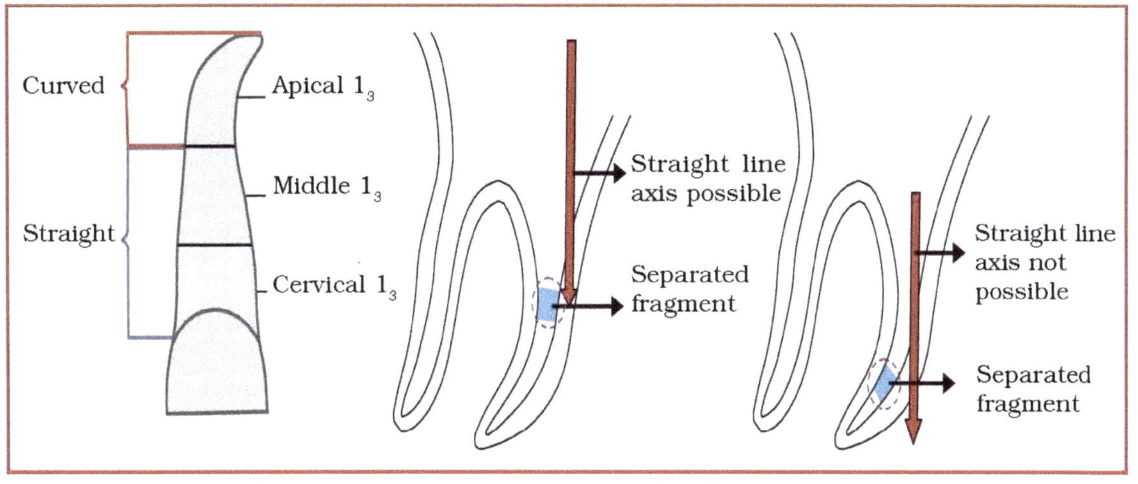

Fig. 10.18:

Diameter of roots in cross section

In cervical 1/3 of all teeth it is almost roughly oval and/or roughly elliptical so when instruments, separation occurs in the body there is space left between separated fragment and canal walls management is less difficult. Apical 1/3 of all teeth is circular, so when any separation occurs in apica, 1/3 there is no space left between separated fragment and canal walls - management is difficult.

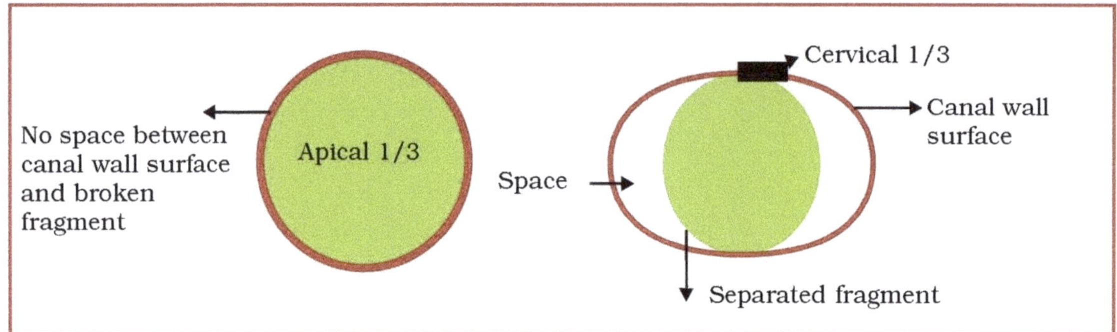

Fig. 10.19: Body of canal (cervical 1/3 and middle 1/3)

Features of instrument separated in the root

All instruments used in endodontics are round in cross section-burs, files, posts, drills. If separated in circular portion of root management is difficult, if separated in elliptical or oval portion of root management is easy.

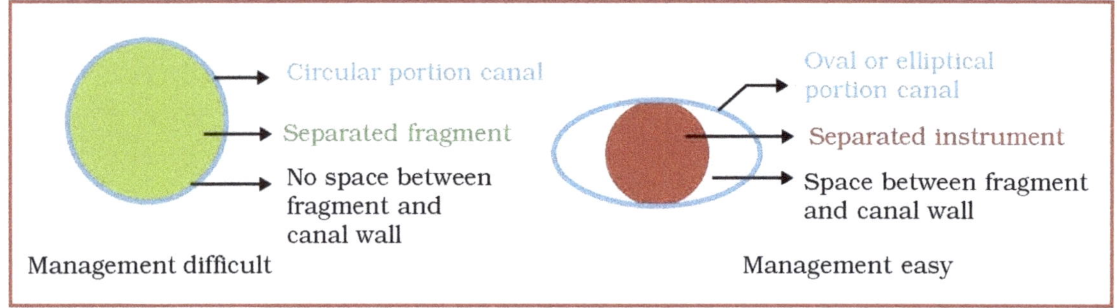

Fig. 10.20:

Files with radial lands occupy more space in canals leaving very less space between separated fragment and canal walls which makes retrieval more difficult. Files without radial lands occupy less space in canals leaving more space between canal wall and separated fragment which makes retrieval less difficult.

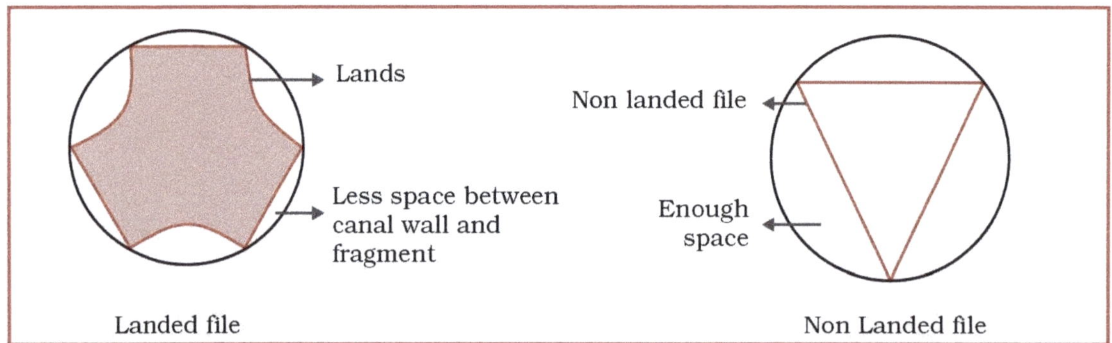

Fig. 10.21:

Posts and GG drills occupy more space—retrieval very difficult. Stainless steel hand files occupy less space—bypassing is easier. Retrieval is less difficult.

Time of separation

Later the instrument separation occurs better would be the prognosis, *i.e.* after using 2 or 3 files. Earlier the instrument separation occurs poorer would be the prognosis. If first file breaks exactly at or beyond the apex in necrotic tooth with draining canals-extract the tooth.

Status of tooth

When the tooth was vital without periapical lesion at the start of treatment

–   Prognosis is better

When the tooth was non vital with preapical lesion at the start of treatment

–   Prognosis is poor

Sites of file breakage

1)   Coronal 1/3rd of root
2)   Middle 1/3rd of root
3)   Apical 1/3rd of root
4)   Beyond the apical 1/3rd

CORONAL 1/3RD

Retrieval or bypass

Middle 1/3rd

Retrieval or Bypass.

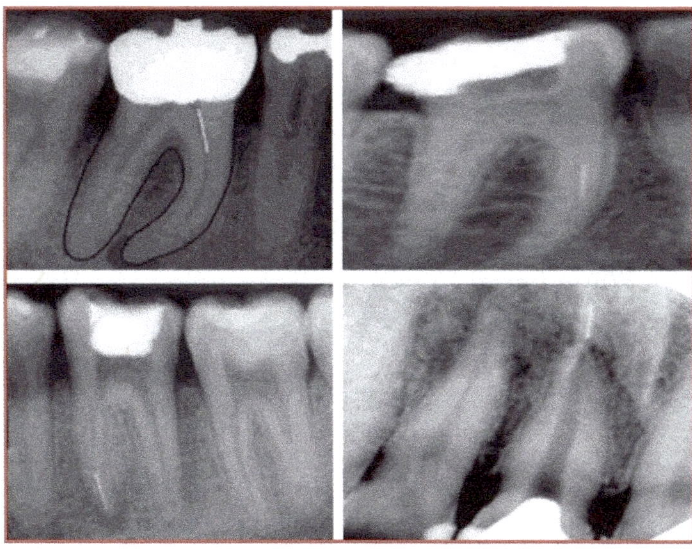

Fig. 10.22: Diffirent sites of file breaking

Apical 1/3rd

Exactly binding to the apex after shaping and cleaning fragment becomes part of obturation-No need of any treatment. If exactly binding to the apical 1/3rd before cleaning & shaping. If it is initial file - Apicectomy in anterior teeth, Hemi section in lower molar, Root resection in upper molar and /or Extraction is considered.

Past the Apex

If separation occurs: Before thorough cleaning & shaping - Apicectomy in anteriors. Root resection in upper molars & hemi section in lower molars.

If separation occurs: After thorough cleaning and shaping - Pain & discomfort is managed by giving steroids in low doses for short period. Wait and watch.

Procedure

Retrieval of separated fragments close to the orifice of canals (from cervical 1/3rd of the root)

Steps

Visualise the head of the separated fragment. Check for the space left between the edge of the fragment and canal walls with the help of sharp probes or files. Create a space between separated fragment and canal walls by removing the dentin with help of narrow long tapering fissure bur or diamond coated ultrasonic tips.

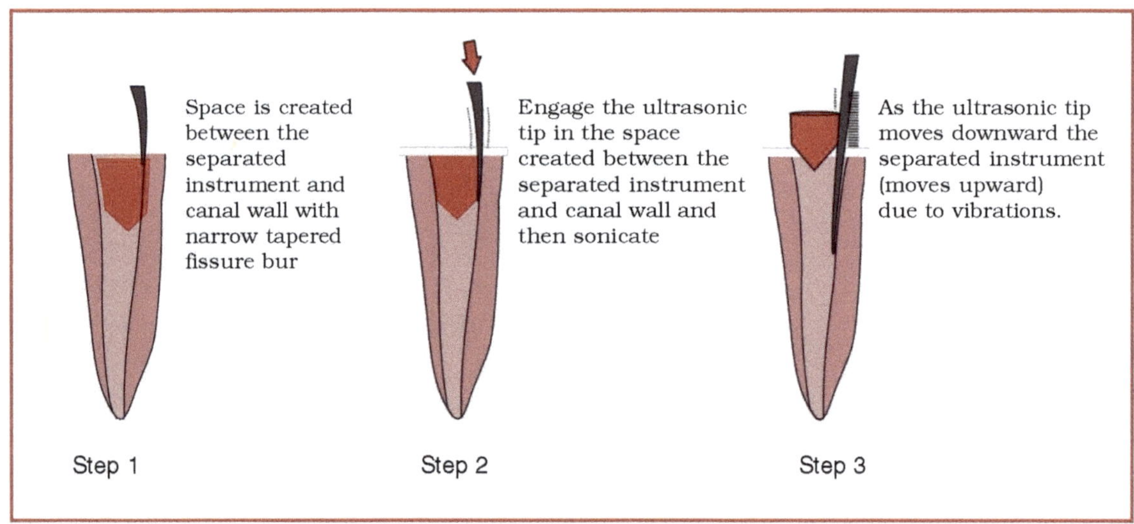

Fig. 10.23. Retrieval from cervical 1/3 of the Root

Note :

If adequate space already exists no need to create space. Engage the ultrasonic tip in the space between canal wall and separated fragment and sonicate all around the head of the fragment. The vibration generated by the tip disengages the fragment from the dentin. As the scalar tip moves more inwards the fragment gets looser and looser and finally dislodges out of the canals.

Retrieval of the separated fragment away from the orifice of canals (from the middle 1/3 of the root)

Steps

Preflaring of cervical 1/3 of root is done with Sx file to get straight line access to the head of fragment Visualise the head of fragment and create a space between the edge of fragment and canal walls with the help of a diamond coated straight narrow ultrasonic tip or with stiff sharp small size hand files. Once the space is created no 15 or 20 u files is passed along the side of the fragment and sonicate. the ultrasonic vibration created by u files disengages the fragment from the dentin and loosens it. Hand stainless steel H files are inserted along the side of the fragment applying lateral and apical pressure. With each in and out stroke of the H file the fragment gets looser and looser finally displaces and dislodged out of canal.

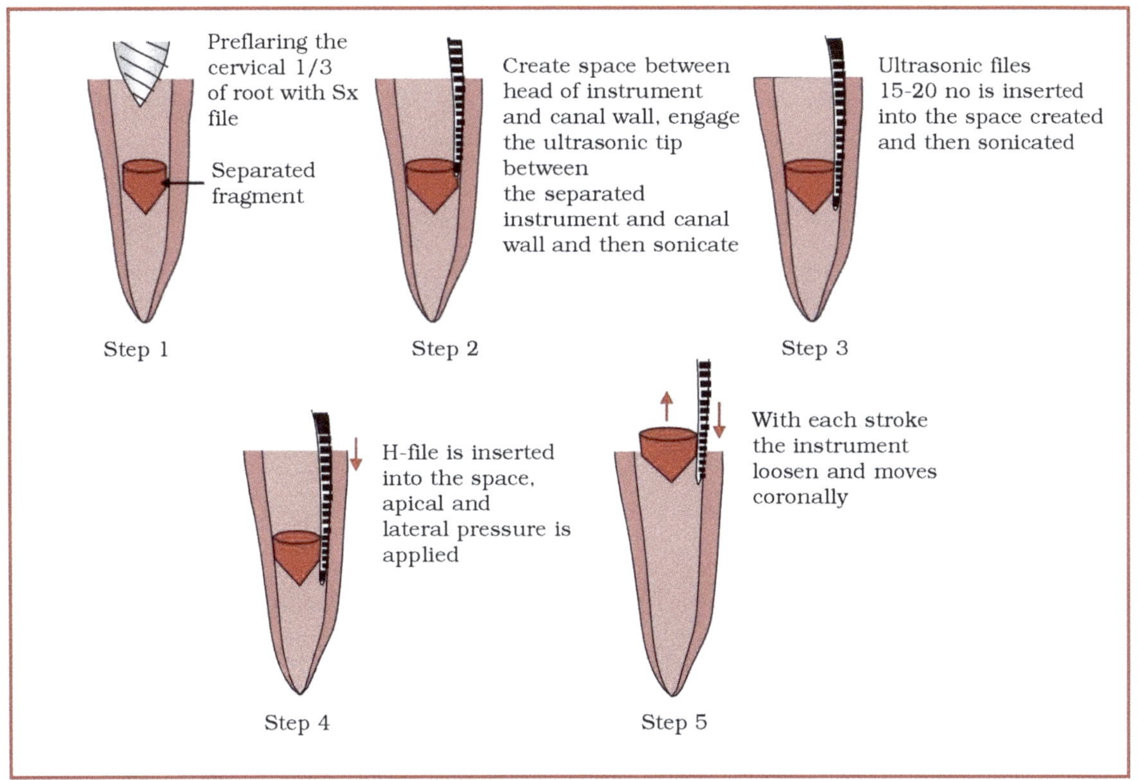

Fig. 10.24. Retrieval from middle 1/3 of the Red

Bypassing the separated instrument

Instruments separated beyond the curvature where Straight line axis to the separated fragment is not possible.

In areas where excessive removal of dentin leads to stripping, perforation and fracture of tooth.

Procedure

Preflaring of cervical 1/3 to widen the radicular axis. Thorough irrigation is done. Pulp chamber is flooded with viscous chelators. Stiff sharpened flex-R file is inserted slowly to make a way between fragment and canal walls.

Once the file is stuck between the canal walls and the fragment, rotate the file in an anticlockwise direction and pull— with each low intensity pull and push strokes the file proceeds forward micron by micron creating the way parallel to the long axis of fragment. The procedure is repeated until the file moves past the fragment. Once the initial file has passed past the separated fragment, the procedure is repeated with serially larger files, canal behind the fragment is shaped and cleaned. Finally the canal is obturated with 2 percent gutta-percha (lateral condensation Tec) Or thermoplastic gutta-percha.

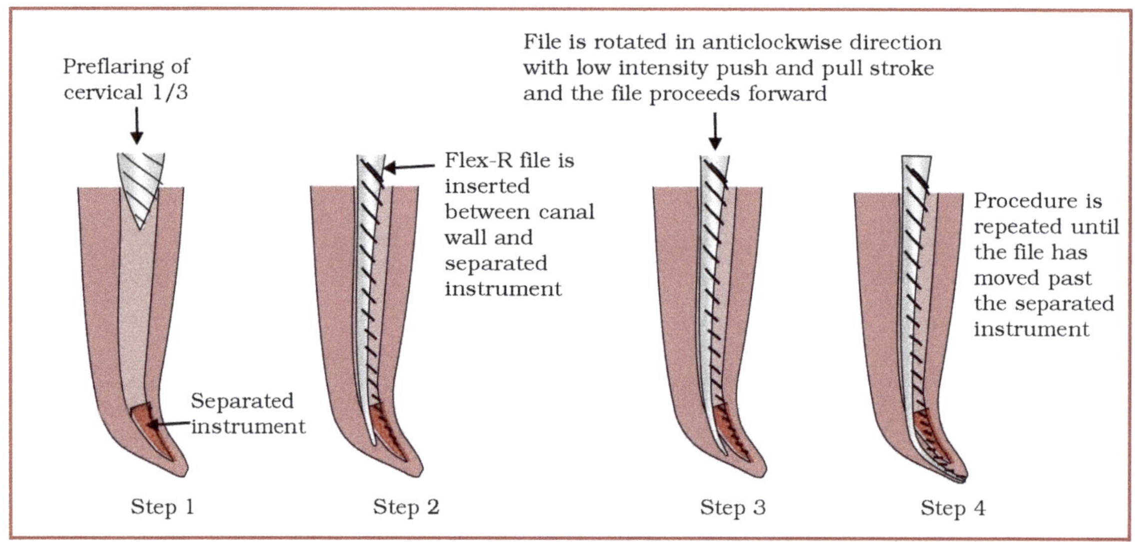

Fig. 10.25: Bypassing the separated instrument

11

Re-root Canal Treatment

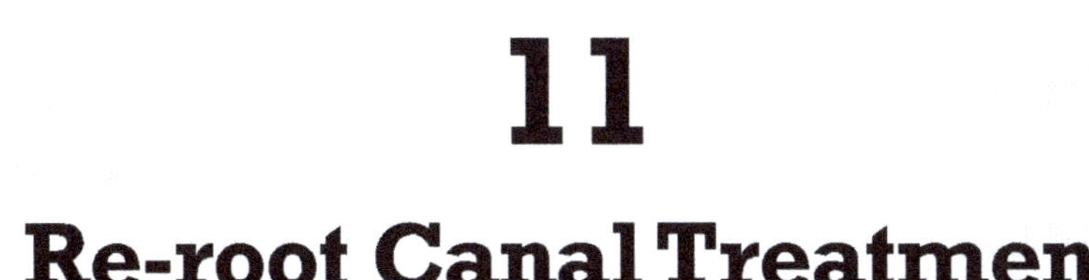

Introduction

It is a challenging and time-consuming procedure compared to the conventional initial root canal treatment however advances in technology has made it less time consuming and less difficult. The semisolid soft flexible nature of gutta percha allows it to retrieve out of canals and make re root canal treatment feasible. Every dental practitioner should consider it as an expensive learning lesson to learn, grow and excel in endodontics.

Definition

The processes of removing all old fillings and new caries if any from the tooth cavity to address the defects and deficiencies that went un noticed during initial conventional root canal treatment.

Case Selection

Not all failed root canal treatment cases are amenable to Re-root canal treatment. Case selection is done analysing the benefits at the expense of risks involved.

Diagnosis

-    X-ray

-    CBCT

-    Microscopic examination

Clinical Findings

1. Persistent continuous pain after obturation
2. Pain on chewing in the concerned tooth after root canal treatment
3. Sensitivity
4. Nocturnal (night) pain
5. Draining fistula
6. Soft tissue swellings

Contraindication

- Transportation
- Zipping
- Complete vertical fractures of root
- Large posts
- Uncontrolled diabetes
- Recent heart surgery
- Periodontally weakened tooth

Indications

Post root canal acute periodontitis or acute periodontal abscess caused due to the following.

1. **Missed canals**
   - Mb2 in maxillary molars
   - Disto lingul canal in mandibular molars
   - Lingual canal in mandibular anteriors
   - Middle mesial canal in lower molars

2. **Missed complex anatomy of tooth**
   Lateral canals, Accessory canals, Furcal canals, Multiple foramen, Isthmuses

3. **Procedural errors:**
   A. Before cleaning & shaping
      - Broken instruments. large perforation.
      - Stripping
      - Zipping
      - Root fractures.
      - Canal transportation only in selected cases

   B. During obturation
      - Under obturation
      - Over obturation specially in nonvital, severely infected, necrotic teeth

Procedure

Removal of all old fillings, defective prosthesis, and new caries if any is done with high speed small straight fissure or round burs. Thorough irrigation is done with 3 percent sodium hypochlorite and hydrogen peroxide to remove remnants of filling materials. Sonicate the pulp chamber with Activated ultrasonic tip to remove fillings and gutta percha from the floor of tooth cavity. Gutta percha in and around the orifice is softened with the help of eucalyptus oil or chloroform. Softened gutta percha is removed with the help of sharp probes or spoon excavators.

Avoid removing remnants of filling materials and gutta-percha lodged in the isthmus area by burs or rotary files, explore the canal orifice with straight probes or ultrasonic tips. Once orifice is explored butt joint of gutta percha is visualized.

De obturation of gutta percha

Steps

1.2 to 5 mm of gutta-percha is removed from the coronal 1/3 of the root by using SX file to create a space for the solvent. Thoroughly clean and dry the created space. Inject or place solvent into the space, wait until the solvent is absorbed by the gutta percha. S1 2% or 4% rotary file is used in a crown down manner to remove. Gutta percha from the body of canal. S2 2% OR 4%. Rotary file is used in a same manner to remove gutta percha from the rest of the canal.

Note:

a)   High torque and high speed is adjected to remove densely compacted filling.

b)   Always start with smaller taper files to avoid excessive removal of dentin from canal walls.

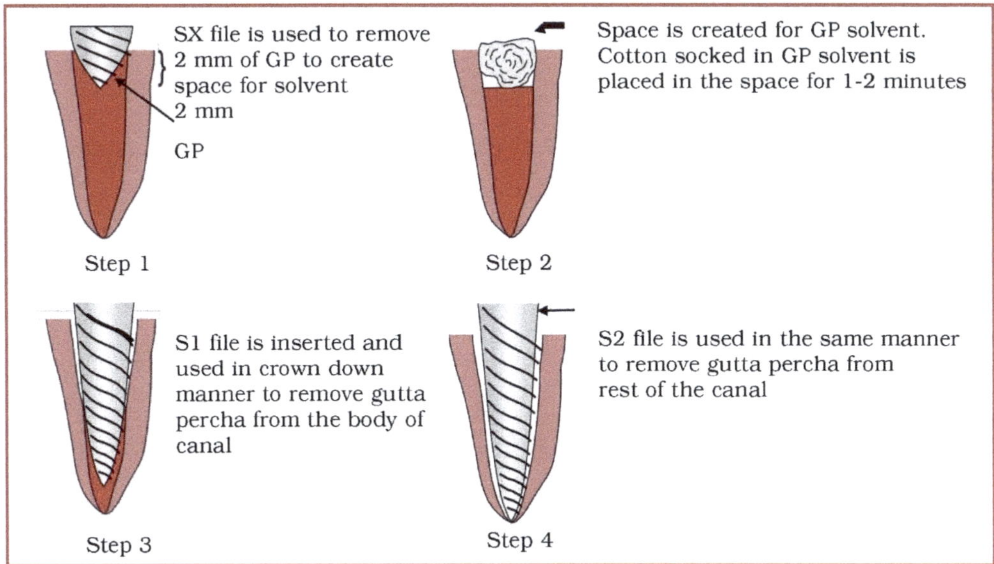

Fig. 11.1: Rotary method.

Sonication with ultrasonic files

High water spray and ultrasonic energy is created by sonic files. It displaces and dissolves the sealer from the canal walls and pushes it out coronally out of the canals avoiding its extrusion in to the periapical area.

NOTE: Excessive use should be avoided as it causes ledges and weakening of root.

Finally, defects are addressed, working length re-established, thorough cleaning and shaping done as usual. Irrigation with chlorhexidine or doxycycline is mandate. Calcium hydroxide intra canal medicament is placed in to the canals. Closed dressing with triple antibiotic paste (metronidazole, ciprofloxacin, doxycycline) is given and patient is recalled after 7 days. If the patient is asymptomatic radiographs are taken to confirm the peri apical radiolucency, if radiolucency is resolving re obturation is done. If the patient is symptomatic, the procedure is repeated and corticosteroid intra canal medicament is placed and patient is called after 15 days. If pain subsides then obturate the canals. If pain has still not subsided then extract the tooth.

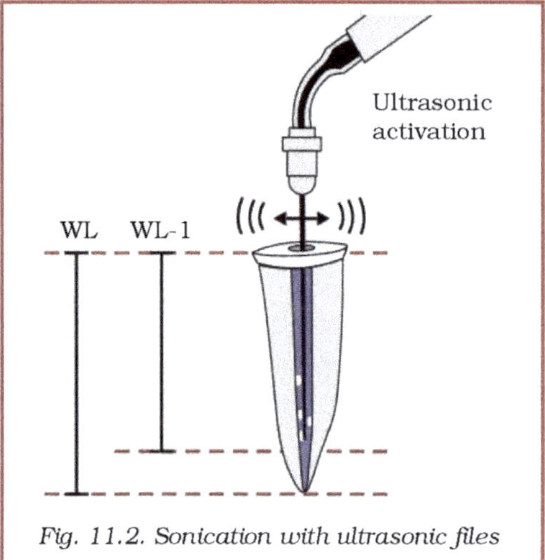

Fig. 11.2. Sonication with ultrasonic files

Manual method of De-obturation

Indications

1. Where there is risk of strip perforation in e.g. in mesial roots Mandibular molars.

2. Risk of lateral transportation in severely curved canals.

3. Where there is risk of excessive removal of dentin from the apical 1/3 of narrow and smaller canals.

Selection of files - stainless steel hand files

Rigid modified sharp ended   K flex - files

H files

Procedure

- Gutta percha is softened either with solvents or heated files or both
- Stiff sharpended flex-R file is inserted slowly to make a way between softened gutta percha and canal walls.

- Once the file is stuck between canal walls and gutta percha, the file is forced inward with high intensity push and pull strokes. With each high intensity pull and push strokes the file proceeds forward micron by micron creating the way parallel to the long axis of gutta percha the procedure is repeated until the file moves till 2 to 3 mm short of apex. Once the initial file has passed till the desired length, the procedure is repeated with sequentially larger files. Finally, H files in a sequential order is used to remove gutta percha. Sometimes gutta percha can be removed by engaging multiple H FILES at a time.

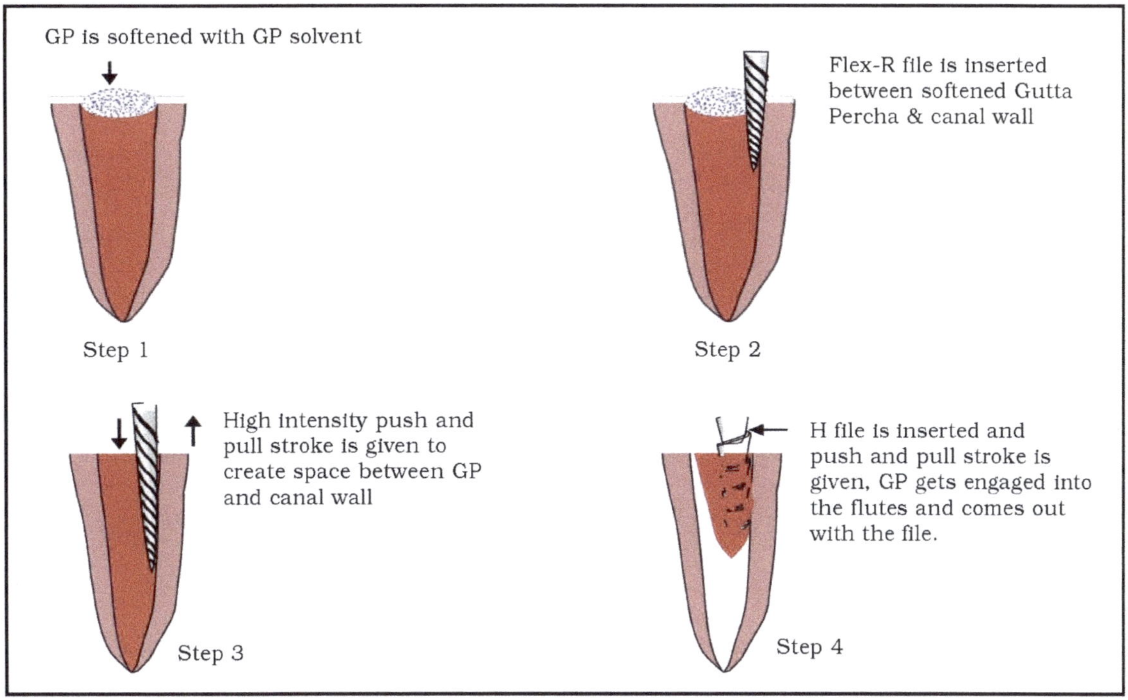

Fig. 11.3: Manual method

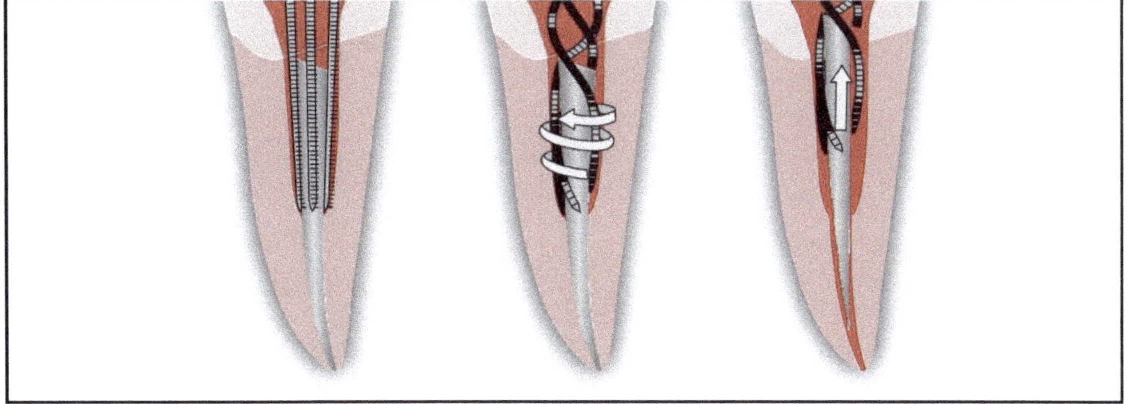

Fig. 11.4: The Headstrom file technique.

12

Non vital Pulp Therapy

a) APEXIFICATION

- "Apex" means root end and "Fication" means causing to make or inducing to develop.

Definition

- It is a clinical procedure performed either to induce innate regenerative potential to develop calcified barrier or to install artificial barrier across the open root end of immature non vital tooth.

Objective

- To provide apical stop for root canal obturating materials to get three-dimensional hermetic apical seal which is critical for endodontic success.

Indication

- Immature non vital or necrotic young permanent tooth with open apex.

Contraindication

- Tooth with incompletely formed short roots
- Tooth with very wide-open apex
- Tooth with compromised periodontium

Material

1) Calcium hydroxide
2) Mineral trioxide aggregate

1) Calcium Hydroxide Apexification

Procedure

Local anaesthesia is given to control the pain, and rubber dam isolation is done to avoid salivary contamination.

- Routine root canal treatment is done following some special precaution, exact working length is established by carrying the initial files (size 25 or 30 OR 40 k file) till the radiographic end of root. Care must be taken to avoid over instrumenting the file past the working length to avoid damage to the residual hertz wig epithelial root sheath which is the main source of pluripotent stem cells responsible for apexification. Complete extirpation of necrotic pulp tissue is done with the help of barbed broaches and H files. After flooding the chamber with EDTA Minimal instrumentation with hand files is carried out to remove biofilm f rom the canal w al l s especi al ly at the api cal 1/3. C opi ous irrigation with hydrogen peroxide, sodium hypochlorite and chlorhexidine is carried out to disinfect the root canals completely which is critical for success of apexification. Dry the canals with larger paper points, completely fill the canals with calcium hydroxide, finger spreaders are used to condense the material till root end. Care must be taken not to extrude excess material in the periapical area.

- Place cotton ball at the root canal entrance and finally restore the tooth completely with interim restoration. Patient is recalled after 6 weeks for second placement of medicament paste, then after 12 weeks for third placement and 18 weeks for fourth placement.

- At 6-month visit: Take a new IOPA of the tooth being treated.

Examine the radiograph for evidence of root end closure and confirm by passing instrument through the apex after removing the intracanal medicament, if results are not satisfactory the procedure is repeated for another 6 to 18 months.

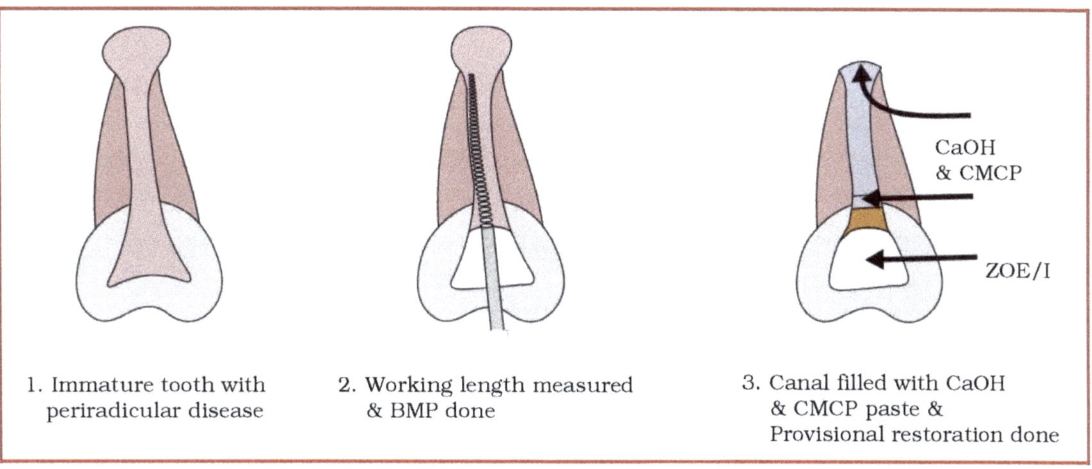

Fig. 12.1: Procedure CaOH Apexifilation

If results of apexification that is root end closure is satisfactory definitive three-dimensional obturation with gutta percha is done followed by permanent restoration with composite. Finally the tooth is covered with prosthetic crown.

Advantages of calcium hydroxide apexification

1) Induces physiologic formation of apical barrier
2) Success rate is good if done properly in appropriate case
3) Less expensive and easily available
4) Gets easily resorbed when extruded in to the periapical area

Disadvantages of calcium hydroxide apexification

1) Multiple visits usually 5 to 6 visits
2) Long treatment may take 6 to 18 months
3) Possibility of contamination due to skippin of visits and too long inter visit interval.
4) Requires replacement at every monthly visit
5) Chances of root fracture of fragile and weakened dentinal walls

2) Apexification With MTA

- Routine root canal treatment is done following some special precaution. Exact working length is established by carrying the initial file (larger size 25 or 30 or 40 k file) till the radiographic end of root Care must be taken to avoid over instrumenting the file past the working length to avoid damage to the residual Hartwig's epithelial root sheath which is the main source of pluripotent stem cells responsible for apexification. Complete extirpation of necrotic pulp tissue is done with the help of barbed broaches and H files. After flooding the chamber with EDTA Minimal instrumentation with hand files is carried out to remove biofilm from the canal walls especially at the apical 1/3. Copious irrigation with hydrogen peroxide, sodium hypochlorite and chlorhexidine is carried out to disinfect the root canals completely which is critical for success of apexification. Dry the canals with larger paper points, completely fill the canals with calcium hydroxide, finger spreaders are used to condense material

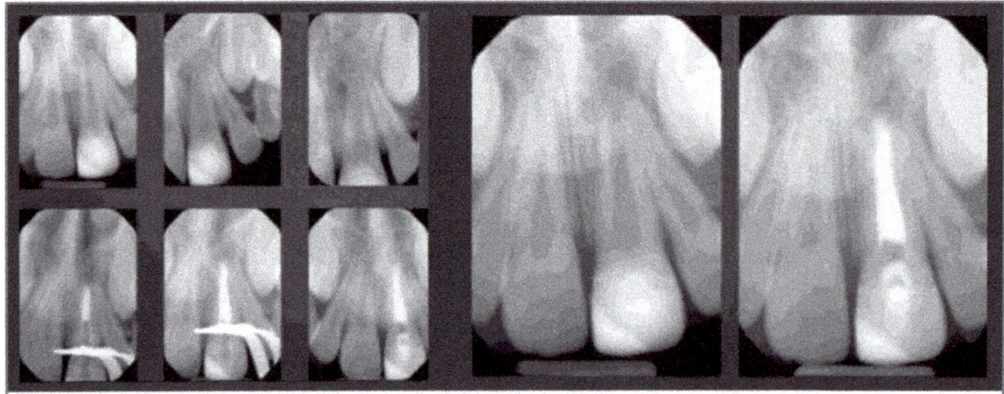

Fig. 12.2: MTA plug as an alternative to apexification

till root end. Care must be taken not to extrude excess material in the periapical area, place cotton ball at the root canal entrance and finally restore the tooth completely with interim restoration. Patient is recalled after 6 days. In the second visit, tooth is re-entered and calcium hydroxide intra canal medicament is completely removed using H-file and broaches. Instrumentation should be carried out 2 to 3 mm short of working length to avoid extrusion of material into the periapical area.

- Irrigation with sodium hypochlorite, normal saline and chlorhexidine is done.

Dry the canals with larger paper points, MTA is mixed with sterile water to a loose sand like consistency, mix is carried in to the canal with the help of MTA carrier and filled in increments till 3 to 4 mm of thickness and then wait for the MTA to set. Once MTA sets, obturation of the remaining canal is carried out with gutta percha followed by placement of reinforced GIC as a sub base and final filling done with composite restoration followed by prosthetic crowns.

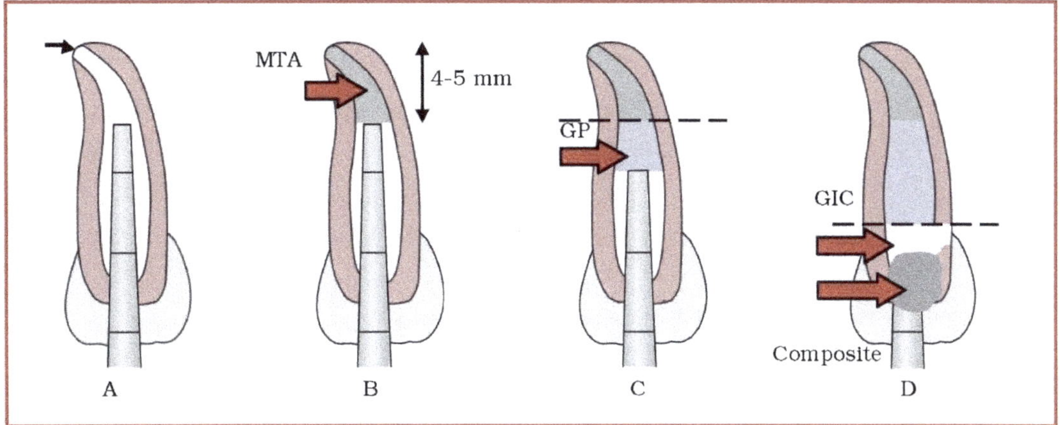

Fig. 12.3 : Apexification with MTA procedure

Advantages...

- Single or two visit procedure
- Treatment duration is short
- Saves lot of time
- No chance for inter visit contamination and fracture tooth
- Excellent sealing property
- Sets in presence of moisture
- Expands while setting
- Adhesion to the dentinal walls is excellent and provides three- dimensional hermetic apical seal.

- Can induce the formation of dentin, cementum and bone and thus provides physiologic seal besides artificial seal.
- Highly biocompatible unlike calcium hydroxide, less soluble and does not easily dissolve in oral fluids.
- Exhibits broad spectrum antimicrobial properties.

Disadvantages...

- High cost
- Too long setting time
- Loose sandy mix difficult to carry and condense in the canals
- Does not increase the length and thickness of root walls, so over time the root becomes brittle and prone to fracture

b) NATURAL OBTURATION VIA BLOOD CLOT

It is an alternative procedure to calcium hydroxide and MTA apexification.

It involves providing a mesh of blood clot in the completely disinfected sterile root canal system in to which cell could grow and revitalise the canal system.

Definition

An extension of endodontic treatment which attempts to bring back the tooth to its natural state by replacing the non-vital necrotic tissue with vital tissue.

Rationale

Periapical area of immature tooth has more cellularity and high vascularity Immature tooth exhibits innate potential to recover and repair.

Revascularisation through Angio neogenesis.

Revitalization through growth, maturation and mitosis of residual pluripotent stem cells of dental papillae and differentiation of undifferentiated ectomesenchyme cells of the dental sac.

Objectives

- Elimination of pulpal necrosis and apical periodontitis.
- Revitalization of pulp
- Increase in the length and thickness of root walls
- Narrowing of root walls
- Closure of apical foramina

Indications

1) Non vital incompletely formed immature permanent tooth with following features

    A) Short roots

    B) Wide open apex

    C) Thin fragile root walls

    D) Bunder buss canals

2) Non vital immature tooth with congenital anomalies where conventional root canal treatment is not possible e.g. dense invaginatous or dense in dente.

3) Immature avulsed tooth

Contraindications

- Non restorable tooth - Tooth with extensive loss of crown or grossly destructed tooth
- Tooth can't be isolated
- Deciduous tooth
- Medically comprised patients-immune compromised and mentally retarded
- Mature permanent tooth whose apical diameter is less than 1 mm
- Patient with bleeding disorders and patient on anticoagulant therapy
- Need for placement of post in canal space

Advantages

- By bringing back the tooth to its natural state, the tooth's natural immune system will be brought back to normal function.
- Simple natural approach to revitalise the tooth
- Preserve vitality of tooth
- Relatively strong and thick dentinal walls formed compared to other methods
- Long term surveillance of tooth is more compared to other methods
- Do not require expensive armamentarium and materials
- Patient satisfaction is great
- Patient compliance and co-operation more despite of multiple visits and long treatment

Disadvantages

- Compared to MTA plug barrier technique, long treatment and multiple visits
- Discolouration of tooth due to minocycline and grey MTA

Causes of Failure

- Poor root development
- Insufficient bleeding
- Pulp calcifications and internal resorptions

Procedure

First visit

Premedication

- If necessary, premedication with anti salivary drugs like propantheline and scopolamine is given to control saliva and promote dry working environment.

Local anaesthesia with vasoconstrictor – 2% lignocaine hydrochloride with adrenalin is given to control the pain.

Isolation with rubber dam

- Completely isolate the tooth from the oral cavity to prevent contamination from oral fluids.

Occlusal or incisal clearance

- A clearance of 0.3 to 0.5 mm is given it aids in removal of superficial Bacteria and healing of tooth. Disinfect the tooth surface with 10% betadine before access opening.

Access opening

- Straight line access to canal orifice is obtained with a small round bur at low speed with adequate coolant.

Disinfection of root canal space

- Totally relys on irrigation as instrumentation is contraindicated to avoid damage to the thin fragile root walls and injury to diaphragm of hertz wig epithelial root sheath. Negative pressure irrigation is recommended to avoid extrusion of irrigating solution in periapical area to avoid damage to delicate stem cells.

- Copious irrigation with 20 ml sodium hypochlorite at conc. of between 1.75% and 3.25% is done followed by normal saline and finally with 2% chlorhexidine

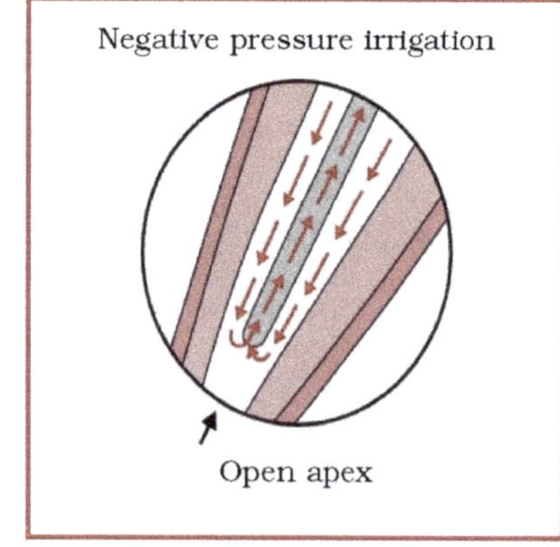

Fig. 11.4. Irrigation

Drying the root canals

- Root canals are thoroughly dried by using larger paper points. Blowing air inside the tooth should be avoided as it may cause dessication or dehydration of delicate stem cells.

Placement of intracanal medicaments

- Done by filling the canals with calcium hydroxide paste or triple antibiotic paste lentilo spiral is used for this purpose. If triple antibiotic paste is used the pulp chamber should be treated with bonding agent to avoid discolouration of crowns due to minocycline. Care must be taken to restrict the placement of paste below the CEJ (cemento enamel junction) that is why usually calcium hydroxide paste is recommended. Finally a cotton ball is placed over the canal entrance. Seal the cavity with

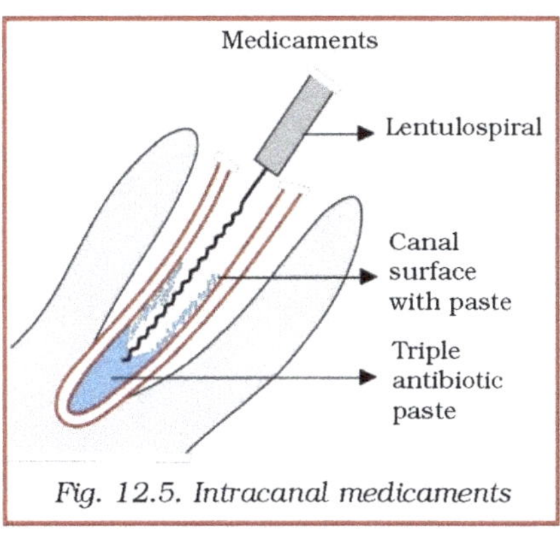

Fig. 12.5. Intracanal medicaments

temporary restoration and patient is recalled after 1 or 3 weeks depending upon the severity of infection the patient had at the start of treatment.

Second visit

Assessment

Repeat the procedure if the patient is symptomatic with signs and symptoms of apical periodontitis.

If the patient is asymptomatic with clinical and radiographic evidence of apical healing.

Local anaesthesia without vasoconstrictor (plain 2% lignocaine or bupivacaine) is used to induce adequate bleeding. As adrenaline is a vasoconstrictor it decreases the blood flow and inhibits bleeding. Induction of adequate bleeding and clot formation in complete aseptic canal system plays a major role in the final outcome.

Isolation with rubber dam

- Completely isolate the tooth from the oral cavity to prevent contamination from oral fluids. This is the key to the success of the procedure.

Removal of intracanal medicament

- The cavity is re-entered after removing the temporary restoration and cotton pellet, thorough irrigation with hydrogen peroxide and sodium hypochlorite is done to remove intracanal medicament if necessary. Large H files or barbed broches are used at a safe distance from the apex and finally gentle irrigation with 20 ml 17% EDTA is done.

- Bleeding is induced by over instrumenting the canal 2 mm past the apex with help of 20 size file. Bleeding should fill the canal to the level of CEJ. Once the blood clot forms resorbable collagen matrix colla plug is packed over the clot. The colla plug stabilizes the clot and provides seat for medicament placement. Calcium hydroxide or 2 to 3 mm thickness of MTA is placed over the colla plug. MTA should cover the entire cavity surface. White MTA is used in anterior tooth to avoid crown discoloration and grey MTA in posterior tooth for more predictable results.

- Thick base of modified high strength glass ionomer cement is placed as a sub base and finally entire cavity is filled with composite filling.

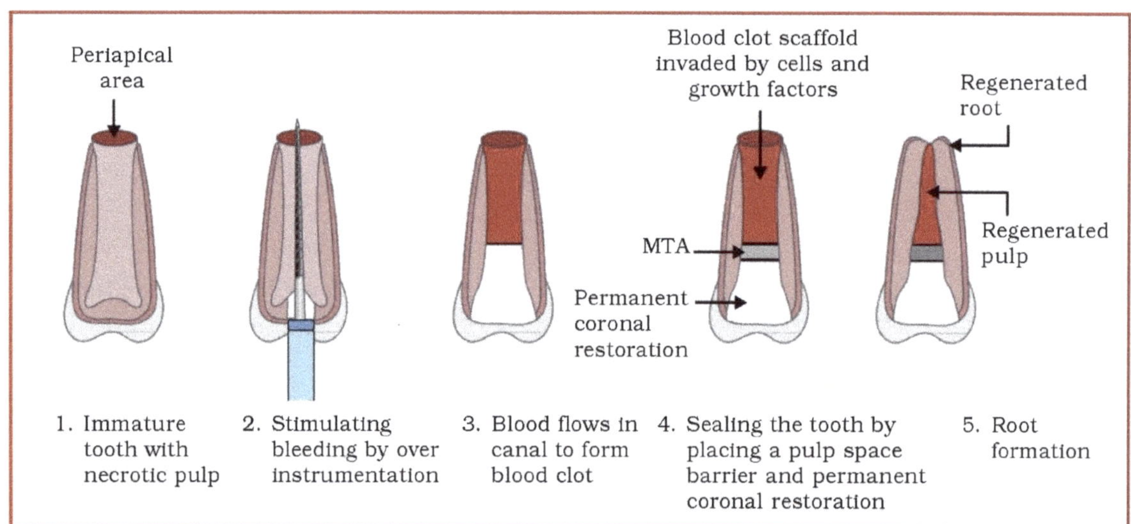

Fig. 12.6. Natural obturation procedure

Follow up visits

Clinical examination

- To assess the pulpal and periodontal status pulp vitality tests and periodontal tests are carried out
- Resolution of periapical radiolucency within 6 to 12 months
- Increase in the length of root walls within 6 to 12 months.
- Increase in the width of root canals from 12 to 24 months.
- Closure or narrowing of apical foramina within 15 to 24 months

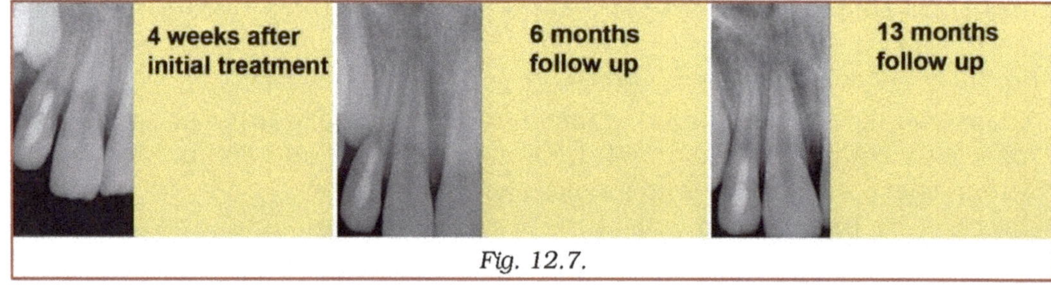

Fig. 12.7.

A

C

N

O

P